2005
YEAR BOOK OF
EMERGENCY MEDICINE®

The 2005 Year Book Series

Year Book of Allergy, Asthma, and Clinical Immunology™: Drs Rosenwasser, Boguniewicz, Milgrom, Routes, and Spahn

Year Book of Anesthesiology and Pain Management™: Drs Chestnut, Abram, Black, Gravlee, Mathru, Lee, and Roizen

Year Book of Cardiology®: Drs Gersh, Cheitlin, Graham, Kaplan, Sundt, and Waldo

Year Book of Critical Care Medicine®: Drs Dellinger, Parrillo, Balk, Bekes, Dries, and Dorman

Year Book of Dentistry®: Drs Zakariasen, Hatcher, Horswell, McIntyre, Scott, Victoroff, and Zakariasen

Year Book of Dermatology and Dermatologic Surgery™: Drs Thiers and Lang

Year Book of Diagnostic Radiology®: Drs Osborn, Birdwell, Dalinka, Gardiner, Levy, Maynard, and Oestreich

Year Book of Emergency Medicine®: Drs Burdick, Cydulka, Hamilton, Handly, Werner, and Quintana

Year Book of Endocrinology®: Drs Mazzaferri, Rubin, Molitch, Leahy, Kennedy, Kannan, Bessesen, Rogol, and Meikle

Year Book of Family Practice®: Drs Bowman, Apgar, Dexter, Miser, Neill, and Scherger

Year Book of Gastroenterology™: Drs Lichtenstein, Dempsey, Drebin, Faust, Ginsberg, Katzka, Kochman, Morris, Reddy, and Stein

Year Book of Hand and Upper Limb Surgery®: Drs Berger and Ladd

Year Book of Medicine®: Drs Barkin, Frishman, Klahr, Loehrer, Mazzaferri, Phillips, Pillinger, and Snydman

Year Book of Neonatal and Perinatal Medicine®: Drs Fanaroff, Maisels, and Stevenson

Year Book of Neurology and Neurosurgery®: Drs Gibbs and Verma

Year Book of Nuclear Medicine®: Drs Coleman, Blaufox, Royal, Strauss, and Zubal

Year Book of Obstetrics, Gynecology, and Women's Health®: Dr Shulman

Year Book of Oncology®: Drs Loehrer, Arceci, Glatstein, Gordon, Hanna, Morrow, and Thigpen

Year Book of Ophthalmology®: Drs Rapuano, Cohen, Eagle, Grossman, Hammersmith, Myers, Nelson, Penne, Sergott, Shields, Tipperman, and Vander

Year Book of Orthopedics®: Drs Morrey, Beauchamp, Peterson, Swiontkowski, Trigg, and Yaszemski

Year Book of Otolaryngology-Head and Neck Surgery®: Drs Paparella, Otto, and Keefe

2005

The Year Book of EMERGENCY MEDICINE®

Editor-in-Chief

William P. Burdick, MD, MSEd

Clinical Professor of Emergency Medicine, Drexel University College of Medicine; Assistant Vice President, Assessment Services, Educational Commission for Foreign Medical Graduates; Director of Education, Foundation for Advancement of International Medical Education and Research; Attending Physician, Hahnemann University Hospital, Philadelphia, Pennsylvania

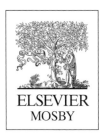

ELSEVIER
MOSBY

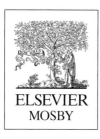

Vice President, Continuity Publishing: Timothy M. Griswold
Managing Editor: David Orzechowski
Developmental Editor: Dana M. Lamparello
Senior Manager, Continuity Production: Idelle L. Winer
Senior Issue Manager: Pat Costigan
Illustrations and Permissions Coordinator: Kimberly E. Denando

2005 EDITION

Printed in the United States of America
Composition by Thomas Technology Solutions, Inc.
Printing/binding by Sheridan Books

Editorial Office:
Elsevier
300 East
170 South Independence Mall West
Philadelphia, PA 19106-3399

International Standard Serial Number: 0271-7964
International Standard Book Number: 0-323-02071-2

Table of Contents

Journals Represented

Mayo Clinic Proceedings
Medical Care
Nephrology, Dialysis, Transplantation
Neurosurgery
New England Journal of Medicine
Pediatric Cardiology
Pediatric Emergency Care
Pediatric Infectious Disease Journal
Pediatrics
Pharmacotherapy
Prehospital Emergency Care
Radiology
Respiratory Medicine
Skeletal Radiology
Southern Medical Journal
Stroke
Transplantation

STANDARD ABBREVIATIONS

The following terms are abbreviated in this edition: acquired immunodeficiency syndrome (AIDS), central nervous system (CNS), cardiopulmonary resuscitation (CPR), cerebrospinal fluid (CSF), computed tomography (CT), deoxyribonucleic acid (DNA), electrocardiography (ECG), emergency department (ED), emergency medical services (EMS), human immunodeficiency virus (HIV), health maintenance organization (HMO), intensive care unit (ICU), intramuscular (IM), intravenous (IV), magnetic resonance (MR) imaging (MRI), ribonucleic acid (RNA), ultrasound (US), and ultraviolet (UV).

NOTE

The YEAR BOOK OF EMERGENCY MEDICINE® is a literature survey service providing abstracts of articles published in the professional literature. Every effort is made to assure the accuracy of the information presented in these pages. Neither the editors nor the publisher of the YEAR BOOK OF EMERGENCY MEDICINE® can be responsible for errors in the original materials. The editors' comments are their own opinions. Mention of specific products within this publication does not constitute endorsement.

To facilitate the use of the YEAR BOOK OF EMERGENCY MEDICINE® as a reference tool, all illustrations and tables included in this publication are now identified as they appear in the original article. This change is meant to help the reader recognize that any illustration or table appearing in the YEAR BOOK OF EMERGENCY MEDICINE® may be only one of many in the original article. For this reason, figure and table numbers will often appear to be out of sequence within the YEAR BOOK OF EMERGENCY MEDICINE®.

Introduction

Welcome to the 2005 YEAR BOOK OF EMERGENCY MEDICINE! Our world on the front lines of medical care continues to evolve as medications with which we were just learning to become comfortable are found to affect more patients with side effects than were anticipated. It now turns out that one of the reasons for this is the over-prescribing of cyclooxygenase-2 (COX-2) inhibitors to patients who would have done just as well with existing nonsteroidal anti-inflammatory drugs. The world of diagnosis and treatment is probabilistic, and if low odds are applied to a larger number of patients, the absolute number of side-effect victims will inevitably increase. Physicians are in part responsible for the alarm about COX-2 inhibitors because we prescribed them to too many patients, many of whom would have done well with less risky (and less expensive) medications. We jumped on the bandwagon.

Jumping on the bandwagon and practicing medicine commensurate with community standards are two concepts that are unfortunately not too far apart. The challenge of making this distinction forces each of us to practice with integrity. Don't just do something because it is the latest thing, or because everyone else is doing it. Practice medicine by the book—the evidence book—and use the medical literature carefully and thoughtfully to make wise decisions.

The energy required to practice evidence-based medicine can be exhausting. Our compilation and analysis of this year's key emergency medicine literature is intended to reduce your exhaustion and help you practice more evidence-based medicine, and not just jump on the bandwagon.

William P. Burdick, MD, MSEd

GENERAL EMERGENCY MEDICINE

1 Trauma

Head Injury

Prehospital Hypertonic Saline Resuscitation of Patients With Hypotension and Severe Traumatic Brain Injury: A Randomized Controlled Trial
Cooper DJ, for the HTS Study Investigators (Alfred Hosp, Melbourne, Victoria, Australia; et al)
JAMA 291:1350-1357, 2004   1–1

Background.—Severe traumatic brain injury (TBI) is a common finding in patients with major trauma, and these patients are usually young adult men. The mortality rate of patients with severe TBI is high (31%-49%), and a large number of survivors have persistent, severe neurologic disability. Patients with severe TBI may experience secondary brain injury as a result of hypoxia, hypotension, or elevated intracranial pressure, and this scenario is associated with a worse neurologic outcome. Aggressive resuscitation with IV fluids is recommended for the management of patients with severe TBI, as patients with hypotension after severe TBI have twice the mortality rate of normotensive patients. There is evidence that prehospital hypertonic saline (HTS) resuscitation of patients with TBI may increase survival, but it is not known whether HTS improves neurologic outcomes. Whether prehospital resuscitation with IV HTS improves long-term neurologic outcomes in patients with severe TBI compared with resuscitation with conventional fluids was determined.

Methods.—A total of 229 patients with TBI who were comatose and hypotensive were randomly assigned to receive a rapid IV infusion of either 250 mL of 7.5% saline (114 patients) or 250 mL of Ringer's lactate solution (115 patients; controls), in addition to conventional IV fluid and resuscitation protocols administered by paramedics. The main outcome measure was neurologic function at 6 months, measured by the extended Glasgow Outcome Score.

Results.—Primary outcomes were obtained in 99% of the patients. Baseline characteristics of the groups were equivalent. At admission to the hospital, the mean serum sodium level was 149 mEq/L for the HTS patients compared with 141 mEq/L for patients in the control group. The proportion of patients who survived to hospital discharge was similar for both groups (55% for HTS patients vs 50% for control patients). The survival rates at 6 months were 55% in the HTS group and 47% in the control group. There was no significant difference between the groups in favorable outcomes or in any other measure of postinjury neurologic function.

Conclusion.—The administration of prehospital HTS for prehospital resuscitation in patients with hypotension and severe TBI provided nearly identical neurologic function at 6 months after injury compared with conventional fluid resuscitation.

▶ The mortality and morbidity associated with severe TBI are high, and the cost of care for survivors is enormous ($100 billion per year in the United States alone). Patients with TBI and initial hypotension generally have the worst outcomes. A cohort analysis of a previous study by Wade et al[1] showed early use of HTS and HTS/dextran improved survival in this group of patients, but did not address the neurologic outcomes associated with increased survival. This study attempted to determine the effect of early HTS on neurologic outcomes in patients with TBI and hypotension. Unfortunately, its results seem to have muddied the water on this issue further. Not only did the authors find no difference in neurologic outcomes with HTS, but also no difference in survival when compared with a standard, aggressive fluid resuscitation protocol. The data should be interpreted with caution, as the study has 2 important limitations in addition to its small size. First is the use of HTS without dextran, which makes its findings somewhat difficult to compare with earlier studies. In addition, the authors do not appear to have evaluated the effects of potential differences in ED and inpatient treatment between the 12 hospitals receiving the study patients. Bottom line, if there are benefits to the use of HTS with or without dextran, they are likely small. While continued efforts in improving the outcomes of patients with TBI are needed, efforts at prevention are more likely to have significant impacts on reducing the overall burden of TBI.

S. L. Werner, MD

Reference

1. Wade CE, Grady JJ, Kramer GC, et al: Individual patient cohort analysis of the efficacy of hypertonic saline/dextran in patients with traumatic brain injury and hypotension. *J Trauma* 42:S61-S65, 1997.

▶ Although initiation of HTS to increase arterial blood pressure and subsequently increase cerebral perfusion pressure in patients with severe TBI and hypotension intuitively makes sense, Cooper and colleagues failed to show improved neurologic outcomes over resuscitation with Ringer's lactate solution. Even though the results are disappointing, hopefully this study will lead to another study evaluating prehospital use of HTS-dextran, another solution currently used regularly in Europe.

R. K. Cydulka, MD, MS

Prospective Validation of a Proposal for Diagnosis and Management of Patients Attending the Emergency Department for Mild Head Injury
Fabbri A, Servadei F, Marchesini G, et al (Ospedale GB Morgagni, Forli, Italy)
J Neurol Neurosurg Psychiatry 75:410-416, 2004   1–2

Introduction.—For patients with mild head injury, predictors are needed to determine the appropriate use of CT and plan management. The strength of evidence of published recommendations is currently inadequate. Diagnostic accuracy and the clinical validity of the proposal of the Neurotraumatology Committee of the World Federation of Neurosurgical Societies on mild head injury were examined from an ED perspective.

Methods.—During a 3-year period, 5578 adolescents and adults were prospectively recruited and managed with the proposed protocol. Outcome measures included any posttraumatic lesion; need for neurosurgical intervention; and unfavorable outcome (death, permanent vegetative state, or severe disability) after 6 months. The predictive value of a model based on 5 variables (Glasgow coma score, clinical findings, risk factors, neurologic deficits, and skull fracture) was evaluated.

Results.—At initial CT examination, 327 patients (5.9%) had intracranial posttraumatic lesions. Previously undiagnosed lesions were identified after re-evaluation within 7 days in 16 cases (0.3%). Neurosurgical intervention was necessary in 71 patients (1.3%), and 39 (0.7%) had an unfavorable outcome. The area under the receiver operating characteristic curve of variables for predicting posttraumatic lesions was 0.906 (0.009) (at best cutoff: sensitivity, 70.0%; specificity, 94.1%), neurosurgical intervention was 0.926 (0.016) (sensitivity, 81.7%; specificity, 94.1%), and unfavorable outcome was 0.953 (0.014) (sensitivity, 88.1%; specificity 95.1%).

Conclusion.—The variables were highly accurate in predicting clinically meaningful outcomes when applied to a consecutive series of patients with mild head injury in the clinical setting of a level I ED.

▶ The authors validate a system to stratify mild head-injured patients into low/medium/high risk for a set of intracranial injuries. Predictive elements were Glasgow coma scale score, clinical findings, risk factors, neurologic deficits, and skull fractures. Validation was done by showing that worse outcomes were associated with higher risk assignment.

It may not be possible to compare the results from this study with those in other practices. First, the authors did not have CT available 24 hours a day and often utilized skull films instead (it is rather rare to use skull films in the setting of trauma at MCP and Hahnemann hospitals). Additionally, CT was performed at least 2 hours after the trauma event. At our hospitals, both level I trauma centers, the trauma team does not wait long after arrival to the ED to send the stable patient for an indicated head CT. (However, it may be good to wait for the first head CT for these lower risk patients to avoid missing delayed bleeds.) The problem for emergency physicians is that the disposition of these patients is postponed for at least 2 hours. In the setting of ED overcrowding, these delays are not going to be welcome.

N. B. Handly, MD, MSc, MS

Retrospective Application of the NEXUS Low-Risk Criteria for Cervical Spine Radiography in Canadian Emergency Departments
Dickinson G, for the Canadian C-Spine and CT Head Study Group (Univ of Ottawa, Ont, Canada; et al)
Ann Emerg Med 43:507-514, 2004   1–3

Background.—Blunt trauma with potential cervical spine injury is a common presentation in the ED. Most of these 1 million or more cases annually in the United States involve soft tissue injuries, but approximately 30,000 patients have cervical spine fractures or dislocations, and about 10,000 patients have spinal cord injuries. The disastrous sequelae of cervical spinal cord injury have led to a low threshold for ordering cervical spine radiographs in trauma patients. Studies have reported that despite the widespread use of cervical spine radiographs in all trauma patients, more than 98% of the results are negative. This inefficient use of cervical spine radiography wastes health care resources, prolongs uncomfortable immobilization with hard collars and back boards, and results in unnecessary exposure to ionizing radiation. Adoption of a widely accepted clinical decision rule for cervical spine radiography that is safe and efficient could reduce the large number of normal radiographic studies. The accuracy, reliability, and potential effects of the National Emergency X-Radiography Utilization Study (NEXUS) low-risk criteria for cervical spine radiography were evaluated in a large cohort of alert blunt trauma patients in Canadian EDs.

Methods.—The Canadian C-Spine Rule derivation study was a prospective cohort study that was conducted in 10 EDs in Canada. The study included alert and stable adult trauma patients. Physicians completed a 20-item data form for each patient and performed interobserver examinations when feasible. The prospective assessments included the 5 individual NEXUS criteria but not an explicit interpretation of the overall need for radiography according to the criteria. The patients were evaluated with plain radiography, flexion-extension views, and CT at the discretion of the treating physician. Patients who did not undergo radiographic examination were followed up with a structured outcome assessment by telephone to determine clinically important cervical spine injury.

Results.—A total of 8924 patients were enrolled, and 151 (1.7%) of them had an important cervical spine injury. The sensitivity and specificity of the combined NEXUS for identification of important cervical spine injury were 92.7% and 37.8%, respectively. Application of the NEXUS criteria would have potentially reduced cervical spine radiography rates by 6.1% from the actual rate of 68.9% to 62.8%. Of the 11 patients who had important injuries not identified, 2 were treated with internal fixation and 3 with a halo.

Conclusions.—The NEXUS low-risk criteria were less sensitive than previously reported. These criteria should be subjected to further prospective evaluation of their accuracy and reliability before they are widely used outside the United States.

▶ This study from the Canadian C-Spine Group shows how much results can change based on a change of a few study details. While NEXUS criteria as tested in the United States yielded a sensitivity of 99.6% for identifying clinically significant C-spine injury, this study found a sensitivity of only 92.7%. This allowed several significant injuries to be missed.

This difference likely occurred because the authors did not apply the exact protocol of the NEXUS study. The difference was how the application of the criteria regarding intoxication and neurologic deficits were used in the Canadian study. The authors noted that their surrogate markers for each were more subjective (their κ values as measures of interobserver agreement were much less than those found in the NEXUS study). In addition, the inclusion criteria in the 2 studies were not the same. However, at least the study samples appeared to have a similar likelihood of significant C-spine injury (1.7%).

The authors suggest that the NEXUS criteria are not as ideal for use in application in Canadian EDs. However, the study needs to be repeated with the specific NEXUS criteria (no surrogates) before it can be truly judged lacking.

It is reasonable to apply the NEXUS criteria, but we need to be a bit obsessive about following the NEXUS protocol precisely.

N. B. Handly, MD, MSc, MS

Whole Spine MRI in the Assessment of Acute Vertebral Body Trauma
Green RAR, Saifuddin A (Royal Natl Orthopaedic Hosp Trust, Middlesex, England)
Skeletal Radiol 33:129-135, 2004   1–4

Background.—The incidence of noncontiguous, multilevel injury is reported to range from 4.2% to 23.8% on the basis of plain radiographic studies of patients with spinal trauma referred to spinal injury units. Serious implications can be present for the management of patients when additional spinal injuries are not diagnosed. Thus, radiographic assessment of the spine has been advocated for all patients who have suffered a spinal fracture to identify noncontiguous vertebral injuries. The incidence and types of multilevel vertebral body injury in association with acute spinal trauma as assessed by whole spine MRI were determined.

Methods.—A whole spine MRI was performed on all acute admissions to a regional spinal injury unit for detection of occult vertebral body injury. During 3 years, 127 cases were prospectively assessed by 2 radiologists. All of the patients were examined with T2-weighted sagittal imaging of the whole spine, with T1-weighted imaging in both sagittal and axial planes covering the primary injury. The main outcome measure was the incidence of secondary spinal injury (bone bruising, wedge compression fracture, or burst fracture) as determined by type, site, and relationship to the primary injury.

Results.—A secondary injury level was identified in 77% of cases. Of these, bone bruising was the most common, but it often occurred in combination with secondary wedge compression fracture or burst fracture. Twenty-seven noncontiguous wedge compression fractures and 16 noncontiguous burst fractures were seen, equal to an incidence of approximately 34% for secondary level, noncontiguous fracture.

Conclusions.—A higher frequency of secondary level vertebral body injury may be identified by MRI than has been reported in previous studies that were based on radiographic evaluation of the whole spine. Whole spine MRI as assessment for occult vertebral body fracture can provide increased confidence in the conservative or surgical management of patients with severe spinal injury.

▶ Green and Saifuddin report a significant number of secondary spinal injuries associated with initial obvious spinal cord injuries. They did not report how many of their findings necessitated a change in management, which would have been interesting to note, but all the injuries they report are associated with significant long-term pain. The authors also did not report whether the patients complained of pain at the site of secondary injury (and thus, why the injury wasn't initially diagnosed after careful examination and attention to detail). I'll be interested to see if routine whole spine MRI becomes standard fare for patients with acute spinal cord injury.

R. K. Cydulka, MD, MS

Extremity Injury

Jumpers and Fallers: A Comparison of the Distribution of Skeletal Injury
Teh J, Firth M, Sharma A, et al (Royal London Hosp, Whitechapel; St Bartholomew's Hosp, West Smithfield, London)
Clin Radiol 58:482-486, 2003   1–5

Introduction.—The multiple injuries sustained in free-falls from heights present complex management problems. In such cases, the distribution of injuries tends to differ from that seen in other causes of polytrauma. The radiological records of patients injured by either jumping or falling from a height were reviewed to determine whether patterns of skeletal injury differ between jumpers and fallers.

Methods.—Patients included in the study had been admitted via the Helicopter Medical Service (HEMS) to the Royal London Hospital. Those injured in falls were classified as jumpers or fallers by their own or eye-witness accounts. Demographic data and the distribution of bony injuries were compared in the 2 groups.

Results.—Of the 2040 patients admitted via HEMS between 1990 and 1998, 342 were fallers and 57 were jumpers. Most jumpers had attempted suicide, whereas most fallers were working at a height on ladders or at construction sites. Sex distribution was similar in the jumper group; men far out-

numbered women in the faller group. The mean number of fractures per person was 5.8 for jumpers and 2.4 for fallers. Jumpers had a higher death rate (28%) than fallers (16%), a higher mean Injury Severity Score (26.1 vs 18.4) than for fallers, and sustained more rib fractures (particularly on the right) and more pelvic and lower limb fractures. There were more skull fractures, however, among fallers.

Conclusion.—This is the first study to document a marked difference in the distribution of injury between jumpers and fallers. Jumpers had more serious injuries and a higher mortality rate, possibly because the distance of their falls was greater. Jumpers also tended to land feet-first and appeared to try to break their falls using their dominant (right) side, thus sustaining greater injury to the right chest wall. The pattern of injury may help the forensic pathologist to distinguish whether a patient has jumped or fallen from a height.

▶ You may have missed this article from the United Kingdom—a comparison of the bones broken when someone jumps as opposed to falls from a height, based on 399 patients with 1244 fractures. It turns out that the awareness that a jumper has while falling makes it more likely that the person will try to break their fall with their extremities, particularly with their dominant side, and will tend to have a marked right-sided predominance of rib fracture. Fallers, who are presumably unprepared, have an even distribution of right and left rib fractures. Useful information? A careful look for lower extremity injury is, of course, warranted in both groups, but knowing the history might cause more scrutiny on the right side and lower extremities. This information can also be added to your emergency medicine trivia collection.

W. P. Burdick, MD, MSEd

Magnetic Resonance Imaging in Bone Bruising in the Acutely Injured Knee—Short-term Outcome
Davies NH, Niall D, King LJ, et al (Westminster Hosp, London)
Clin Radiol 59:439-445, 2004   1–6

Background.—The frequency and pattern of bone bruising associated with different injuries have been well documented. However, the short-term clinical significance, time to resolution, and long-term implications of bone bruising are not known. The short-term radiologic outcome of bone bruising in patients with acutely injured knees was determined.

Methods.—The study included 30 patients, 17 to 39 years old. All had bone bruising detected by MRI after acute knee injury. The patients were rescanned 12 to 14 weeks after the initial injury. The volume of bone bruising was measured on coronal short R1 inversion recovery (STIR) images. Findings were correlated with the presence and types of ligamentous and osteochondral injuries.

Findings.—In all patients, bone bruises were seen on repeat MRI. Sixty-seven percent of the patients had associated anterior cruciate ligament

(ACL) injuries. Twenty-three percent had collateral ligament injuries, and 10% had no associated ligamentous injuries. Eighty percent of the patients had a more than 50%-reduction in bone bruise volume at repeat scanning, and 17% had a less than 50%-reduction. In 1 patient, bone bruising volume was increased at follow-up. Initial size and size reduction of bone bruising were not associated with the presence or type of associated injury. Bone bruises resolved from the periphery in 21 patients. In 8 patients, all of whom had associated osteochondral injuries, bone bruises resolved toward the joint margins. Seventeen patients had bone bruising extending to the joint margin, including 10 with associated osteochondral injuries on MRI. At clinical review, all but 1 patient still had some knee pain. The 1 patient with complete symptom resolution was 1 of 3 with isolated bone bruising.

Conclusions.—These data suggest that bone bruises persist for at least 12 to 14 weeks, which is longer than has been appreciated. Two discrete patterns of bone bruise resolution were identified. The size and persistence of bone bruising is not associated with the presence or type of associated ligamentous injury.

▶ I must admit that prior to reading this article, bone bruising was a clinical entity that I didn't really know existed. I suppose I haven't kept my finger on the pulse of orthopedics as closely as I could have. Sure, I've used the term for many years to explain to patients why they were having so much pain in the absence of a radiographic fracture, but now I can say it and know that I'm describing a real entity. Although this study deals with a skewed population, that is, patients already undergoing MRI for acute knee injuries and therefore, can't be generalized to everyone with bony trauma, the take-home message from this article is that bone bruises persist for several months and may lead to ongoing pain.

R. K. Cydulka, MD, MS

Pain Management After Discharge From the ED
McIntosh SE, Leffler S (Univ of Vermont, Burlington)
Am J Emerg Med 22:98-100, 2004   1–7

Background.—Pain management is an important aspect of emergency medical care that has not been well studied. Some studies have evaluated the use of analgesic medication during the ED visit, but few studies have specifically addressed the topic of pain control after a patient has been discharged from the ED. This is of particular concern because ED physicians seldom have an opportunity to follow-up a patient through scheduled visits. It is assumed by physicians that the analgesic is efficacious for the particular patient, the patient will fill the prescription, take the medication as prescribed, and use the medication safely, and that patients who continue to experience pain will return to the ED or to their primary care physician. However, it is not known whether these assumptions are true. The management of pain after patients are discharged from the ED was examined. It was hypothesized

that pain management after discharge would be adequate and that patients would use their medications as prescribed.

Methods.—A total of 144 patients were surveyed by telephone after treatment in the ED for common orthopedic complaints. A standardized questionnaire was used to assess prescription-filling practices, side effects of medications, interventions by other health care professionals, and the adequacy of pain relief.

Results.—Survey results indicated that most patients (77%) discharged from the ED were satisfied with their pain relief. Of the patients who did not fill their prescriptions, only 67% were satisfied with their pain relief. Side effects were reported by 26% of patients, but most were minor. Medication prescriptions went unfilled by 13% of patients. Of the patients for whom narcotic analgesics were prescribed, 7% drove vehicles while taking medications.

Conclusions.—Most of these patients after discharge from the ED were satisfied with their pain control. Most filled their prescriptions and did so in a timely manner. Patients who did not fill their prescriptions reported the lowest level of satisfaction with their pain control.

▶ This is an interesting problem for emergency physicians. The Joint Commission of Accreditation of Healthcare Organizations expects us to document pain scores and response to treatment in the hospital. But what happens when the patients leave the ED? Were the plans effective?

There may be some sampling problems with this study. The authors say they contacted 150 patients, of which 144 consented to the survey. However, we are not told how many met the inclusion criteria of orthopedic injury. We have no way of knowing whether the uncontacted group is described by the results of the 144.

Utilizing their results, it is interesting that satisfaction with pain relief was present in 88% of those not given take-home medications or not receiving a a prescription. Seventy-seven percent of those given medications or filling their prescriptions were satisfied, as were 67% of those who did not fill their prescriptions. (I entered these values into Stata 7 [StataCorp LP, College Station, Texas] software and found that there was no statistical difference between these values of satisfaction.)

While there are a number of limitations to this work, this article raises some interesting points to pursue. If pain is defined by the patient, from both physiologic and psychologic mechanisms, what is our role in giving or not giving medications? Clearly, we have to ensure safe use of the medications. This study reveals that a number of patients did use narcotics while driving, which is potentially dangerous. What constitutes effective medication for pain relief? We do pretty well according to this study. Note that those who did not fill their prescriptions generally fell into 2 groups: those who did not like the effects of narcotics, and those who felt that the nonsteroidal anti-inflammatory drugs (NSAIDs) would be inadequate for managing their pain. (Should patients' statements that certain pain medications do not work for them always be interpreted as drug-seeking behavior? Shouldn't a patient be seeking effective pain relief? What is abusive drug seeking?) How do we identify those patients who do not need further medications? These patients had the highest frequency of satisfaction with their pain management. Was this accomplished by establishing a satisfactory relationship in the ED?

It would be interesting to look at prescribing behaviors of emergency physicians to see which cases are identified as severe (likely to receive narcotics), as intermediate (likely to be managed with NSAIDs), and as mild (likely to be managed without further medication).

N. B. Handly, MD, MSc, MS

Emergency Department Analgesia for Fracture Pain

Brown JC, Klein EJ, Lewis CW, Johnston BD, et al (Univ of Washington, Seattle)

Ann Emerg Med 42:197-205, 2003   1–8

Background.—Research on the use of analgesia in EDs has demonstrated that patients often do not receive medication for painful conditions. The use

TABLE 2.— Proportion of Patients Who Had Closed Clavicle or Extremity Fractures and Received Pain and Narcotic Analgesia (Adjusted for Survey Design, Fracture Type, Year, Hospital Admission, Orthopedic Care, and Geographic Location)

Population/ Age, y	No. of Patients (% Total)*	Proportion Receiving Any Analgesic Agents (95% Confidence Limits)	Proportion Receiving Narcotic (95% Confidence Limits)
All patients			
0-3	102	0.54 (0.41, 0.67)	0.21 (0.11, 0.31)
4-8	232	0.63 (0.57, 0.68)	0.30 (0.22, 0.37)
9-15	487	0.60 (0.57, 0.64)	0.27 (0.23, 0.32)
16-29	514	0.67 (0.62, 0.73)	0.47 (0.40, 0.54)
30-69	1,039	0.68 (0.64, 0.72)	0.51 (0.46, 0.56)
≥70	454	0.58 (0.52, 0.65)	0.41 (0.35, 0.48)
Patients with any pain score recorded			
0-3	46 (47)	0.56 (0.40, 0.72)	0.32 (0.17, 0.46)
4-8	141 (62)	0.63 (0.56, 0.71)	0.28 (0.18, 0.39)
9-15	277 (57)	0.61 (0.56, 0.66)	0.32 (0.26, 0.39)
16-29	287 (58)	0.67 (0.60, 0.74)	0.49 (0.41, 0.57)
30-69	604 (60)	0.73 (0.67, 0.79)	0.56 (0.48, 0.64)
≥70	268 (61)	0.60 (0.52, 0.67)	0.43 (0.35, 0.52)
Patients with moderate to severe pain recorded			
0-3	28 (25)	0.62 (0.41, 0.84)	0.45 (0.24, 0.66)
4-8	85 (35)	0.76 (0.63, 0.88)	0.43 (0.26, 0.59)
9-15	150 (28)	0.68 (0.59, 0.77)	0.41 (0.30, 0.51)
16-29	149 (38)	0.79 (0.71, 0.87)	0.59 (0.48, 0.89)
30-69	380 (42)	0.78 (0.71, 0.85)	0.63 (0.55, 0.70)
≥70	185 (35)	0.62 (0.51, 0.72)	0.47 (0.39, 0.55)

*Adjusted for survey design only.

(Courtesy of Brown JC, Klein EJ, Lewis CW, et al: Emergency department analgesia for fracture pain. *Ann Emerg Med* 42:197-205, 2003.)

of analgesics among patients with extremity or clavicular fractures seeking ED care was analyzed retrospectively.

Methods.—Data were obtained from the National Center for Health Statistics National Hospital Ambulatory Medical Care Survey done between 1997 and 2000. The analysis included 2828 patients with isolated closed fractures of the extremities or clavicle.

Findings.—Any analgesic was given to 64% of the patients, and a narcotic analgesic was received by 42%. Pain severity scores had been documented in 59% of visits overall, including 47% of children younger than 4 years and 34% of those younger than 1 year. An analgesic was given to 73% of patients with documented moderate or severe pain, and a narcotic was given to 54%. A smaller proportion of children received an analgesic or narcotic compared with adults. After adjusting for confounders and survey design, any analgesic was received by 54% of patients, 0 to 3 years old; 63% of patients, 4 to 8 years old; 60% of patients, 9 to 15 years old, 67% of patients, 16 to 29 years old; 68% of patients, 30 to 69 years old; and 58% of patients, 70 years and older. The respective proportions of patients receiving a narcotic analgesic were 21%, 30%, 27%, 47%, 51%, and 41%. Children treated in pediatric EDs were about as likely as those treated in other EDs to receive any analgesia or a narcotic analgesia (Table 2).

Conclusions.—Pain medications are often not given to children and adults with extremity or clavicular fractures seen in an ED, even when the pain is documented to be moderate or severe. Frequently, pain severity scores are not noted. Children are least likely to receive analgesics.

► Brown and colleagues remind us (again) of our failure to provide analgesia to our patients with clavicular and extremity fractures, conditions obviously associated with a lot of pain. Clearly, we need to pay closer attention to our patients' comfort. However, at the risk of incurring the wrath of some of my closest colleagues, I must take exception to our national preoccupation with pain scores. Personally, I don't give a hoot what my patients' pain scores are. I ask them if they're having pain and are uncomfortable and if they would like an analgesic. I then provide them with an analgesic and return a short while later to determine if they've obtained pain relief. I continue this process until the patient is comfortable. No scores—just common sense. Go ahead and report me to the pain police. At least my patients are comfortable.

R. K. Cydulka, MD, MS

A Novel Pain Management Strategy for Combat Casualty Care
Kotwal RS, O'Connor KC, Johnson TR, et al (Univ of Texas, Galveston; Command and Gen Staff College, Fort Leavenworth, KS; Uniformed Services Univ of Health Sciences, Bethesda, Md; et al)
Ann Emerg Med 44:121-127, 2004   1–9

Background.—The effective management of severe pain in a traditional hospital setting is often challenging; managing such pain in an out-of-hospital, combat, or austere setting is even more demanding. Opiates have for many years been the foundation of treatment for moderate to severe pain. However, it takes 20 to 30 minutes to achieve pain relief with opiates in pill, capsule, or liquid form. Transdermal patches are suboptimal because of their delay in pain relief, and IM or subcutaneous opiates can be inadequate because of uncertainty regarding their absorption. In light of these limitations, IV morphine is recommended for combat casualties requiring analgesia. However, the insertion of a simple IV catheter can often be delayed by tactical requirements and environmental limitations. The effectiveness of a novel application of oral transmucosal fentanyl citrate, currently indicated for the management of chronic cancer pain, in the amelioration of acute pain in soldiers wounded in a combat environment was evaluated.

Methods.—Oral transmucosal fentanyl citrate was administered in doses of 1600 μg by medical personnel during combat operations in Operation Iraqi Freedom from March 3, 2003, to May 3, 2003. Hemodynamically stable casualties presenting with isolated, uncomplicated orthopedic injuries or extremity wounds who would not have otherwise required an IV catheter were eligible for treatment and evaluation. The verbal 0 to 10 numeric rating scale was used to quantify pretreatment, 15-minute posttreatment, and 5-hour posttreatment pain intensity.

Results.—A total of 22 patients age 21 to 37 years were enrolled in the study. The mean difference in verbal pain scores was found to be statistically significant between the mean pain rating at 0 minutes and the rating at 15 minutes. However, the mean difference was not statistically different between 15 minutes and 5 hours, which is indicative of the sustained action of the intervention without the need for redosing. Hypoventilation was experienced by 1 patient, but the episode was quickly resolved with the administration of naloxone. Other adverse effects were minor and included pruritis (22.7%), nausea (13.6%), emesis (9.1%), and lightheadedness (9.1%).

Conclusions.—Oral transmucosal fentanyl citrate was found to be an effective alternative for pain management, providing rapid-onset and noninvasive pain management in a combat, out-of-hospital, or austere environment.

▶ This is mandatory reading for anyone engaged in the practice of disaster medicine or tactical EMS, military or civilian. Although this was a small study and its results are not terribly surprising, it shows that research can be done in a war or mass casualty setting and should encourage others in this area. The study is also important because it examines the use of nonparental opiate administration in the out-of-hospital environment, an idea warranting further study in both the EMS and disaster medicine fields.

S. L. Werner, MD

Rapid Onset of Cutaneous Anethesia With EMLA Cream After Pretreatment With a New Ultrasound-Emitting Device

Katz NP, Shapiro DE, Herrmann TE, et al (Brigham and Women's Hosp, Boston)
Anesth Analg 98:371-376, 2004   1–10

Introduction.—Topical anesthetics such as EMLA cream, a eutectic mixture of the local anesthetics lidocaine and prilocaine, take approximately 60 minutes to induce local anesthesia of the skin, a waiting period that is impractical in many clinical situations. Sonophoresis, in which sound energy is used to enhance drug transport, may be able to accelerate the transdermal delivery of lidocaine. A prototype device for sonophoresis was tested in a randomized, double-blinded, placebo-controlled trial.

Methods.—The treatments compared in a group of volunteers used low-frequency (55 kHz) US pretreatment or no pretreatment followed by application of 1 g of EMLA or placebo cream for 5, 10, 15, and 60 minutes. Both creams were applied to various sites on the ventral forearms in a crossover manner in which each volunteer received both EMLA and placebo cream for a given treatment time. Pain was tested by pricks with a 20-g needle, and volunteers were asked to state their treatment preference.

Results.—The EMLA cream was significantly better than the placebo cream at each time point for both pain score and arm preference. When EMLA cream was compared with and without US pretreatment, the estimates of difference in treatment effect favored US pretreatment at 60 minutes, but the difference did not reach statistical significance. No significant side effects were attributed to either US or EMLA cream, although pallor, a known effect of EMLA cream, was more common with EMLA than with placebo cream.

Conclusion.—After only 5 minutes, EMLA cream with US pretreatment provided cutaneous analgesia at a level that was not significantly different from that of EMLA cream without pretreatment at 60 minutes. Low-energy US may be useful in hastening the analgesic effect of EMLA cream when used in patients undergoing procedures such as IV cannulation and venipuncture.

▶ Sonophoresis is a new word in my vocabulary, and it means the enhancement of drug transport using sound energy. Topical anesthetic therapy makes so much sense; the duration of onset, however, is often longer than some clinicians are willing to wait. This study, supported by the manufacturer of the product, unfortunately, doesn't solidly answer the question of interest—namely: does the device speed up the onset of anesthesia? The authors used historic evidence of duration of EMLA onset to make the claim that the device worked, since they report that at 5 minutes participants felt the level of anesthesia with US expected at 60 minutes without US. It would have been more convincing to look at the level of anesthesia with and without the device at each time interval. In addition, a potential placebo effect should be been controlled for with a sham US. Despite the drawbacks with the current study, if a simple, cheap, small delivery system can be developed, this concept may have a future.

W. P. Burdick, MD, MSEd

Sterile Versus Nonsterile Gloves for Repair of Uncomplicated Lacerations in the Emergency Department: A Randomized Controlled Trial
Perelman VS, Francis GJ, Rutledge T, et al (Univ of Toronto; McMaster Univ, Ont, Canada)
Ann Emerg Med 43:362-370, 2004   1–11

Introduction.—Sterile technique continues to be recommended for treating lacerations in the ED, although evidence to support this practice is lacking. Some studies, in fact, report that tap water is safe for cleansing traumatic wounds in the ED and that infection rates are not increased when masks or sterile gloves are not used during laceration repair. The infection rate of lacerations was compared in patients randomly assigned to receive repair with the use of sterile versus clean, nonsterile gloves.

Methods.—The study was conducted in 3 large community hospitals in the greater Toronto area. A total of 816 patients agreed to take part in the trial and were randomly designated in strata according to the site of laceration. Data recorded included age and sex of the patient, type of injury, time from injury to repair, and technique of repair. Physicians who provided follow-up care were asked to complete a questionnaire related to the presence or absence of wound infection. Neither these physicians nor the patients were aware of whether sterile or nonsterile gloves had been used.

Results.—The clean-boxed and sterile glove groups were similar in baseline characteristics. Most patients were men (72.9%) and most lacerations were located on the extremities (61.8%). Lacerations were typically treated approximately 3 hours after the injury, and treatment was similar in the 2 groups. Follow-up was obtained for 98% of the sterile group and 96.6% of the clean gloves group. There were 24 wound infections in the sterile gloves group (6.1%) and 17 in the clean-boxed gloves group (4.4%), not a statistically significant difference.

Conclusion.—Infections are not more common when lacerations are repaired with clean, nonsterile gloves instead of sterile gloves. Routine use of boxed gloves rather than sterile gloves and strict sterile technique would be more convenient and reduce the cost of supplies.

▶ Sometimes we do things because we have always done it that way. Here is a gutsy article that challenges the assumption that the use of sterile gloves is necessary to prevent wound infections. Wrong. In fact, probably the most important intervention is vigorous mechanical irrigation with water, and guess what—the water doesn't need to be sterile either. I routinely bring patients with minor hand injuries to the sink and direct a reasonably strong stream of water onto the wound. In addition to cleaning and debriding the wound, it teaches patients the right thing to do for the lacerations we never see.

W. P. Burdick, MD, MSEd

Tetanus Immunity and Physician Compliance With Tetanus Prophylaxis Practices Among Emergency Department Patients Presenting With Wounds
Talan DA, Abrahamian FM, Moran GJ, et al (Olive View-Univ of California, Sylmar, Calif; Univ of California, Los Angeles; Long Island Jewish Med Ctr, New Hyde Park Island, NY; et al)
Ann Emerg Med 43:305-314, 2004   1–12

Introduction.—There is widespread availability of a safe and effective vaccine, yet tetanus continues to occur in the United States. No seroprevalence data exists regarding ED patients seeking wound care. There is concern that many patients treated for wounds do not receive adequate tetanus immunizations. Tetanus seroprotection rates and physician compliance with tetanus prophylaxis recommendations were examined among patients seeking wound care.

Methods.—Patients aged 18 years or older who received wound care at 5 university-affiliated EDs were evaluated between March 1999 and August 2000 in a prospective observational trial. Serum antitoxin levels were measured via enzyme immunoassay. Seroprotection was defined as over 0.15 IU/mL. Seroprotection rates, risk factors for lack of seroprotection, and rates of physician compliance with tetanus prophylaxis recommendations by the Advisory Committee on Immunization Practices were ascertained.

Results.—The rate of seroprotection for 1988 patients was 90.2% (95% confidence interval, 88.8%-91.5%). Groups that had significantly lower seroprotection rates were persons aged 70 years or older, 59.5% (risk ratio [RR], 5.2); immigrants from outside North America or Western Europe, 75.3% (RR, 3.7); individuals with a history of inadequate immunization, 86.3% (RR, 2.9); and persons with no education beyond grade school, 76.5% (RR, 2.5). They had a history of adequate immunization, but 18% of immigrants lacked seroprotection. Of the 60.9% of patients who needed immunization, 57.6% did not receive recommended immunization. Among patients with tetanus-prone wounds, appropriate prophylaxis (ie, tetanus immunoglobulin and toxoid) was not provided to any of the 504 patients who gave a history of inadequate primary immunization (15.1% had nonprotective antibody titers). Among the 276 who required only a toxoid booster, 218 (79%) received appropriate prophylaxis.

Conclusion.—Seroprotection rates are usually high in the United States, but the risk of tetanus remains among the elderly, immigrants, and persons without education beyond grade school. Underimmunization is substantial in the ED—particularly concerning use of tetanus immunoglobulin—leaving many patients unprotected, especially those in high-risk groups.

▶ A startlingly high proportion of patients who need tetanus prophylaxis leave the ED without getting it. This is clearly a preventable system failure, since there are many checks along the way that should be invoked to make sure this doesn't happen. Computerized discharge instructions that force the physician to question whether a patient needs prophylaxis is one way, but several members of the team—including the triage nurse, admitting clerk, floor nurse, aide—can easily become involved in a system that prevents this from happening.

I have only seen one case of clinical tetanus, but it was one I will never forget. The patient survived, probably because he presented to the ED for a subcutaneous broken needle (used for heroin) and proceeded to develop opisthotonus while waiting for an x-ray. Sometimes simple interventions that have been highly successful, like tetanus prophylaxis, are taken for granted and awareness of the consequences of infection relegated to medical history books.

W. P. Burdick, MD, MSEd

▶ I was stunned when I read this study. My gut impression was always that we overimmunize rather than underimmunize. I wonder how much of the underimmunization in 2000 reported by Talan and colleagues was contributed to by the shortage of tetanus vaccines, which may have resulted in some emergency physician's reluctance to order the vaccine.

Regarding tetanus: I've now diagnosed and cared for 3 patients in my career with tetanus. All 3 patients were older and unimmunized. Two of the three had wounds that they thought to be too inconsequential to seek medical care at the time of injury. All 3 patients required mechanical ventilation, prolonged hospital stays, and suffered a great deal of morbidity. All 3 cases could have been prevented with adequate immunization. The Advisory Committee on Immunization Practices, 1991, recommendations seem firmly straightforward: (1) Learn the recommendations. (2) Ask patients about immunization status. (3) Apply the recommendations.

R. K. Cydulka, MD, MS

Cyclobenzaprine With Ibuprofen Versus Ibuprofen Alone in Acute Myofascial Strain: A Randomized, Double-blind Clinical Trial
Turturro MA, Frater CR, D'Amico FJ (Univ of Pittsburgh, Pa; Duquesne Univ, Pittsburgh, Pa)
Ann Emerg Med 41:818-826, 2003   1–13

Background.—Emergency physicians often treat conditions involving acute muscular spasm. Centrally acting muscle relaxants are commonly used to ameliorate loss of function and the discomfort associated with traumatic and atraumatic muscular spasm. The use of cyclobenzaprine in addition to ibuprofen in ED patients with acute myofascial strain was evaluated.

Methods.—One hundred two patients, aged 18 to 70 years, with acute myofascial strain caused by minor trauma in the preceding 48 hours were enrolled in the randomized, prospective, double-blind study. Seventy-seven patients completed the protocol. Each was given 1 dose of 800 mg ibuprofen in the ED and a vial of 6 capsules containing 800 mg ibuprofen to take every 8 hours as needed at ED discharge. Fifty-one patients also received 1 dose of 10 mg cyclobenzaprine and a vial of 6 capsules containing 10 mg cyclobenzaprine to take every 8 hours as needed after ED discharge. The remaining 51 patients were given an identical placebo and vial of placebo capsules. Patients rated their pain intensity on a 100-mm visual analog scale (VAS) periodically up to 48 hours after treatment. Data on adverse effects were collected at 24 and 48 hours by open-ended questioning.

Findings.—Diagnoses and baseline pain scores were similar in the 2 groups. The mean VAS score for the combination therapy group declined from 60.4 to 35.6 during the 48-hour protocol, compared with a decline from 62.2 to 35.4 in the ibuprofen-only group. The mean VAS scores between groups across time were not significant statistically. At 24 and 48 hours, CNS side effects were more frequently reported in the cyclobenzaprine group than in the ibuprofen-only group.

Conclusions.—Adding cyclobenzaprine to ibuprofen in the treatment of ED patients with acute myofascial strain does not improve analgesia. Furthermore, adding cyclobenzaprine is associated with a higher prevalence of adverse CNS effects.

▶ This small underpowered study reported no benefit to adding cyclobenzaprine to ibuprofen in patients with acute myofascial strain. Although the methodologic flaws with this study are too numerous to mention, I like the conclusion because it supports the way I've always practiced and what I've been teaching residents—adding a muscle relaxant to an nonsteroidal anti-inflammatory drug for patients with acute myofascial strain will not improve analgesia but will probably make them too tired to care or function.

R. K. Cydulka, MD, MS

Panoramic Versus Conventional Radiography of Scaphoid Fractures
Berná JD, Chavarria G, Albaladejo F, et al (Univ Gen Hosp, Murcia, Spain; Univ of Murcia, Spain)
AJR 182:155-159, 2004   1–14

Background.—Scaphoid fractures are the most common fractures of the carpal bones and are often difficult to diagnose. Conventional radiography remains the most commonly used diagnostic tool. The role of panoramic radiography (orthopantomography) in the diagnosis of scaphoid fracture of the wrist was examined in this retrospective study.

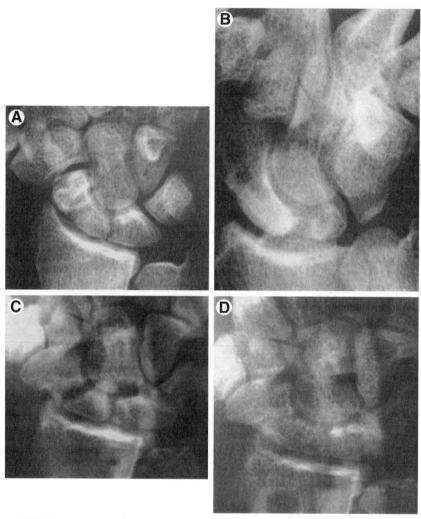

FIGURE 2.—A 20-year-old man who underwent bone graft because of nonunion of scaphoid fracture. A and B, Conventional radiographs obtained 12 months after trauma show doubtful fracture union. C, Panoramic radiograph obtained at same time as A and B shows nonunion (fracture type D_1). D, Panormaic radiograph obtained 4 months after implant shows fracture union. (Courtesy of Berná JD, Chavarria G, Albaladejo F, et al: Panoramic versus conventional radiography of scaphoid fractures. *AJR* 182: 155-159, 2004. Reprinted with permission from the *American Journal of Roentgenology*.)

Study Design.—The study group consisted of 70 male and 20 female patients, aged 11 to 72 years, with acute or chronic wrist trauma seen at 1 hospital between February 1994 and April 2000. These patients all had both conventional and panoramic radiography. The images were independently and retrospectively assessed by 4 observers to compare results between imaging modalities and to evaluate interobserver and intraobserver agreement.

Findings.—Panoramic radiography was superior to conventional radiography of the wrist for determining scaphoid fracture, delayed union, nonunion, and union (Fig 2). Interobserver and intraobserver agreement was higher for panoramic than for conventional radiographs of the wrist.

Conclusion.—Panoramic radiography of the wrist is a simple, rapid, cost-effective procedure for examination of scaphoid fracture. This procedure is useful for clarification of inconclusive conventional radiographic studies of the wrist.

▶ Sometimes the older technology is best. Panoramic views of the scaphoid, like panoramic views of the mouth, make sense because of the curvilinear aspect of the object of interest. The resulting radiographs are also easy to read, and the equipment is readily available and far less expensive to obtain than a CT or MRI machine. In low-resourced or remote locations, this may be an important addition to a plain x-ray.

W. P. Burdick, MD, MSEd

Prevalence and Patterns of Occult Hip Fractures and Mimics Revealed by MRI
Oka M, Monu JUV (Univ of Rochester, NY)
AJR 182:283-288, 2004   1–15

Background.—The prompt and early diagnosis of minimally displaced fractures of the femoral neck is important because delayed diagnosis and treatment can result in significant displacement of the fracture fragment. However, the diagnosis of hip fractures can be difficult on radiography alone. MRI is frequently used to confirm or deny the presence of a minimally displaced hip fracture. The patterns of injury seen on MRI that are difficult to diagnose on radiography were evaluated.

Methods.—The MRIs of 73 patients who were examined for possible fractures of the hip and whose radiographic findings were negative or equivocal for hip fracture were reviewed. A total of 76 studies was performed in 73 patients who were between 24 and 102 years old. The MRIs were evaluated for the presence and location of bone or soft tissue injury. Muscle injuries were classified on the basis of location and type of injury.

Results.—Of the 76 studies, 35 (46%) showed subtle fractures, of which 17 were in the proximal femur and 18 in the innominate bone (Fig 2). Soft tissue abnormalities were found in 65% of the studies. MRI findings were considered normal in 20% of the studied because there was no apparent finding on the images that could explain the patients' symptoms.

Conclusions.—This study of the patterns of hip injury seen on MRI demonstrated that soft tissue abnormalities are commonly observed alone or in association with subtle fractures observed on MRI in patients who are evaluated for a clinical suspicion of hip fracture. It is recommended that MRI ex-

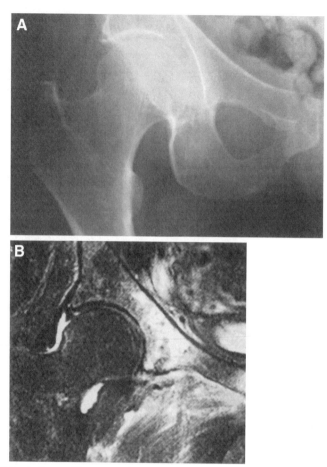

FIGURE 2.—A 67-year-old woman with persistent right hip pain after fall 3 weeks earlier. **A,** Frontal radiograph of right hip shows unremarkable findings. **B,** Coronal T2-weighted image shows abnormally high signal in anterior column of hip and in area of superior pubic ramus, consistent with trabecular fracture. Linear abnormally high signal is seen in adductors and obturator externus and is compatible with presence of interstitial edema or hemorrhage. (Courtesy of Oka M, Monu JUV: Prevalence and patterns of occult hip fractures and mimics revealed by MRI. *AJR* 182:283-288, 2004. Reprinted with permission from the *American Journal of Roentgenology.*)

aminations be performed for all symptomatic patients in whom radiographic findings are negative for hip fracture.

▶ In the past, a negative plain radiograph of the hip meant obtaining a bone scan in several days to look for indirect evidence of fracture. MRI has changed all that. As the figure demonstrates, MRI will literally light up immediately in areas of subtle trabecular fracture and clearly show other fractures that are simply not visible on plain films. Muscle injury, previously a diagnosis of exclusion, is also well defined on MRI, with areas of edema and hemorrhage prominently displayed.

W. P. Burdick, MD, MSEd

Fractures in Access to and Assessment of Trauma Systems
Vassar MJ, Holcroft JJ, Knudson MM, et al (Univ of California, San Francisco; Case Western Reserve Univ, Cleveland, Ohio; Natl Quality Forum, Washington, DC)
J Am Coll Surg 197:717-725, 2003   1–16

Introduction.—The implementation of organized systems of trauma care substantially reduces trauma-related deaths, but few studies have examined deaths at non–trauma center hospitals or compared patient outcomes for trauma center versus non–trauma center hospitals. To determine whether dedicated trauma centers are optimally used in California, discharge records for all acute care hospitals in the state for a 3-year period were reviewed.

Methods.—From 1995 through 1997, a total of 483,997 records were related to trauma (diagnosis codes of 800 to 959 and external cause of injury codes E800 to 999); 400,487 records met inclusion criteria. During this period, 32 (55%) of California's 58 counties were served by 41 designated trauma centers. The 360,743 records used in the final analysis were those of 352,559 survivors and 8184 nonsurvivors who had Abbreviated Injury Scale (AIS) scores assigned. Severity of the trauma and the need for trauma center care were defined by 8 AIS criteria combined with patient age and type of injury.

Results.—Fourteen level I trauma centers treated 22.0% of the discharges; 27 level II and III centers treated 19.3%, and 395 non–trauma center hospitals treated 58.7%. At both trauma centers and non–trauma centers, most study admissions (89% and 82%, respectively) came directly from the ED. According to study criteria, 67,718 patients needed trauma center care and 56% of these patients were treated at a trauma center. Patients 55 years or older who needed trauma center care were less likely than younger patients to receive treatment at a trauma center (40% vs 62%). Of the 29,849 patients who fulfilled AIS criteria but were not treated at a trauma center, 59% were in counties with designated trauma centers and 41% were in counties without trauma centers.

Conclusion.—Most of the serious injuries included in this review occurred in the catchment areas of designated trauma care systems, but only 56% of patients who met AIS severity of trauma criteria were treated at trauma centers. There appears to be substantial undertriage to trauma centers, especially for patients 55 and older and patients with brain injuries. This problem is not explained by a lack of nearby trauma centers in some areas.

▶ "Build it and they will come." Well, not to California trauma centers according to the study by Vassar et al. Trauma centers have been shown to generate better outcomes for trauma victims of all ages; however, this report suggests that even in California regions that have trauma centers, not all patients who "need" trauma care are being transported to trauma centers. Additionally, and perhaps more concerning, there appears to be a significant difference in the fraction being treated at trauma centers based on age, ie, a victim older than 55 years needing trauma care is statistically less likely to receive transport to a trauma center than one less than 55 years old. This is certainly concerning to us in the ED whether we practice in trauma centers or not. (Consider that these elderly patients are thus more likely to show up at non–trauma centers and may need transfer to a trauma center to provide a level of resources that non–trauma centers may not have.)

The determination of "need" for trauma care is the major weakness of this work. The authors use hospital discharge data to construct a list of injuries based on the AIS. They then define a serious injury category, based on the AIS (see Table 1 in the original article), in which any patient satisfying the AIS criteria should need trauma care. The problem with this method is that the discharge diagnoses do not tell us what the paramedics or emergency physicians observed, such as mechanism of injury or unstable vital signs, which are important parts of the triage system for trauma centers. Some of the injuries identified at discharge may not have been detected by the paramedics and thus could have played a role in their triage decision making.

The authors also report levels of overtriage: patients with injuries that did not meet the AIS criteria proposed for trauma center care yet were still transported to trauma centers. We are unable to sort out whether these patients were inappropriately brought to the trauma centers or were among those who came to the ED for general trauma care.

This is an important study with significant results. However, it needs to be redone using paramedic and ED admission data to really answer the possible undertriage issue and how age may play a role.

N. B. Handly, MD, MSc, MS

Should the Routine Wrist Examination for Trauma Be a Four-View Study, Including a Semisupinated Oblique View?

Russin LD, Bergman G, Miller L, et al (Sutter Amador Hosp, Jackson, Calif; Mark Twain St Joseph's Hosp, San Andreas, Calif; American College of Radiology, Reston, Va)
AJR 181:1235-1238, 2003   1–17

Background.—With the exception of navicular bone fractures, fractures of the distal radius are more frequently missed on initial radiographs than any other fracture. Routine radiographic examination of the injured wrist usually includes posteroanterior, posteroanterior oblique, and lateral views. A semisupinated oblique projection is suggested as an additional view when the routine study is inconclusive. The subjective experience at 1 community hospital at which the semisupinated oblique view is part of the routine examination has suggested that this view is particularly sensitive for the detection of distal radius fractures. The relative sensitivity of each of these 4 views for fracture detection was documented, and whether there is a benefit to the routine use of 4 views in the radiographic examination of the wrist for trauma was determined.

Methods.—All wrist examinations performed over a 7-month period at a community hospital that routinely uses the 4-view radiographic examination were collected, and all cases in which an acute fracture of any type was diagnosed were included in this review. The radiographic examinations were reviewed by 3 radiologists at another community hospital and an ED physician with 20 years of experience.

Results.—A total of 54 examinations were reviewed. The reviewers did not find fractures of any bone in 2 of 54 examinations originally reported as positive for fracture. However, the true number of radial fractures in the 54 examinations could not be determined because follow-up examinations and clinical information were not available for confirmation of the diagnoses.

Conclusions.—The semisupinated oblique view of the wrist is the most sensitive view for detection of radial fractures. It is suggested that the routine wrist radiographic examination for trauma should be a 4-view study that includes the semisupinated oblique view.

▶ This study suggests that the semisupinated oblique (SSO) wrist view may provide the best sensitivity for identifying distal radius fractures and thus should be added to the typical 3-view (posteroanterior, lateral, and posteroanterior oblique) wrist series. Suggesting is the correct word, and the authors recognize the limitations of their study. The authors illustrate with a selected set of images the ability of this view to identify a distal radius fracture that each of the other classic 3 views do not. It is the authors' contention that this SSO view allows better visualization of the dorsal distal radius since in this position there is no overlap with the ulna.

This report describes that effort to determine the sensitivity of each of the individual views to diagnose a wrist fracture. The individual views were separated and read randomly to prevent a bias of information from one view to another (this is not the way we normally read films series, however). The reading of a distal radius fracture was observed at a significantly greater frequency in the SSO view than in the other 3. To equate this frequency with sensitivity is not appropriate since the gold standard was a unanimous diagnosis of fracture by the 4 test readers instead of an external objective measure. The false-negative readings of the SSO views (which were all positive for fracture in the other views from the same patient's wrist) demonstrate the importance of multiple views.

Clearly, the SSO view gives information that the other views do not. It is unclear what the cost of adding this image to a routine wrist series would be versus the time and cost of sending the patient back to the radiologic suite for a single SSO view if the standard 3 do not find the fracture.

The problem for the ED physician is to recognize an injury as significant, immobilize it sufficiently, and refer the patient for follow-up. A more appropriate study would be to compare outcomes and costs of the standard 3 views plus clinical evaluation to those with 4 views and clinical evaluation.

N. B. Handly, MD, MSc, MS

Randomized Clinical Trial of Propofol Versus Methohexital for Procedural Sedation During Fracture and Dislocation Reduction in the Emergency Department

Miner JR, Biros M, Krieg S, et al (Hennepin County Med Ctr, Minneapolis)
Acad Emerg Med 10:931-937, 2003   1–18

Background.—Procedural sedation in the ED is intended to minimize perceived pain while maintaining cardiorespiratory function and minimizing the risk of adverse events. However, the risk of cardiorespiratory suppression increases as patients are more deeply sedated. Thus, it is important to determine how deeply a patient is sedated to establish the safety of procedural sedation in the ED. Methohexital has been well studied for use in ED procedural sedation, but propofol has been evaluated less extensively for ED use. The hypothesis that there is no difference in the depth of sedation and the rate of respiratory depression between propofol and methohexital in procedural sedation during the reduction of fractures and dislocations in the ED was investigated.

Methods.—A total of 103 patients were included in this randomized prospective study of nonintoxicated adult patients undergoing procedural sedation for fracture or dislocation reduction in the ED from July 2001 to March 2002. The patients were randomly assigned to either propofol or methohexital 1 mg/kg IV, followed by repeat boluses of 0.5 mg/kg every 2 minutes until adequate sedation was obtained.

Results.—Of the 103 patients, 52 received methohexital and 51 received propofol. Reduction was successful in 94% of patients in the methohexital group and in 98% of patients in the propofol group. There were no cardiac rhythm abnormalities or significant (>20%) declines in systolic pressure. Bag-valve-mask–assisted ventilation was required in 6 patients during the procedure, all for less than 1 minute. Two of these patients received methohexital and 4 received propofol. Respiratory depression was observed in 48% of patients in the methohexital group and 49% of patients in the propofol group. Patients responses on visual analog scales regarding pain associated with the procedure, recall of the procedure, and satisfaction showed similar rates of reported pain, recall, and satisfaction for the 2 agents.

Conclusions.—Methohexital and propofol are safe in the ED. There were no significant differences between the 2 agents in the level of subclinical respiratory depression or the level of sedation by bispectral electroencephalogram analysis.

▶ The authors report a randomized clinical trial of propofol versus methohexital in the ED for procedures of fracture or dislocation reduction. Both agents are notable for rapid onset and short duration. The outcomes measured were respirator depression, depth of sedation (measured by bispectral electroencephalographic analysis [BIS]), duration of sedation, and a postanesthesia recall of pain and satisfaction by the patient. Respiratory depression was measured by early changes such as oxygen saturation to less than 90%, change in end-tidal carbon dioxide greater than 10 mm Hg, or a loss of the end-tidal carbon dioxide waveform from the monitor. Because propofol is an opaque solution and methohexital is not, the treating physician was not blinded to the study drug. Power analysis was used to find the number of patients (n = 44 in each group) so that a 20% difference in fraction having respiratory depression could be found (α = .05; β = .2). The end point of drug delivery was not specified; it is not clear if the end point was objectively based on BIS (it was not stated if the physician giving the drug was aware of the BIS score) or subjectively made by the treating physician based on clinical experience.

No significant differences in outcome were found except that patients requiring multiple doses of either medication were more likely to have respiratory depression and that a single dose of propofol at 1 mg/mL was less likely to cause respiratory depression (1 of 11 patients) than a single dose of methohexital at 1 mg/mL (10 of 23 patients). It seems that methohexital needs to be given in smaller doses or that methohexital is a riskier medication to use.

It is interesting that lowest BIS scores for either drug were not significantly different for either drug. Again, if the physician ordering the sedative was aware of the BIS score, this would not be very surprising. If the physician ordering propofol or methohexital was blinded to BIS score, then that judgment similarity could be based on similarity of training to recognize undescribed factors such as the "Tim sign" (named after one of our nurses) when the eyes roll back. Identifying these factors and comparing them to objective measures such as BIS scores would be interesting.

This study suggests several thoughts about the use of these agents. First, it is difficult to really compare dosing of sedatives without objective measures of sedation. Second, the initial bolus dose of methohexital may be too high; however, the time interval between additional doses (approximately 3 to 5 minutes) may add significantly to the time to complete a procedure. We want to deliver rapid, safe, and effective sedation; having to give multiple doses takes time and, as shown in this study, is more apt to cause respiratory depression. Third, it would be valuable to map the temporal patterns of respiratory depression to understand better how cumulative doses of sedative lead to respiratory depression. This would be helpful in determining if there is an optimal time between multiple doses.

N. B. Handly, MD, MSc, MS

Evaluation

Consequences of Delayed Diagnoses in Trauma Patients: A Prospective Study
Vles WJ, Veen EJ, Roukema JA, et al (St Elisabeth Hosp, Tilburg, The Netherlands)
J Am Coll Surg 197:596-602, 2003   1–19

Background.—A structured approach to the management of injured patients is needed to improve quality of trauma care. Despite recent improvements in trauma care, delays in diagnosis still occur. The prevalence and consequences of delayed diagnoses in 1 European trauma center were described.

Methods.—Complications among all 3879 injured patients hospitalized between January 1996, and January 2000 were registered prospectively. The physicians entered all relevant data into a hospital-wide trauma database with client server architecture. Patients underwent a tertiary survey. All radiographs and CT scans were reassessed within 24 hours after admission.

Findings.—Of the 3879 injured patients, 1016 complications were documented. Fifty-five complications in 49 (1.3%) of the total injured patients were related to delayed diagnoses. In 57.1% of these patients, tertiary survey and re-evaluation of radiographs and CT scans enabled detection of the delayed diagnoses within 24 hours. A delay in diagnosis resulted in delayed treatment in 55.1%. Surgery was needed in 24.5%. None of the diagnosis delays resulted in a patient's death.

Conclusions.—A prospective trauma and complication registration provided an effective method for evaluating delays in diagnosis. More than half of the delayed diagnoses were detected by a tertiary survey and reassessment of radiographs and CT scans. Reducing the number of diagnosis delays can be expected to improve quality of trauma care.

▶ I suspect that using a trauma registry to estimate delayed diagnoses in trauma patients underestimates the designated outcome but doesn't negate the important message that Vles and colleagues present: Physicians must actively investigate their shortcomings in medical care to correct them. Vles et al suggest 2 methods in which trauma care may be improved: (1) Tertiary survey within 24 hours of admission combined with standardized reevaluation of x-rays and CT scans; (2) use of prospective trauma and complication registry databases to elucidate consequences of delayed diagnoses and determination of effects of standardized procedures. I agree and would add 1 more—ongoing daily tertiary surveys. Most of the missed injuries described were associated with changes in care plans, and several were associated with significant morbidity that may have been prevented had the diagnoses been made sooner.

R. K. Cydulka, MD, MS

Prevention of Contrast-Induced Nephropathy With Sodium Bicarbonate: A Randomized Controlled Trial
Merten GJ, Burgess WP, Gray LV, et al (Carolinas Med Ctr, Charlotte, NC)
JAMA 291:2328-2334, 2004   1–20

Introduction.—Contrast-induced nephropathy continues to be a frequent complication in patients undergoing radiographic procedures. Pretreatment with sodium bicarbonate is more protective, compared to sodium chloride, in animal models of acute ischemic renal failure. Acute renal failure from both ischemia and contrast are believed to occur due to free-radical injury. No trials in humans or animals have assessed the efficacy of sodium bicarbonate for prophylaxis against contrast-induced nephropathy. The efficacy of sodium bicarbonate for preventive hydration before and after radiographic contrast was evaluated in a prospective, single-center, randomized trial.

Methods.—Between September 16, 2002, and June 17, 2003, 119 patients with stable serum creatinine levels of at least 1.1 mg/dL (97.2 µmol/L or greater) were randomly assigned to receive a 154 mEq/L infusion of either sodium chloride or sodium bicarbonate before and after iopamidol administration (370 mg iodine/mL). Serum creatinine levels were determined at baseline (bolus of 3 mL/kg/h for 1 hour preprocedure, followed by 1 mL/kg/h for 6 hours postprocedure) and 1 and 2 days after contrast. The primary outcome measure was contrast-induced nephropathy, defined as an increase of 25% or more in serum creatinine within 2 days of contrast.

Results.—No significant group differences were observed in age, gender, incidence of diabetes mellitus, ethnicity, or contrast volume. The baseline serum creatinine level was slightly higher, yet not statistically different, in patients undergoing sodium chloride treatment (mean, 1.71 mg/dL for sodium chloride vs 1.89 mg/dL for sodium bicarbonate; $P = .09$). The primary end point of contrast-induced nephropathy was realized in 8 patients (13.6%) in the sodium chloride group versus 1 (1.7%) in the sodium bicarbonate group (mean difference, 11.9%; 95% confidence interval, 2.6%-21.2%; $P = .02$). A follow-up registry of 191 consecutive patients receiving prophylactic sodium bicarbonate and meeting the identical inclusion criteria resulted in 3 cases of contrast-induced nephropathy (1.6%; 95% confidence interval, 0%-3.4%).

Conclusion.—Hydration with sodium bicarbonate before contrast exposure is more effective compared with hydration with sodium chloride for prophylaxis for contrast-induced renal failure.

▶ There are very few studies that I read that lead me to change my practice. This may be one. Dramatically reducing the incidence of contrast-induced nephropathy by infusing sodium bicarbonate for an hour before contrast exposure seems to make sense after reading Merten and colleagues' report. Of course, like any new therapy, caution must be exercised, and I will await confirmatory studies.

R. K. Cydulka, MD, MS

Sensitivity in Detecting Free Intraperitoneal Fluid With the Pelvic Views of the FAST Exam
von Kuenssberg Jehle D, Stiller G, Wagner D (State Univ of New York, Buffalo)
Am J Emerg Med 21:476-478, 2003   1–21

Background.—The American College of Surgeons has recommended the use of either an abdominal focused assessment with sonography for trauma (FAST) examination or a diagnostic peritoneal lavage (DPL) for the detection of intraperitoneal fluid at the bedside in patients with blunt abdominal trauma. It has been shown that US approaches the accuracy of DPL in determining the need for surgical intervention in blunt abdominal trauma. FAST has also been shown to be a cost-effective bedside procedure that can be rapidly and easily used early during resuscitation in an unstable patient. The recommended use of FAST in blunt abdominal trauma involves 4 examination sites: pericardial, perihepatic, perisplenic, and pelvic. The multiple-view FAST examination has an overall sensitivity of 93%, specificity of 99%, and accuracy of 98% for detection of hemoperitoneum. An average of 2.9 minutes is needed to perform this multiple-view examination, but a single-view FAST examination requires less than 1 minute to perform. The average minimum volume of detectable intraperitoneal fluid with the pelvic views of the FAST examination was evaluated.

Methods.—A prospective observational study was conducted from October 1999 to May 2001 in the ED of a regional level I trauma center. All adult patients who presented to the ED in that period with blunt abdominal trauma and who underwent a clinically indicated DPL were eligible for the study. Patients were placed in the supine position and were administered lavage fluid in 100-mL increments until the fluid was detected on US. Hard-copy US images were also examined for fluid detection. Patients were excluded if they had a positive DPL for hemoperitoneum or a positive initial US for free fluid or lacked sufficient hard-copy US images.

Results.—Seven patients were enrolled. The mean minimal volume of fluid needed for pelvic US detection by the examiner and reviewer was 157 mL and 129 mL, respectively. The median quantity of fluid needed for US detection by both the examiner and reviewer was 100 mL.

Conclusions.—The pelvic views of the FAST examination identified a significantly smaller quantity of intraperitoneal fluid than previous studies of the right upper quadrant single-view examination.

▶ In a study that might be difficult to reproduce with large numbers of patients, these authors infused 100-mL increments of lavage fluid into stable victims of blunt abdominal trauma who had indicated DPLs. Infusion was stopped when the ultrasonographer detected free fluid in the pelvis.

The ultrasonographers were able to find as little as 100 mL (average, 157 mL). Independently, a blinded expert overreader was able to detect an average amount of 129 mL from the US images (the authors do not report, but I have calculated by a paired student *t* test, that these 2 values are not significantly different; $P = .36$). It probably does not matter that the overreader can detect a different amount since the ultrasonographer's reading would be used to direct trauma care.

This study reveals that pelvic views can be more sensitive for detecting free fluid in the peritoneum than right upper quadrant views. Besides the high sensitivity of the pelvic view, the authors remind us that it is easier learned and obtained in the midst of a trauma evaluation. Yet blood in the pelvis may not reflect the typical pattern of bleeding caused by blunt abdominal trauma (which is more likely to come from the liver or spleen and fills other spaces prior to filling the pelvis).

There is no need to change the 4 views of the FAST exam. However, the order in which the views are gathered depends on patient presentation. We often do cardiac views first in unstable views and pelvic views prior to Foley catheter placement. The finding of free fluid by FAST exam should help direct that patient to the operating room. Negative FAST scans alone do not rule out an injury, and further evaluations should occur (including repeated FAST scans).

N. B. Handly, MD, MSc, MS

FAST (Focused Assessment With Sonography in Trauma) Accurate for Cardiac and Intraperitoneal Injury in Penetrating Anterior Chest Trauma
Tayal VS, Beatty MA, Marx JA, et al (Carolinas Med Ctr, Charlotte, NC)
J Ultrasound Med 23:467-472, 2004   1–22

Background.—Evaluation of the patient with penetrating anterior chest trauma is complex and time sensitive because of the critical nature of the organs in that region and the need to identify or exclude the presence of hemorrhage in several cavities simultaneously. Before the introduction of sonography, invasive and surgical procedures were often required to evaluate these patients. The focused assessment with sonography in trauma (FAST) is used to evaluate 3 dependent peritoneal spaces and 1 pericardial view, which allows rapid evaluation of more than 1 torso cavity with sonography. The FAST examination has been widely accepted for the initial evaluation of patients with blunt abdominal trauma and isolated penetrating cardiac injury. The effectiveness of the FAST examination for determining traumatic pericardial effusion and intraperitoneal fluid indicative of injury was evaluated in patients with penetrating anterior chest trauma.

Methods.—This observational prospective study was conducted over a 30-month period at an urban level I trauma center. FAST was performed in the ED by emergency physicians and trauma surgeons. FAST results were recorded before review of patient outcome as determined by one or more of the following: thoracotomy, laparotomy, pericardial window, cardiologic echocardiography, diagnostic peritoneal lavage, CT, and serial examinations.

Results.—FAST was performed in 32 patients with penetrating anterior chest trauma, including 20 with stab wounds and 12 with gunshot wounds. The sensitivity of FAST for cardiac injury (n = 8) in patients with pericardial effusion was 100%. The presence of pericardial effusion determined by FAST was found to be correlated with the need for thoracotomy in 7 of 8 patients (87.5%). Nonsurgical treatment was used in 1 patient with a pericardial blood clot on cardiologic echocardiography. FAST demonstrated a sensitivity of 100% for intraperitoneal injury in 8 patients with views indicating intraperitoneal fluid without pericardial effusion, also with no false-positive results, yielding a specificity of 100%. Necessary laparotomy was prompted by these findings in all 8 patients. Representative FAST examination images show patients in this series with positive pericardial subcostal and hepatorenal windows.

Conclusions.—The FAST examination was sensitive and specific in the determination of both traumatic pericardial effusion and intraperitoneal fluid indicative of injury in this series of patients with penetrating anterior chest trauma, and effectively guided surgical decision making in an emergency setting.

▶ The authors found 100% sensitivity and specificity for traumatic pericardial effusion and for intraperitoneal injury after penetrating anterior chest trauma. Seven of 8 patients with traumatic pericardial effusion required thoracotomy. This is a small number of patients in this series, but a positive study indicates the need for a significant emergent response. Keep in mind that a negative study does not guarantee that there is no injury.

This article reminds us that FAST is not just for abdominal sonography in trauma. It is possible and should be expected that an emergency physician will view pericardial and pleural spaces as well.

N. B. Handly, MD, MSc, MS

▶ This study is important for 2 reasons. It is the first study to examine the efficacy of the FAST examination specific to penetrating chest trauma. The role of the FAST examination in blunt trauma is widely accepted. Plummer et al[1] previously demonstrated that emergency department echocardiography improves outcomes in penetrating cardiac trauma, but this study shows that the FAST examination, when performed by emergency physicians and trauma surgeons in the case of penetrating anterior chest trauma, can identify both cardiac and abdominal injuries requiring emergent operative intervention. This study confirms and adds to the pool of evidence supporting the use of bedside emergency US by emergency physicians. This article is also important in that it was published by the American Institute of Ultrasound Medicine (AIUM). Publication of emergency medicine US research by the AIUM and its creation of a section of Emergency Medicine Ultrasound would seem to signal the growing acceptance of emergency physician use of point of care limited US.

S. L. Werner, MD

Reference

1. Plummer D, Brunnette D, Asinger R, et al: Emergency department echocardiography improves outcome in penetrating cardiac injury. *Ann Emerg Med* 29:357-366, 1997.

Performance of Abdominal Ultrasonography in Blunt Trauma Patients With Out-of-Hospital or Emergency Department Hypotension
Holmes JF, Harris D, Battistella FD (Univ of California-Davis, Sacramento)
Ann Emerg Med 43:354-361, 2004   1–23

Background.—After sustaining blunt trauma, patients with hypotension must be evaluated rapidly to identify and treat the source or sources of hypotension. The initial identification of hemorrhagic sources of hypotension is a priority during initial resuscitation because hypotension caused by hemorrhaging requires urgent volume replacement and specific therapy to stop further hemorrhaging. External sources of hemorrhaging are readily identified on physical examination, and hemorrhaging from pelvic fractures or into the thoracic cavity may be assessed first with pelvic and chest radiography. However, the unreliability of the abdominal examination and limitations of acceptable diagnostic testing in the hemodynamically unstable patient have made intra-abdominal hemorrhages a challenge for the clinician to identify. The test performance of abdominal US for the detection of hemoperitoneum in patients with blunt trauma and out-of-hospital or ED hypotension was determined.

Methods.—A review was conducted of the medical records of all patients with blunt trauma who were hospitalized at a level I trauma center. The patients were included in the study if they were older than 6 years and had out-of-hospital or ED hypotension (systolic blood pressure, ≤90 mm Hg) and had undergone US in the ED. The initial interpretation of the abdominal US scan was recorded and included the presence or absence of intraperitoneal fluid and the specific location of such fluid. The presence or absence of an intra-abdominal injury was determined by an abdominal CT scan, laparotomy, or clinical follow-up.

Results.—The study group was composed of 447 patients whose mean age was 36.0 ± 27.5 years. Of these patients, 148 (33%) had intra-abdominal injuries, and 116 (78%) of these patients had hemoperitoneum. Abdominal US had the following test performance for the detection of patients with intra-abdominal injuries and hemoperitoneum: sensitivity, 79%; specificity, 95%; positive predictive value, 86%; and negative predictive value, 93%. The positive likelihood ratio was 15.8, and the negative likelihood ratio was 0.22. Of the 116 patients with intra-abdominal injuries and hemoperitoneum, 105 underwent therapeutic laparotomy. Abdominal US demonstrated intraperitoneal fluid in 87 of these 105 patients.

Conclusions.—Among patients with out-of-hospital or ED hypotension, abdominal US identified most patients with hemoperitoneum and intra-abdominal injuries. However, further evaluation, including an abdominal evaluation, is needed in patients with hypotension and negative abdominal US results to determine the sources of their hypotension as soon as they are hemodynamically stable.

▶ Diagnostic interventions in all settings need to be iterative and complementary. Very rarely does a single test or examination at a single point in time reveal the diagnosis. This is particularly true in patients with blunt abdominal injuries. US is useful, but as this study points out, it is far from perfect. A combination of US, repeated examinations, and clinical judgment is required to make the decision to proceed to surgery.

W. P. Burdick, MD, MSEd

▶ This study is significantly hampered by its retrospective design. It is not possible to tell whether the subset of patients found to have hemoperitoneum at laparotomy or on CT had hemoperitoneum at the time of the focused abdominal sonography for trauma (FAST) examination. While the authors presume that the sensitivity of the FAST exam may be higher for trauma patients with hypotension than in all trauma patients, it should be noted that many of the patients with hemoperitoneum at laparotomy or on CT had additional significant injuries that may have accounted for their hypotension. It would be interesting to see this study done as a prospective investigation. The study does serve as a reminder as to the limitations of US. It cannot reliably detect solid organ injury or bowel injury—both of which may lead to delayed presentation of hemoperitoneum.

S. L. Werner, MD

Blunt Abdominal Trauma: Clinical Value of Negative Screening US Scans
Sirlin CB, Brown MA, Andrade-Barreto OA, et al (Univ of California, San Diego)
Radiology 230:661-668, 2004   1–24

Background.—US is the primary screening examination for blunt abdominal trauma in a number of centers in Europe and Asia and in select centers in the United States. The advantages of US are that it is nonionizing and portable and can be performed during ongoing resuscitation without interference. However, the use of screening US for detection of blunt abdominal trauma is controversial. The sensitivity of US for detection of abdominal injury ranges from 63% to 99% in published series and compares favorably with that for CT. The concern is that injuries may be missed in patients with negative findings on US; thus, the clinical value of negative screening US is unclear. The clinical and surgical outcomes in patients with blunt abdominal trauma and negative findings on screening US were assessed.

Methods.—A database of 4000 patients who underwent screening US for suspected blunt trauma at a level 1 trauma center was used to retrospectively identify 3679 patients with negative findings on US. The outcome in these patients was determined by a retrospective review of the trauma registry and all radiologic, surgical, and autopsy reports. All imaging studies and medical charts in patients with false-negative findings at screening US were also reviewed.

Results.—Among the 3679 patients with negative findings at screening US, 99.9% had no injuries (true-negative findings). The differences in true-negative rates as a function of year or time of day were not significant. Among the 3641 patients with true-negative findings, 93.7% required no additional tests, and 6.4% underwent CT or other tests. The percentage of patients who underwent additional tests was significantly higher in the first year of the study (19.2%) than in subsequent years. Thirty-eight patients had false-negative US findings for abdominal injury. The injuries that were missed in 24 patients were nonsurgical, and those in 14 patients were surgical. Overall, 65 injuries were missed. The 6 most common injuries were retroperitoneal hematoma (n = 13) and injuries in the spleen (n = 10), liver (n = 9), kidney (n = 8), adrenal gland (n = 8), and small bowel (n = 7). No or trace hemoperitoneum was found in 25 of the 38 patients with false-negative US findings for abdominal injury. The mean diagnostic delay until recognition of missed injury was 16.8 hours. The missed injury was identified within 12 hours in 19 (50%) of 38 patients and within 24 hours in 24 (70%) of 34 patients.

Conclusions.—Negative findings on US in combination with negative clinical observations are virtually exclusive of abdominal injury in patients who are admitted and observed for at least 12 to 24 hours.

▶ This article from the radiology literature uses a large database that is a nice confirmation that a negative US really does exclude pathology. The results are somewhat limited by the retrospective nature of the study design, and the study's generalizability assumes comparable operator skill levels. It is interesting to note that at the authors' institution, radiology residents apparently do the trauma US; after they go home, according to the article, only CT is performed.

W. P. Burdick, MD, MSEd

Blunt Trauma to the Gastrointestinal Tract and Mesentery: Is There a Role for Helical CT in the Decision-Making Process?
Scaglione M, de Lutio di Castelguidone E, Scialpi M, et al ("A Cardarelli" Hosp, Naples, Italy; Santissima Annunziata Hosp, Taranto, Italy; Univ of Naples, Italy)
Eur J Radiol 50:67-73, 2004   1–25

Background.—Early diagnosis of bowel perforation is difficult in patients who have previously had upper abdominal trauma. Clinical diagnosis of mesenteric injuries, and the differentiation of these injuries requiring surgery from those that can heal clinically, is often difficult. CT of the bowel and mesenteric injuries is difficult, and optimal technique and skilled interpretation are needed to accurately assess the spectrum of findings provided. The diagnostic capabilities and limitations of CT in the detection of bowel and mesenteric injuries were investigated, the CT findings of bowel and mesenteric injuries were evaluated in light of the clinical and surgical observations, and the effects of CT findings on clinical management decisions were assessed by reviewing experience during the past 3 years.

Methods.—A retrospective review was conducted of 36 consecutive patients with blunt traumatic injuries to the bowel and mesentery at one regional level I trauma center during the past 3 years. Physical examination, laboratory findings, and CT and intraoperative findings were compared.

Results.—Surgically proved bowel injuries (13 patients) occurred in the duodenum (3 patients), the ileum (2 patients), the jejunum (2 patients), the colon (3 patients), and the stomach (3 cases). CT findings considered specific for bowel rupture were observed in 5 of 13 patients. CT findings considered suggestive of bowel injury were observed in the remaining 8 patients. Mesenteric injury was surgically observed in 23 patients. CT findings considered specific for mesenteric laceration were active extravasation of contrast material from the mesenteric vessels. CT findings suggestive of mesenteric injury were observed in 13 patients.

Conclusions.—Helical CT was shown to be sensitive in the identification of bowel and mesenteric injury after blunt trauma and can provide a wide spectrum of findings. However, CT cannot be used as the only indicator of bowel and mesenteric injury in patients with isolated thickened bowel wall, mesenteric hematoma, bowel, hematoma, pneumoperitoneum, or gas bubbles.

▶ As we develop more sophisticated tools to make diagnoses, the question should be asked: do we need or want to, and what is the cost? The cost must be liberally construed to include not just the money it takes to obtain and use the equipment and the cost of the personnel to perform and interpret the results, but also the "opportunity cost." This is the term economists use for "what else could we be doing with our time or money?" In the case of trauma patients, this may mean less opportunity for clinicians to perform serial exams or, for the facility, longer waits for patients who "really" need a CT. The majority of findings (eg, thickened bowel wall, hematomas) do not require surgical intervention unless the clinical status deteriorates, raising the question of any significant effect on outcome. It is true, however, that as these new tools become even more advanced and testing times, risks, and false-positive results go down, the opportunity costs may go down as well. The challenge then will be knowing what to do with all the information.

W. P. Burdick, MD, MSEd

Miscellaneous

Trauma Team Activation Criteria as Predictors of Patient Disposition From the Emergency Department
Kohn MA, Hammel JM, Bretz SW, et al (Univ of California, San Francisco; New York Univ; San Francisco Gen Hosp)
Acad Emerg Med 11:1-9, 2004   1–26

Background.—First-tier physiologic criteria, such as abnormal vital signs, and second-tier criteria related to mechanism and location of trauma are often used to determine whether to activate the trauma team in response to an out-of-hospital call. However, use of some of these second-tier criteria can result in a high volume of unnecessary team activations while identifying a small number of additional patients requiring immediate surgical intervention. Under evaluation was the incremental predictive value of specific first-tier and second-tier trauma team activation criteria for severe injury as they are reflected by patient disposition from the ED.

Methods.—A prospective cohort study was conducted to evaluated the association between individual trauma team activation criteria and disposition from the ED. Activation criteria were collected on all adult patients for whom the trauma team was activated over a period of 5 months at an urban level I trauma center. Severe injury disposition, and thus "appropriate" team activation, was defined as immediate operative intervention, admission to the ICU, or death in the ED. Recursive partitioning and multiple logistic regression were used for data analysis.

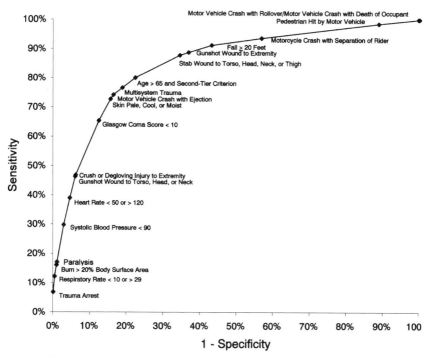

FIGURE 1.—Receiver operating characteristic curve showing each trauma team activation criterion's incremental contribution to both sensitivity and false-positive rate (1–specificity.) (Courtesy of Kohn MA, Hammel JM, Bretz SW, et al: Trauma team activation criteria as predictors of patient disposition from the emergency department. *Acad Emerg Med* 11:1-9, 2004.)

Results.—There were 305 activations for mainly first-tier physiologic criteria, of which 157 (51.5%) resulted in severe injury disposition. The first-tier criterion that caused the greatest increase in inappropriate activations for the lowest increase in appropriate activations was "age greater than 65 years." Of the 34 additional activations caused by this criterion, 7 (20.6%) resulted in severe injury disposition. Of the 700 activations for second-tier criteria, which related to mechanism of injury, 54 (7.7%) resulted in admission to the ICU or operating room, and none resulted in ED death.

The 4 least predictive second-tier criteria were "motorcycle crash with separation of rider," "pedestrian hit by motor vehicle," "motor vehicle crash with rollover," and "motor vehicle crash with death of occupant." Of the 452 activations for these criteria, only 18 activations (4%) resulted in ICU or operating room admission.

Conclusion.—The 4 least predictive second-tier criteria noted above were found to add little sensitivity to the trauma team activation rule at the cost of significantly decreased specificity (Fig 1). It is recommended that these criteria be modified or eliminated. The first-tier criteria evaluated in this study were all found to be useful in predicting the need for an immediate multidisciplinary response. Increased specificity of the first-tier criteria can be obtained by first eliminating the criterion "age greater than 65 years."

▶ This is an elegant study that others may wish to replicate to assess the validity of their own trauma team activation criteria. By simply using patient disposition as criteria for the "true" diagnosis, the sensitivity and specificity for various criteria could be assessed and summarized in a receiver operator characteristic curve. While a careful history and physical examination need to be performed in elderly patients with any trauma, those with stable vital signs and without a central gunshot wound or substantial burn do not need activation of the trauma team.

W. P. Burdick, MD, MSEd

Reliability and Validity of Scores on the Emergency Severity Index Version 3
Tanabe P, Gimbel R, Yarnold PR, et al (Evanston Northwestern Health Care, Ill; Northwestern Univ, Chicago)
Acad Emerg Med 11:59-65, 2004   1–27

Introduction.—Accurate triage category assignment is of particular importance in overcrowded EDs, but the 3-level triage systems used in the United States have shown poor interrater reliability and validity. The Emergency Severity Index (ESI), a 5-level triage system that appears to be superior to 3-level systems, was evaluated in a population-based, cross-sectional, retrospective study.

Methods.—The setting was a large academic urban medical center with an overall ED hospital admission rate of 25%. In August 2000, an ESI replaced the typical 3-level triage system. The records of 199 admitted and 204 discharged patients seen at the ED from May through October 2001 were selected for inclusion. Twenty-seven variables were abstracted, including triage level assigned, admission status, site, and death. Interrater reliability between true triage level and triage score assigned by the registered nurse was calculated using weighted kappa and Pearson correlation. Relationships between the true ESI level and admission, admission site, and death were analyzed.

Results.—The median patient age was 46 years; only 14 patients were younger than 18 years; 51% of the patients were male. Males and females were admitted to hospital in equal proportions, but admitted patients were significantly older than discharged patients (mean, 51.2 vs 38.3 years). Interrater reliability was assessed for 359 patients with complete data. The triage nurse had excellent concordance with the true ESI score (weighted kappa, 0.89; Pearson r, 0.83). There were only 4 cases of marked discordance. The likelihood of admission clearly increased as the ESI score decreased.

Admissions by ESI level were as follows: 1 (80%), 2 (73%), 3 (51%), 4 (6%), and 5 (5%). Admissions to the ICU for these ESI levels were 40%,

12%, 2%, 0%, and 0%, respectively. Three of the 4 patients who died were ESI level 1 or 2.

Conclusion.—Scores on the ESI versus 3 triage algorithm showed excellent reliability and validity and were able to predict admission and location of admission. In this latest version of the ESI, the triage nurse should only consider up-triaging patients with abnormal vital signs.

▶ An ideal triage system would(1) be be easy to use, (2) give similar results no matter who is using it, (3) determine the final disposition of the patient, (4) predict the amount of resource needed to care for the patient, and lastly (5) the method should work in any hospital setting (community and academic).

The ESI had been previously shown to be easy to teach and use (criterion 1), to have good interrelater reliablity (criterion 2, above), and predict disposition of patients (criterion 3). The method has been modified (now version 3) to allow the triage agent to use discretion when confronted by abnormal vitals to upgrade level 3 patients to level 2, instead of rigorously requiring this upgrade in previous versions. These authors tested the new method in an academic center outside the derivation hospitals.

It is clear that the ESI versus 3 seems to work like previous versions in meeting criteria (1-3), even though it now includes an additional subjective step. The authors' work suggests that criterion 5 is also supported by this method.

Determining the amount of resources needed to care for patients with this method is still elusive. Unfortunately, estimates of resources needed is a subjective input to this method, so that ESI in its current form cannot generate logically an output measure of resources needed. Further refinement to help predict these resource needs would be welcome. We often care for patients requiring extensive workup, even though those patients would ultimately be discharged (consider, for example, those who come with right lower quadrant abdominal pain for whom a suspicion of appendicitis must be ruled out before discharge occurs).

Much is made of how important the number of triage levels is to the final product. Tanabe et al find that levels 1 and 5 are so sparsely populated that the system behaves more as a three-level system. Three-level systems have been claimed to be deficient; however, closer looks at the original studies suggest that they failed not because of the number of levels but because of a subjective process for assigning the patients to these levels that the ESI corrects.

N. B. Handly, MD, MSc, MS

Personal Watercraft Injuries: 62 Patients Admitted to the San Diego County Trauma Services
Kim CW, Smith JM, Lee A, et al (Univ of California, San Diego; Sharp Mem Hosp, San Diego, Calif; Children's Hosp, San Diego, Calif; et al)
J Orthop Trauma 17:571-573, 2003   1–28

Background.—It is estimated that more than 1 million personal watercraft, more popularly known as jet skis or waverunners, are in use in the

United States. The percentage of accidents related to personal watercraft is much higher than expected compared with personal watercraft registration totals. Although statistics from California indicate that personal watercraft account for only 16% of all vessels registered in that state, they accounted for 45% of all accidents, 55% of all injuries, 14% of all deaths, and 23% of all property damage in 1997. Most accidents have involved collisions between 2 vessels, and 71% have involved collisions with another personal watercraft. The types and patterns of injuries seen in personal watercraft accidents were determined.

Methods.—A retrospective review of medical records and imaging studies was conducted at level 1 and level 2 trauma centers in San Diego County, California. The study enrolled all trauma patients treated for personal watercraft–related injuries between 1984 and 1997. The main outcome measures were evaluation of injury patterns by chart review and imaging studies.

Results.—A total of 62 patients were included in the study. The average age of the patients was 23 years (range, 2 to 59 years), and the group included 41 male and 21 female patients. Collisions with another personal watercraft were involved in 56% of the injuries. Among the patients, 24 lost consciousness and 8 suffered closed head injuries. There were 17 chest injuries, with 10 cases of pneumothorax, and 16 lower extremity fractures.

Conclusions.—There has been a dramatic increase in recent years in the number of injuries related to personal watercraft, which are now one of the leading causes of recreational water sports injuries. These findings support a high level of awareness for significant blunt trauma to the chest and lower extremities in patients involved in personal watercraft accidents.

▶ In this retrospective study of patients admitted to trauma centers in San Diego, the authors describe the type and frequency of injuries to individuals related to personal watercraft (PWC) injuries. These vehicles could be thought of as motorcycles on water; passengers sit on the vehicle and the craft provides no protection on collision.

The value to us as emergency physicians is that we can increase our suspicion of possible injuries if we know our patient was involved in a PWC accident. Head, chest, and lower extremity injuries were among the most common. Additionally, we can advocate for measures to prevent injuries such as helmets, padding, and flotation jackets.

N. B. Handly, MD, MSc, MS

Community Characteristics and Demographic Information as Determinants for a Hospital-Based Injury Prevention Outreach Program
Chang D, Cornwell EE III, Phillips J, et al (Johns Hopkins Med Institution, Baltimore, Md)
Arch Surg 138:1344-1346, 2003   1–29

Background.—A publication from the American College of Surgeons has stipulated that level I trauma centers are expected to have major activity in prehospital management, education, and injury prevention. Injury prevention activities make take many forms and may include activities such as the promotion of seat belt use in automobiles or helmet use for cyclists as well as a broad range of violence-prevention activities. However, information on patient demographics, characteristics of the community, and types of injuries is needed to focus the efforts of any hospital-based injury prevention outreach program toward designing a program that is relevant to the specific clinical experience of that trauma center. Prospectively collected data in the trauma registry or a level I university-based trauma center were evaluated.

Methods.—Demographic data and data on mechanism of injury, mortality rate, and home ZIP codes of patients admitted to a trauma service at 1 university-based hospital in Baltimore, Maryland, were compared for 2 separate calendar years, 2 years before (1995) and 2 years after (2000) the implementation of a dedicated trauma program that included an injury-prevention program.

Results.—There was only minimal variation in the list of common patient ZIP codes from 1995 to 2000. The 18 most common ZIP codes were found to represent 80% of patients, a total area of 99 square miles, and a region with a mean household income that is 67% of the statewide median. An increasingly disproportionate percentage of patients with gunshot wounds were the youngest patients (18 to 24 years) treated by the trauma service. Although the overall survival of trauma patients improved in 2000, there was no improvement among patients with gunshot wounds. More than half the patients (57%) seen in 2000 who did not survive and more than two thirds of patients with lethal gunshot wounds were declared dead in the ED, which is suggestive of nonpreventability from a standpoint of clinical care.

Conclusions.—The catchment area that comprised the majority of patients admitted to a level I urban trauma center is compact and economically disadvantaged. This study found that although there had been a decline in overall trauma mortality rate, gunshot wounds are now more lethal and have increased in prevalence among teenagers and young men, indicating that violence prevention is an area of emphasis for an injury prevention outreach program in this urban area.

▶ Trauma care delivered by emergency physicians and surgical colleagues has reduced the overall mortality rate in Baltimore over the study period of 1995 to 2000. However, the GSW (gunshot wound) mortality rate has not changed, and the frequency of deaths declared in the ED remains high for GSW victims. (The data from Baltimore also confirm the pattern of young men being very frequent victims of GSW.) Thus, it remains clear that primary prevention is critical to prevent the deaths and morbidity rates further.

Mapping software has made it possible to identify geographic areas of events and, as used in this report, the home addresses of trauma victims. The authors stated that there were no adequate data to identify the location where the injury occurred; however, for the purposes of designing prevention programs, the home addresses are more important so that the programs can be brought to those most at risk.

The hard work ahead is to show that programs can reduce morbidity and mortality rates of trauma and stop the individuals from becoming victims in the first place.

N. B. Handly, MD, MSc, MS

Diabetes and Driving Mishaps: Frequency and Correlations From a Multinational Survey

Cox DJ, Penberthy JK, Zrebiec J, et al (Univ of Virgina, Charlottesville; Joslin Diabetes Ctr, Boston; Univ of Chicago; et al)
Diabetes Care 26:2329-2334, 2003   1–30

Background.—Intensive treatment to obtain strict glycemic control in diabetic patients is associated with an increased incidence of hypoglycemia. Hypoglycemia while driving is hazardous and may result in more driving mishaps. Whether having diabetes correlates with an increased risk of mishaps while driving was determined.

Methods.—The study included 341 adults with type 1 diabetes, 332 adults with type 2 diabetes, and 363 nondiabetic spouse control subjects. These participants completed an anonymous questionnaire about diabetes and driving during routine visits to diabetes specialty clinics in 7 US and 4 European cities.

Findings.—Patients with type 1 diabetes reported significantly more crashes, moving violations, episodes of hypoglycemic stupor, required assistance, and mild hypoglycemia while driving compared with those of the other 2 groups. Drivers with type 2 diabetes had rates of driving mishaps comparable to those of the nondiabetic spouses. The use of insulin or oral agents did not affect the occurrence of driving mishaps. Crashes among type 1 diabetic drivers correlated with more frequent hypoglycemic stupor episodes while driving, less frequent monitoring of blood glucose before driving, and insulin injection therapy compared with pump therapy. One half of the type 1 diabetes group and three fourths of the type 2 diabetes group had never talked with their physicians about hypoglycemia and driving.

Conclusions.—Drivers with type 1 diabetes are at increased risk for driving mishaps. Drivers with type 2 diabetes, even those receiving insulin therapy, do not appear to be at increased risk. Risk appears to be increased by more frequent hypoglycemia while driving, method of insulin delivery, and infrequent self-testing before driving. Physicians should discuss hypoglycemia and driving with their type 1 diabetic patients.

▶ The findings of Cox et al serve as a reminder to discuss driving issues with our type 1 diabetic patients. At the very least, we should bring up the dangers of hypoglycemia when driving when discharging patients who come to the ED with hypoglycemic episodes. Cox and colleagues' suggestions seem sound and could be considered for incorporation into the standard ED discharge sheets as follows: (1) Measure blood glucose before driving and at intervals during long drives. (2) Do not begin driving when blood glucose is less than 5 mmol/L (90 mg/dL). (3) If hypoglycemia is suspected while driving, immediately discontinue driving, consume fast-acting carbohydrates, and do not resume driving until blood glucose levels and cognitive motor functioning return to normal. This is another case where an ounce of prevention can go a long way.

R. K. Cydulka, MD, MS

Violence and Substance Use Among an Injured Emergency Department Population

Cunningham R, Walton MA, Maio RF, et al (Univ of Michigan, Ann Arbor; Department of Veterans Affairs (FCB), Ann Arbor, Mich)
Acad Emerg Med 10:764-775, 2003   1–31

Background.—Approximately 17% of all ED visits are related to violence. Twenty-percent of all fatal injuries are violence-related. A sample of ED patients was evaluated for a history of violence and substance abuse.

Methods.—The study included 320 injured patients who completed questionnaires during an urban ED visit after acute injury. The refusal rate was 14%. Data elicited included whether the injury was related to acute violence (AV), whether there was a past-year history of violence (VH), including victimization and perpetration in partner and nonpartner relationships, and substance abuse.

Findings.—AV-related injuries were reported by 14% of the patients. VH was reported by 53%. Of the AV patients, 89% reported VH. The AV and VH groups did not differ in demographic data, substance abuse, or substance-related consequences. When compared with non-AV and non-VH patients, men were significantly more likely than women to report AV or VH. Being in the AV or VH group correlated significantly with substance abuse and substance-related consequences. Patients reporting illicit drug use were 6.2 times more likely to report AV or VH. Patients drinking any alcohol were 2 times as likely to report AV or VH.

Conclusions.—A high proportion of injured patients in this urban ED reported violence in the previous year. The use of alcohol and illicit drugs appears to be associated with violence.

▶ Cunningham and colleagues demonstrate an association between violence and substance abuse. Although they are careful to point out that because of their study design, the findings cannot be extrapolated to indicate cause and effect, most of us who work in similar environments suspect that the link is indeed present. They also note that violence is frequently a chronic problem, rather than an acute, isolated occurrence for many of our injured patients. So now there is another reason to screen for both substance abuse and violence in our patient populations. Now what do we do with the information once we obtain it? That's another conundrum that needs a solution.

R. K. Cydulka, MD, MS

The Incidences of Positive Kleihauer-Betke Test in Low-Risk Pregnancies and Maternal Trauma Patients

Dhanraj D, Lambers D (Good Samaritan Hosp, Cincinnati, Ohio)
Am J Obstet Gynecol 190:1461-1463, 2004   1–32

Background.—The Kleihauer-Betke (KB) test is a laboratory test that differentiates fetal from maternal erythrocytes. Fetomaternal hemorrhage can be quantified on the basis of the difference in stability of hemoglobin F compared with hemoglobin A in an acidic environment. The incidence of positive KB tests in low-risk, third-trimester patients was investigated and compared with that of patients undergoing KB testing after maternal trauma.

Methods.—One hundred low-risk gravid women gave informed consent for KB testing at the time of their routine glucose challenge tests. The Clayton modification was used to analyze fetal hemoglobin. A review of the medical charts of 583 patients seen for maternal trauma between 1998 and 2001 was performed. One hundred fifty-one women with KB testing at comparable gestations made up the historical control group.

Findings.—The incidence of a positive KB test was 5.1% in the low-risk group compared with 2.6% of the maternal trauma control group. None of the positive findings was associated with a clinical abruption or fetal distress. A low-risk patient with sickle cell trait had a KB finding of 40 mL.

Conclusions.—The incidence of a positive KB test in women with low-risk pregnancies is comparable to that in women evaluated after maternal trauma. Thus a positive KB test alone does not necessarily indicate pathologic fetal-maternal bleeding in pregnant women with trauma.

▶ I hope this article prompts a prospective observational study, as it will better clarify the usefulness of the routine use of the KB test in pregnant patients with trauma. Of course, the KB test must still be used in patients who are Rh⊖, as its results will significantly affect therapy.

I have a few issues with this study: (1) Dhanraj and Lambers neglect to mention how fetal injury was ruled out among trauma patients; (2) they fail to report the odds ratio of significant fetal injury among trauma in patients with a positive KB test versus those with a negative test; and (3) they do not note whether abruption was routinely ruled out in all patients presenting for a routine visit who were found to have a positive KB test.

R. K. Cydulka, MD, MS

Perflubron Emulsion in Prolonged Hemorrhagic Shock: Influence on Hepatocellular Energy Metabolism and Oxygen-Dependent Gene Expression

Paxian M, Rensing H, Geckeis K, et al (Universität des Saarlandes, Hamburg, Germany; Centre Hospitalier Universitaire Vaudois, Lausanne, Switzerland)
Anesthesiology 98:1391-1399, 2003   1–33

Background.—Hemorrhagic shock in association with trauma is the leading cause of death in those aged 40 years and younger in most Western countries. These patients are at risk for multiple organ failure because microvascular failure and depression of energy metabolism may persist despite seemingly adequate resuscitation. Among the failing organ systems, the liver is the second most frequently affected organ after severe and prolonged hemorrhagic shock, and liver dysfunction in these patients contributes to delayed death. Studies have suggested that artificial oxygen carriers may improve oxygen supply to vital organs while also eliminating the need for allogeneic transfusion. Perflubron emulsion (PFE), a second-generation artificial oxygen carrier, was compared with stored blood in terms of hepatocellular adenosine triphosphate (ATP) content, hepatocellular injury, and expression pattern of glutamine synthetase 1 (GluS-1).

Methods.—Rats were subjected to hemorrhage hypotension and then resuscitated with stored whole rat blood, pentastarch, or pentastarch com-

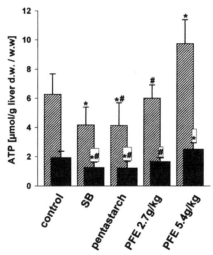

FIGURE 3.—ATP concentrations in liver homogenates after shock and resuscitation. ATP content in liver homogenates was assessed enzymatically at the end of each experiment for wet (*solid bar*) and dry (*hatched bar*) tissue. ATP concentrations remained significantly below controls after resuscitation with stored blood or pentastarch. ATP concentrations completely recovered in animals after resuscitation with low-dose PFE and were significantly increase after administration of high-dose PFE. Data are mean ± SD for n = 8 animals per group. *$P < .05$ compared with control; †$P < .05$ compared with 5.4 g/kg PFE. *Abbreviation: SB*, Stored blood. (Courtesy of Paxian M, Rensing H, Geckeis K, et al: Perflubron emulsion in prolonged hemorrhagic shock: Influence on hepatocellular energy metabolism and oxygen-dependent gene expression. *Anesthesiology* 98:1391-1399, 2003. Copyright American Society of Anesthesiologists, Inc. Used with permission of Lippincott Williams & Wilkins Publishers.)

bined with PFE. The recovery of liver ATP, hepatocellular injury, and expression of GluS-1 were evaluated at 4 hours of resuscitation.

Results.—Stored whole blood or pentastarch did not restore liver ATP concentrations after prolonged shock compared with sham controls, resulting in increased gene expression of GluS-1. The addition of PFE (2.7 g/kg) restored liver ATP to control levels, and the addition of PFE 5.4 g/kg resulted in ATP concentrations that were significantly above control (Fig 3). Improved hepatocellular oxygen supply was confirmed by restoration of the physiologic expression pattern of GluS-1. Serum enzyme concentrations were highest after resuscitation with stored blood, and the addition of PFE did not further decrease enzyme concentrations compared with pentastarch alone.

Conclusions.—Resuscitation with PFE is superior to stored blood or asanguineous resuscitation regarding restoration of hepatocellular energy metabolism, as reflected in normalization of oxygen-dependent gene expression. However, this improved oxygen availability did not ameliorate early hepatocellular injury.

▶ Demonstrating adequacy of oxygen to key organs should be the key variable in assessing techniques for management of shock. This study graphically depicts the hepatic ATP concentrations in the liver, an indirect measure of adequate oxygen delivery. The authors also assessed the degree and pattern of induction of a hypoxia-sensitive gene. The superiority of PFE against stored blood and pentastarch was impressive.

Perfluorochemicals dissolve large amounts of oxygen and carbon dioxide and are able to load and unload them at more than twice the rate of blood. Stored blood has the problem of 2,3-diphosphoglycerate depletion, which leads to difficulty unloading oxygen from hemoglobin. Although there is a long way from this rat model to clinical use in human beings, this second generation of artificial oxygen carriers shows significant promise.

W. P. Burdick, MD, MSEd

New Needle Cricothyroidotomy Setup
Gaufberg SV, Workman TP (Cambridge Health Alliance, Mass; Harvard Med School, Boston)
Am J Emerg Med 22:37-39, 2004   1–34

Background.—Needle cricothyroidotomy is a lifesaving emergency procedure with a number of advantages but a major disadvantage: air flow to the lungs is limited by the diameter of the catheter used for the procedure. Because the diameter is small (14- or 12-gauge), adequate ventilation cannot be provided for a long time. The standard recommended ventilation equipment, a jet insufflator connected to a source of oxygen with 50 psi of pressure, is not always available in emergency situations. Several alternative setups use bag-valve ventilation, but these are too bulky or rigid and increase the risk of cricothyroidotomy catheter dislodgement. The new setup de-

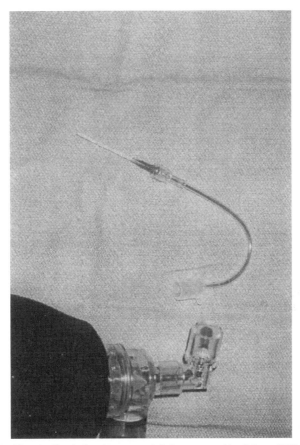

FIGURE 5.—The cut-off end of an intravenous infusion system tubing-2.5 mm ETT connector-bag-valve. *Abbreviation: ETT*, endotracheal tube. (Courtesy of Gaufberg SV, Workman TP: New needle cricothyroidotomy setup. *Am J Emerg Med* 22:37-39, 2004.)

scribed here is a flexible system consisting of the cut-off end of an IV infusion system tubing and a 2.5-mm endotracheal tube (ETT) connector (Fig 5).

Discussion.—Previously suggested bag-valve setups provide a sealed connection between the needle cricothyroidotomy and a bag-valve, but the rigid connection significantly increases the chance of dislodgement of the needle cricothyroidotomy catheter. The new setup is easily available because all EDs and advanced life support ambulances have IV infusion tubing and pediatric size 2.5-mm ETT. Additional advantages are low cost and fast assembly. Most importantly, however, the flexibility of this system provides easier stabilization and control of emergency needle cricothyroidotomy.

▶ In addition to providing an additional option for connecting a bag-valve-mask with a 12-gauge angiocatheter, the authors review 2 other very pragmatic, previously described arrangements. Knowing your connection sizes is the key to success—if you can remember that a 7-mm endotracheal tube connector fits into a 3-mL syringe, or that a 2.5-mm connector fits into cut IV infusion tubing, you can create this setup in a crisis airway management situation. If you use the IV tube setup, remember that resistance increases with tube length (although not as dramatically as with tube radius).

W. P. Burdick, MD, MSEd

2 Resuscitation

Airway

Laryngeal Mask Airway Insertion by Anesthetists and Nonanesthetists Wearing Unconventional Protective Gear: A Prospective, Randomized, Crossover Study in Humans
Flaishon R, Sotman A, Friedman A, et al (Tel Aviv Univ, Israel)
Anesthesiology 100:267-273, 2004   2–1

Introduction.—Rapid and reliable emergent airway control is needed in mass casualty situations, whether injuries are associated with trauma or toxic damage to the respiratory system. There is concern that optimal airway management may be difficult to provide in chaotic situations, particularly when initial medical providers may be nonanesthetists wearing unconventional protective gear. The laryngeal mask airway, popular in emergency situations, was assessed for the speed and success rate by which it could be inserted by inexperienced medical personnel.

Methods.—Twenty-two general surgery residents and 20 anesthesia residents participated in the prospective, randomized, crossover study. Within the 12 months before starting their residency, all had passed the Israeli Defense Forces Medical Corps' Advanced Cardiac Life Support and Advanced Trauma Life Support courses. The duration of residency experience ranged from 2 to 5 years. These physicians and 6 novice physicians with no experience in inserting laryngeal masks in anesthetized patients were tested for their ability to insert the masks while wearing either surgical attire or full antichemical protective gear. The duration of time required for insertion was measured as the time at which the device was first grasped until a normal capnography was obtained.

Results.—For anesthetists, the mean time required to insert the masks was 39 seconds while wearing surgical attire and 40 seconds with protective gear. The mean times required for surgery residents in these situations were 64 seconds and 102 seconds, respectively. Anesthetists inserted masks in a single attempt, but as many as 4 attempts were needed by surgeons. Three of 6 novices reached the mean performance time of the anesthetists after 4 (protective gear) and 2 (surgical attire) trials, with only 1 occurrence of hypoxia and a failure rate similar to that of the surgeons. Butyl rubber gloves considerably lengthened the time required by all physicians to secure the mask.

NON-CONVENTIONAL MASS CASUALTY EVENT

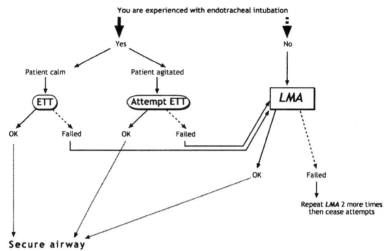

FIGURE 3.—Recommendations for acute airway management by caregivers during unconventional mass casualty conditions. Unlike the situation in conventional mass casualty situations, caregivers might not be informed of the exact type of the toxic agent or the number and severity of the victims. They must protect themselves as best they can. With rare exceptions, victims will not have an IV line, and forceful management of their airway can pose further risk to the patient. Confirmation of successful airway management will be obtained exclusively by observing bilateral equal chest movement. *Abbreviations: LMA*, Laryngeal mask airway; *ETT*, endotracheal tube. (Courtesy of Flaishon R, Sotman A, Friedman A, et al: Laryngeal mask airway insertion by anesthetists and nonanesthetists wearing unconventional protective gear: A prospective, randomized, crossover study in humans. *Anesthesiology* 100:267-273, 2004. Copyright American Society of Anesthesiologists, Inc. Used with permission of Lippincott Williams & Wilkins Publishers.)

Conclusion.—The laryngeal mask airway is a suitable device for initial airway control when the medical provider has limited expertise in ventilatory support and when tracheal intubation is not applicable. Anesthesia residents were able to insert the mask rapidly while wearing both surgical attire and antichemical protective gear, whereas surgeons were slower in both situations. Novices showed a quick learning curve. An algorithm describes the steps that should be taken by caregivers in cases of gas-intoxicated victims (Fig 3).

Antichemical Protective Gear Prolongs Time to Successful Airway Management: A Randomized, Crossover Study in Humans
Flaishon R, Sotman A, Ben-Abraham R, et al (Tel Aviv Univ, Israel)
Anesthesiology 100:260-266, 2004   2–2

Introduction.—Medical personnel responding to an exposure of civilian populations to airborne toxic agents must be prepared to provide rapid and reliable emergent airway control. The chaotic environment of mass casualty situations and the need to wear antichemical protective gear impose special difficulties, even for experienced caregivers. Anesthesia residents participated in a study that examined the effect of such gear on their ability to achieve successful airway control with either an endotracheal tube or a laryngeal mask airway.

Methods.—Fifteen anesthetists with 2 to 5 years of residency training were included in the randomized crossover study. None had previously attempted to intubate a patient while wearing the gear. Sixty consecutive adult patients scheduled to undergo various surgical or orthopedic interventions under general anesthesia gave informed consent to participation. A size 4 laryngeal mask airway was used for all patients. Women were intubated with a 7.5-mm-ID cuffed endotracheal tube and men with an 8.5-mm-ID cuffed tube. The duration of intubation/insertion was measured from the time the device was grasped to the time a normal capnography recording was obtained.

Results.—The protective antichemical gear consisted of butyl rubber boots and gloves, a nylon shirt and pants covered by khaki, and an antigas mask with active filter. Anesthetists also inserted the devices while wearing usual surgical attire. None of the patients required the addition of any drug to facilitate insertion of either device, and none experienced adverse intraoperative events. The protective gear lengthened the time needed for tracheal intubations, but times to laryngeal mask insertion were similar for surgical attire and protective gear conditions. Endotracheal tubes were introduced in a mean of 31 seconds with surgical attire and a mean of 54 seconds with protective gear. For laryngeal mask insertion, the mean times were 44 seconds and 39 seconds, respectively.

Conclusion.—When wearing antichemical protective gear, anesthetists were able to insert a laryngeal mask airway faster than they could perform tracheal intubation. Tracheal intubation is the definitive standard for airway management, but the laryngeal mask airway might be preferable in an unconventional mass casualty event.

▶ Anyone whose hospital or prehospital disaster plan calls for providing medical care while wearing protective personal equipment (PPE) should take note of these 2 studies (Abstracts 2–1 and 2–2). Progress has been made in developing plans for dealing with weapons of mass destruction (WMD) threats, but this is some of the first research I have seen on how the use of PPE may affect our ability to provide patient care. I encourage every EMS and ED whose plans call for the use of PPE, while providing patient care as part of their mass casualty/WMD response, to practice donning and using PPE while performing simulated or actual procedures. Where possible, we should follow the lead of our Israeli colleagues and examine our ability to perform medical care while wearing PPE in a controlled environment before, rather than during, the chaos of an actual incident.

S. L. Werner, MD

Prepared Endotracheal Tubes: Are They a Potential Source for Pathogenic Microorganisms?

Rasic NF, Friesen RM, Anderson B, et al (Foothills Hosp, Calgary, Alta, Canada)
Anesth Analg 97:1133-1136, 2003   2–3

Background.—It is common practice for anesthesiologists and ED physicians to prepare back-up airway equipment for use in an unanticipated difficult intubation, which means that the endotracheal tube (ETT) is removed from its sterile package and often cut. After the integrity of the cuff is tested, the tube is replaced in the original package. There is no standardized protocol for processing and storing prepared ETTs, and their storage time is highly variable and institution dependent. Whether open, unused, prepared ETTs are a potential source of pathogenic microorganisms was investigated and if prepared ETTs can provide a medium for bacterial survival after deliberate contamination.

Methods.—A stylet was inserted into a 7-mm ETT and the system was sterilized with ethylene oxide. In the first phase of the study, the prepared ETTs were placed in 20 different locations and sampled 8 times over the 4-week study period. Growth was determined after 48-hour incubation, and the microorganism was identified. In the second phase of this study, 40 prepared ETTs were swabbed with a fresh suspension of *Haemophilus influenzae*, *Pseudomonas aeruginosa*, *Staphylococcus aureus*, and *Enterococcus faecium* or a negative control.

Results.—Nonvirulent bacteria were cultured from 13 (8.1%) of 60 samples in phase 1 and from 15 (4.7%) of 320 samples in phase 2. None of the prepared ETTs grew the same bacteria more than once. In the second phase of the study, after 24 hours only *E faecium* was recovered.

Conclusions.—The pathogenic potential of prepared ETTs is very small, and they can be safely used for up to 1 month. The use of prepared ETTs in this manner could result in significant cost savings for operating rooms.

▶ How long should an open ETT be kept in your ED? These authors look at the level of bacterial contamination over time of prepared ETTs either left open in hospital environments or deliberately contaminated.

The first phase of this study measured the contamination of ETTs left open in relatively clean areas (operating rooms, labor and delivery suites, and epidural carts). Over 4 weeks, 11 of 20 ETTs had no growth, and no sample had the same bacteria cultured more than once. Of the bacteria cultured, none was considered a virulent species.

In phase 2, ETTs were deliberately contaminated with bacteria to determine whether the ETT would provide a good environment for growth. All deliberately contaminated samples showed decreasing numbers of bacteria with time. While *E faecium* was the most hardy and was recovered in all samples more than 4 weeks after contamination, no *S aureus*, *P aeruginosa*, or *H influenzae* were found after 8 hours. Noninnoculated bacteria (similar to types grown in phase 1) were found in about 5% of the phase 2 samples.

This study suggests that contamination of open ETTs is rare and unlikely to cause nosocomial infection. They determined that open ETTs could be left for up to 4 weeks.

Is the ED as clean as the sites in this study? In our ED, the open ETTs are kept in the code carts and we do not sterilize the prepared ETTs, as was done after placing the stylet in this study. We do not know if our handling the stylet and tube might contaminate the ETT with a hardy or more virulent bacteria that would then make the ETT become a hazard.

This would be an easy and economically meaningful study to be repeated in the ED. We should review our disposal procedures for "opened" equipment to see if we could also save money while delivering quality care.

N. B. Handly, MD, MSc, MS

Cardiac Arrest

A Comparison of Vasopressin and Epinephrine for Out-of-Hospital Cardiopulmonary Resuscitation

Wenzel V, for the European Resuscitation Council Vasopressor During Cardiopulmonary Resuscitation Study Group (Leopold-Franzens Univ, Innsbruck, Austria; Free Univ, Berlin; Philipps Univ, Marburg, Germany)
N Engl J Med 350:105-113, 2004   2–4

Background.—There are more than a half million cases of sudden death annually in Europe and North America. More than half of these deaths occur in persons younger than 65 years, which is evidence of the need for optimal CPR strategies to improve the chances of survival. Epinephrine has been used during CPR for more than 100 years. In recent years, however, its use has become controversial because epinephrine is associated with increased myocardial oxygen consumption, ventricular arrhythmias, and myocardial dysfunction in the period after resuscitation. Vasopressin is an alternative to epinephrine for vasopressor therapy during CPR, but the clinical experience with vasopressin in this setting is limited. Current international guidelines have recommended the use of epinephrine during CPR and advise that vasopressin should be considered a secondary alternative. The effects of vasopressin and epinephrine on survival were assessed in patients who had an out-of-hospital cardiac arrest.

Methods.—A total of 1186 adult patients who had an out-of-hospital cardiac arrest were randomly assigned to receive 2 injections of either 40 IU of vasopressin (589 patients) or 1 mg of epinephrine (597 patients) followed by additional treatment of epinephrine as necessary. The main outcome measure was survival to hospital admission, and the secondary outcome measure was survival to hospital discharge.

Results.—The clinical profiles of the 2 groups were similar. There was no significant difference between the 2 groups in the rates of hospital admission either among patients with ventricular fibrillation or among those with pulseless electrical activity. However, among patients with asystole, the use of vasopressin was associated with significantly higher rates of hospital admission (29% vs 20.3%) and hospital discharge (4.7% vs 1.5%). Among

732 patients in whom spontaneous circulation was not restored after 2 injections of the study drug, additional treatment with epinephrine resulted in significant improvement in survival to hospital admission and hospital discharge in the vasopressin group but not in the epinephrine group (hospital admission rate, 25.7% vs 16.4%; hospital discharge rate, 6.2% vs 1.7%). The groups were similar in terms of cerebral performance.

Conclusions.—This assessment of vasopressin and epinephrine in the setting of out-of-hospital CPR found that the effects of these drugs were similar in terms of management of ventricular fibrillation and pulseless electrical activity; however, vasopressin was shown to be more effective than epinephrine in patients with asystole. Vasopressin followed by epinephrine may be more effective than epinephrine alone in the treatment of refractory cardiac arrest.

▶ This European study compared vasopressin to epinephrine as the initial medication in nontraumatic, out-of-hospital cardiac arrests with ventricular fibrillation, asystole, or pulseless electrical activity as the presenting rhythm. Overall, vasopressin was not superior to epinephrine. However, in the subset of patients with asytole as the presenting rhythm, the use of vasopressin resulted in significant improvement in both the primary and secondary end points: survival to hospital admission and hospital discharge. The current American Heart Association advanced cardiac life support guidelines recommend vasopressin as an alternative to epinephrine in ventricular fibrillation arrests, but it is not currently recommended in patients presenting with asystole. While this study has a number of limitations, as discussed by the authors, its results seem to justify further investigation of vasopressin as the initial vasopressor, particularly in asystolic arrest.

These results should be interpreted with caution, however. While this study did show a significant increase in survival in asystolic arrest, the survival rate in the vasopressin group was still less than 5%, an improvement from 1% but still miserable. Also, discharge with intact cerebral function was not used as an end point, and, in fact, was poor in all categories of patients surviving to hospital discharge. Only 30% of the patients in both the epinephrine and vasopressin groups were discharged with good cerebral performance. In addition, other factors, including suffering a witnessed arrest and receiving basic life support within 10 minutes, had a much greater impact on survival than the use of vasopressin. Take-home message: further study of vasopressin may be warranted, but we still need to improve delivery of the factors repeatedly shown to increase survival—early recognition, early access, early CPR, and early defibrillation.

S. L. Werner, MD

▶ Survival to hospital discharge, the key end point in a CPR study, is clearly higher after treatment of asystole with vasopression instead of epinephrine. Unfortunately, this comes at the expense of discharging comatose or vegetative patients. If vasopression really does do a better job of reviving the heart, it needs to be used in the first few minutes and not as a last ditch effort, so that the brain has a chance to be revived too.

W. P. Burdick, MD, MSEd

Impact of Age on Long-term Survival and Quality of Life Following Out-of-Hospital Cardiac Arrest
Bunch TJ, White RD, Khan AH, et al (Mayo Clinic, Rochester, Minn)
Crit Care Med 32:963-967, 2004   2–5

Background.—Early defibrillation programs have yielded improvements in long-term outcomes for patients who experience out-of-hospital cardiac arrest from ventricular fibrillation. The collective long-term quality of life and survival are favorable for these patients, but there are subsets of these patients who may be predisposed to worse outcomes. Elderly patients in particular are apt to have more comorbid medical conditions affecting their outcome. However, the effects of age on mortality rate and quality of life after rapid defibrillation are unknown.

Methods.—This observational study was conducted among all patients at one hospital with out-of-hospital cardiac arrest between November 1990 and January 2001 who received rapid defibrillation for ventricular fibrillation. The main outcome measures were long-term outcome and quality of life. Survival was estimated with the Kaplan-Meier method. The quality of life was established with an SF-36 survey.

Results.—A total of 200 patients had ventricular fibrillation out-of-hospital cardiac arrest. Of these patients, 138 (69%) survived in the ED, and 79 (39%) were discharged neurologically intact. The average age of the patients was 62 ± 16 years, with 51% of the population aged 65 or older. The average length of follow-up was 4.8 ± 3.0 years. The 5-year survival rate was 94% in patients younger than 65, and 66% in patients aged 65 and older. The observed survival in the younger group was no different from that expected in an age- and gender-matched population in the United States. However, the expected survival in the older group was significantly lower in comparison with an age-, gender-, and disease-matched US population but was similar to an age-, gender-, and disease-matched cohort of patients from the study region who were not experiencing an arrest. A direct comparison between the 2 patient groups showed that the older cohort reported lower levels of physical functioning, role-emotional score, and role-physical score. Other scores on the SF-36 were not different between the 2 groups. In patients younger than 65 years, 65% returned to work, compared with 56% of patients aged 65 and older.

Conclusion.—The survival rate for ventricular fibrillation out-of-hospital cardiac arrest is increased significantly by the presence of a rapid defibrillation program.

▶ Several articles have shown worse outcomes in elderly patients resuscitated from cardiac arrest, but this is the first study I have read that focused on quality of life in the elderly after out-of-hospital cardiac arrest. Impressive in the article is the high survival and high quality of life in both elderly and nonelderly populations, attesting to the success of an aggressive early defibrillation program. In addition, it should be noted that the survivors aged 65 or older did not have decreased survival when compared with an age- and disease-matched population in the same locality. In addition, while the authors did find a reduction in 3 of 9 quality-of-life scores, they found no difference in neurologic function in the elderly survivors, and most returned to work. The authors note that the data were not stratified by place of residence, so some of the elderly survivors may have been nursing home residents, who generally have poorer outcomes.

Overall, this article supports aggressive early out-of-hospital defibrillation, even in the elderly. Interestingly, more than one half of the survivors aged 65 or older returned to work. Given the trend toward longer and healthier lives, I wonder when we will begin to revise our arbitrary transition point to becoming elderly upward from 65.

S. L. Werner, MD

Evaluation of Isoproterenol in Patients Undergoing Resuscitation for Out-of-Hospital Asystolic Cardiac Arrest (the Israel Resuscitation With Isoproterenol Study Prospective Randomized Clinical Trial)

Jaffe R, Rubinshtein R, Feigenberg Z, et al (Lady Davis Carmel Med Ctr, Haifa, Israel; Magen David Adom, Tel-Aviv, Israel; Rambam Med Ctr, Haifa, Israel; et al)

Am J Cardiol 93:1407-1409, 2004   2–6

Background.—Evidence suggests that increasing cardiac β-adrenergic agonism by adding isoproterenol to epinephrine may improve the recovery of cardiac function and spontaneous circulation (ROSC) in patients with out-of-hospital cardiac arrest (OOHCA). The effects of adjunct isoproterenol were examined in patients with asystolic OOHCA.

Methods.—Participants were 79 adults with witnessed asystolic OOHCA (71% men; mean age, 67 years). All patients received conventional basic life support and advanced cardiac life support via the IV infusion of epinephrine (1 mg every 3-5 minutes) and atropine (1 mg every 3-5 minutes until 3 mg had been administered). Patients were randomly assigned to receive either IV isoproterenol (200 μg every 3-5 minutes until 600 μg had been administered) or no isoproterenol. Rates of ROSC (primary end point) and survival to hospital admission (secondary end point) were compared between the 2 groups.

Results.—Doses of IV epinephrine were similar in the isoproterenol and control groups (mean, 7.1 vs 6.5 mg, respectively). The incidence of ROSC was also similar in the 2 groups (17 of 37 patients [46%] vs 19 of 42 patients [45%], respectively). Survival to hospital admission occurred in 9 patients (24%) receiving isoproterenol and in 12 patients (29%) in the control group

(P = not significant). Survival to hospital discharge and 6-month survival were also similar in the 2 groups.

Conclusion.—Isoproterenol infusion in addition to epinephrine and atropine does not improve ROSC or other outcomes in patients experiencing asystolic OOHCA.

▶ Although an open-label study with negative results, this is an example of the quality research that can be conducted in the prehospital environment. Clearly, the best treatment of asystole remains its prevention. Interestingly, the only significant univariate predictor of survival in this study was a shorter interval from arrest to intervention. A large portion of the interval likely represents the time to advanced life support intervention, stressing the importance of early intervention in OOHCA.

S. L. Werner, MD

Shock

A Comparison of Albumin and Saline for Fluid Resuscitation in the Intensive Care Unit
Finfer S, for the SAFE Study Investigators (ANZICS CTG, Carlton, Australia; et al)
N Engl J Med 350:2247-2256, 2004   2–7

Background.—The administration of IV fluids to maintain or increase intravascular volume is a common intervention in the ICU. However, it is unclear whether patients' outcomes are significantly influenced by the choice of fluid. The conflicting results of several meta-analyses have fostered confusion among many clinicians as to the effect of albumin-containing fluids on survival in critically ill patients. In a multicenter, randomized, double-blind trial, the effects of fluid resuscitation with albumin or saline on mortality were compared in a heterogeneous population of patients in the ICU.

Methods.—Patients admitted to the ICU of 16 tertiary care hospitals in Australia and New Zealand from November 2001 to June 2003 were evaluated for eligibility for study entry. Eligible patients were randomly assigned to receive either 4% albumin or normal saline for intravascular fluid resuscitation during the next 28 days. The randomization was stratified according to institution and whether there was a diagnosis of trauma on admission to the ICU. The main outcome measure was death from any cause during the 28 days after randomization.

Results.—Of the 6997 patients enrolled in the study, 3497 were randomly assigned to receive albumin and 3500 to receive saline. Baseline characteristics were similar for the 2 groups. There were 726 deaths in the albumin group and 729 deaths in the saline group. The proportion of patients with new single-organ and multiple-organ failure was similar for both groups. There were no significant differences between the groups in the mean ($\pm$SD) numbers of days spent in the ICU (6.5 ± 6.6 in the albumin group and 6.2 ± 6.2 in the saline group); days spent in the hospital (15.3 ± 9.6 and 15.6 ± 9.6, respectively), days of mechanical ventilation (4.5 ± 6.1 and 4.3 ± 5.7, respectively), or days of renal replacement therapy (0.5 ± 2.3 and 0.4 ± 2.0, respectively).

Conclusion.—Patients in the ICU had similar outcomes at 28 days when intravascular fluid resuscitation was performed with 4% albumin or normal saline.

▶ This is a very large study attempting to put to rest the decades-long dispute over the use of albumin for fluid resuscitation. The economic implications of this debate are significant—albumin was at one point the largest in-hospital drug expenditure. The study was designed to have enough power to detect a 3% difference in mortality. Not only was there no difference found in mortality, but there was no detected difference in proportion of patients with organ failure, duration of ventilator dependence, use of dialysis, or duration of hospital stay. There is simply no advantage to albumin, and it is far more expensive than saline. This study should shift the focus from use of IV albumin to enteral and parenteral nutrition, where the desired outcome of higher plasma protein and consequently less interstitial edema might be better achieved.

While we are not often tempted to use albumin in the ED, the management of critically ill patients is increasingly a shared responsibility as patients stay longer in the department. Understanding the arguments for and against the use of expensive and transiently fashionable therapies in critical care should be our responsibility.

W. P. Burdick, MD, MSEd

Meta-analysis: The Effect of Steroids on Survival and Shock During Sepsis Depends on the Dose
Minneci PC, Deans KJ, Banks SM, et al (NIH, Bethesda, Md; Massachusetts Gen Hosp, Boston)
Ann Intern Med 141:47-56, 2004   2–8

Background.—Septic shock has continued to be the most common cause of death in the ICU, despite the availability of effective antibiotics. The mortality rate from septic shock has been reported to range from 30% to 50%. Several therapies that target the upregulated inflammatory pathways of sepsis have been studied for the purpose of improving survival rates, but few of these therapies have proved beneficial. Previous meta-analyses have shown that high-dose glucocorticoids were not beneficial in sepsis. Recent studies have investigated the effectiveness of lower dose glucocorticoids in sepsis. Recent trials of glucocorticoids for sepsis were compared with previous glucocorticoid trials.

Methods.—A systematic MEDLINE search was conducted for studies published between 1988 and 2003. The studies selected for this review were randomized controlled trials of sepsis that examined the effects of glucocorticoids on survival or vasopressor requirements. Data were collected by 2 independent investigators on patient and study characteristics, treatment interventions, and outcomes.

Results.—Five trials were included in this study. These trials showed a consistent and beneficial effect of glucocorticoids on survival and shock reversal. These effects were the same regardless of adrenal functioning. However, 8 trials published before 1989 showed a survival disadvantage with steroid treatment. When compared with earlier trials, the more recent trials involved administration of steroids later—after patients met enrollment criteria (median, 23 hours vs <2 hours), for longer courses (6 days vs 1 day), and in lower total dosages to patients with higher control group mortality rates (mean, 57% vs 34%) who were more likely to require vasopressor administration (100% vs 65%). The relationship between the steroid dose and survival was linear and was characterized by a benefit at low doses and increasing harm at higher doses.

Conclusions.—Short courses of high-dose glucocorticoids were found to decrease survival rates during sepsis; however, a 5- to 7-day course of physiologic hydrocortisone doses with subsequent tapering was shown to increase the survival rate and shock reversal in patients with vasopressor-dependent septic shock.

▶ The power of a meta-analysis is that it allows small and sometimes subtle differences in interventions to be teased apart. Steroids have come and gone in the treatment of septic shock and now, on the basis of this study, may be back again. It turns out that blasting the patient for a short time is not beneficial and may actually cause harm, but physiologic doses given over a week appear to improve survival rates. This has significant implications for our practice in the initial management of these patients. A small dose of hydrocortisone should be administered, not the multi-gram dose of methylprednisilone we may have given in the past.

W. P. Burdick, MD, MSEd

Nontraumatic Out-of-Hospital Hypotension Predicts Inhospital Mortality
Jones AE, Stiell IG, Nesbitt LP, et al (Carolinas Med Ctr, Charlotte, NC; Univ of Ottawa, Ont, Canada; Univ of Arizona, Tucson)
Ann Emerg Med 43:106-113, 2004   2–9

Background.—Hypotension is often an indicator of a state of circulatory insufficiency and critical illness that necessitates recognition, diagnosis, and resuscitation. The in-hospital mortality rate of ED patients with no history of trauma and an initial systolic blood pressure of less than 100 mm Hg has been reported to be 18%. The significance of out-of-hospital hypotension in nontrauma patients who are transported to the ED by ambulance was studied, and the hypothesis that nontraumatic out-of-hospital hypotension is a significant risk factor for in-hospital death was investigated.

Methods.—This was a multicenter study of ambulance-transported, nontrauma, non-CPR patients at a cross-sectional risk assessment study of high-priority medical transports at a metropolitan county in the United States and in a Canadian prospective multicenter cohort study of patients with respiratory distress. Data from both studies were extracted, and independent analyses were performed. Exposures to hypotension were defined as age older than 17 years, systolic blood pressure less than 100 mm Hg during transport, and 1 or more of 10 predefined symptoms of circulatory insufficiency. The definition of nonexposure to hypotension was similar to that of exposure, with the exception that the systolic blood pressure had to be more than 100 mm Hg during the entire out-of-hospital transport. The primary outcome measure was in-hospital death.

Results.—In the US study of 3128 transports, 395 (13%) exposures and 395 nonexposures were identified. The in-hospital mortality rate of exposures was 26% compared with 8% for nonexposures. In the Canadian study of 7679 transports, 532 exposures (7%) and 7147 nonexposures were identified. The out-of-hospital exposure to hypotension conferred a mortality rate of 32% compared with 11% for nonexposures, for a sensitivity of 18% and a specificity of 95%.

Conclusions.—The in-hospital mortality rate after out-of-hospital, nontraumatic hypotension is high and reproducible. The focus of future research in this area should include ED clinical protocols to ensure appropriate resuscitation and investigation of the cause of out-of-hospital hypotension.

▶ Poor perfusion can be a cause or effect of illness that needs our attention. Much of the design of advanced traumatic life support is based on resuscitating poor perfusion to prevent morbidity and death. But what happens in nontraumatic (NT) patients?

For NT patients whose ED arrival systolic blood pressure (SBP) is less than 100 mm Hg, the in-hospital mortality rate can be 18%.[1] It is important to begin the proper resuscitation for the patients promptly. Can we get a handle on the risk of in-hospital mortality rate for patients whose low SBP could be recognized in the prehospital environment? That is the subject of this study.

With data from prehospital registries in North Carolina and Ottawa, 2 independent tests of the hypothesis that prehospital hypotension (an episode of SBP measuring less than 100 mm Hg) yields higher mortality rates were made.

In North Carolina, the sample consisted of a case-control cohort of patients identified as priority I or II (the top 2 levels of 4 levels, life threatening or potentially life threatening), without trauma and having at least 1 SBP measure of less than 100 mm Hg. The control group was an "adjusted" set to include those patients who better matched the case group—with all prehospital SBP measures greater than 100 mm Hg. All patients in both groups had at least 1 symptom of poor perfusion documented (list of symptoms in the article).

In Ottawa, the samples were made up of patients transported by ambulance with respiratory distress (1 of the symptoms of poor perfusion in the North Carolina sample). The case and control cohorts were divided by prehospital SBP always greater than 100 mm Hg or at least 1 SBP less than 100 mm Hg. These 2 samples were not statistically different in demographic makeup.

In North Carolina, those patients having at least 1 SBP measurement less than 100 mm Hg yielded an odds ratio for in-hospital death of 4.6 when compared to the nonhypotensive patients. The odds ratio for the Ottawa patients with at least 1 SBP measurement less than 100 mm Hg was 3.0 compared with the nonhypotensive patients.

Both study sites had sampling biases. In North Carolina, only the more acute patients were included in the study. The priority levels are somewhat nebulous. Consider how this might affect the results: imagine there were many patients in the lower 2 acuity levels who had an episode of symptomatic SBP measure less than 100 mm Hg who also might be expected to be less likely to die in the hospital. Including these patients in the study might reduce the odds ratio. In Ottawa, only patients with respiratory distress were included. We cannot necessarily apply these results to patients who have other symptoms of poor perfusion.

Nevertheless, the suggestion of this work is that hypotension less than 100 mm Hg is, in fact, a risk factor for in-hospital death for NT patients. The authors suggest that we in the ED need to be ready to resuscitate these hypotensive patients more aggressively. Might it be better to begin resuscitation in the prehospital setting?

N. B. Handly, MD, MSc, MS

Reference

1. Moore CL, Rose GA, Tayal VS, et al: Determination of left ventricular function by emergency physician echocardiography of hypotensive patients. *Acad Emerg Med* 9:186-193, 2002.

Prospective Study of Accuracy and Outcome of Emergency Ultrasound for Abdominal Aortic Aneurysm Over Two Years
Tayal VS, Graf CD, Gibbs MA (Carolinas Med Ctr, Charlotte, NC)
Acad Emerg Med 10:867-871, 2003   2–10

Background.—The majority of patients (60%) with rupture of an abdominal aortic aneurysm (AAA) die before ever reaching the hospital. However, patients who survive to presentation at the hospital have an operative mortality rate of more than 50%. In contrast, the mortality rate in elective repair of AAA ranges from 1% to 5%. The mortality rate is directly related to the timeliness of diagnosis before rupture and definitive repair. Diagnosis of AAA is often delayed because the clinical symptoms are nonspecific (syncope and abdominal, flank, and back pain). Other less emergent diagnoses may be pursued when AAA is excluded. Thus, determination of the presence of an AAA is essential in the management of the symptomatic ED patient. Whether emergency US of the abdominal aorta (EUS-AA) in the ED could accurately identify the presence of AAA and guide ED disposition was identified.

Methods.—This prospective observational study was conducted at an urban ED with more than 100,000 annual patient visits. Consecutive patients were enrolled over a 2-year period. All patients with suspected AAA underwent standard ED evaluation, which consisted of EUS-AA followed by a confirmatory imaging study or laparotomy. AAA was defined as any measured diameter greater than 3 cm. Demographic data, results of confirmatory testing, and patient outcome were collected.

Results.—EUS-AA was performed in 125 patients over a 2-year period. The patients had an average age of 66 years; 54% were male, 56% had hypertension, 395 had coronary artery disease, 22% had diabetes, and 14% had peripheral vascular disease. Confirmatory tests consisted of radiology US in 22%, abdominal CT in 76%, abdominal MRI in 1%, and laparotomy in 1%. AAA was diagnosed in 29 (23%) of 125 patients, of whom 27 of 29 had AAA on confirmatory testing. The sensitivity of EUS-AA was 100%, specificity was 98%, and positive and negative predictive values were 93% and 100%, respectively. The overall admission rate for the study group was 70%. Immediate operative repair was considered in 17 (63%) of 27 patients with AAA, and 10 patients were taken to the operating room.

Conclusions.—EUS-AA was shown to be sensitive and specific for abdominal aortic aneurysm in a symptomatic population, and emergency physicians were able to exclude AAA regardless of disposition from the ED. The presence of AAA on EUS should guide urgent consultation.

▶ US studies of the aorta can be learned rapidly to determine aneurysmal pathology. At our residency in Philadelphia, we find the study of the aorta one of the easiest for our residents to learn and perform well.

Tayal et al report the sensitivity and specificity of emergency US to diagnose AAA. They used radiologic US, CT imaging, and operative reports as gold standards. Sensitivity was 100% and specificity was 99%, which means that US can be effectively used.

The authors acknowledge that they have not examined the effect of EUS-AA on workflow and timing. The patterns of how EUS-AA will change care for patients with suspected AAA will probably be different from place to place. However, we can expect that the time from suspicion to rule in/rule out will significantly decrease. Our surgeons still request a CT study on stable patients with AAA to further characterize the aneurysm, but patients who need immediate operative care move quickly.

N. B. Handly, MD, MSc, MS

Arterial Blood Gas Results Rarely Influence Emergency Physician Management of Patients With Suspected Diabetic Ketoacidosis

Ma OJ, Rush MD, Godfrey MM, et al (Univ of Missouri, Kansas City)
Acad Emerg Med 10:836-841, 2003   2–11

Background.—Diabetic ketoacidosis (DKA) is considered the most common acute, life-threatening complication of diabetes. Arterial blood gas (ABG) sampling is considered by most clinicians to be essential in the initial evaluation of patients with suspected DKA. However, ABG sampling is invasive and potentially difficult and may be accompanied by risks or complications. Venous pH sampling has been proposed as an alternative to ABG sampling; venous pH has been shown to be well correlated with arterial pH in the diagnostic evaluation of patients with DKA. It is possible that ABG data may not be needed by physicians who manage patients with suspected DKA. The hypothesis that ABG results for patients with suspected DKA have no influence on the management of emergency physicians was tested and the correlation and precision between venous pH and arterial pH was validated.

Methods.—The prospective observational study was conducted among physicians in the ED of an urban teaching hospital with an annual volume of 55,000 visits. Patients included in the study were those with capillary blood glucose levels 200 mg/dL or greater, ketonuria, and clinical signs and symptoms of DKA. Venous pH, chemistry panel, and ABG readings were obtained before treatment. The attending emergency physicians indicated planned management and disposition on a standardized form before and after reviewing ABG and venous pH results. The study was designed to detect a 10% difference in management decisions.

Results.—In 200 cases included in the study, results of ABG analysis changed the emergency physicians' diagnosis in 2 cases (1%), altered treatment in 7 cases (3.5%), and changed the disposition of 2 cases (1%). The pH value of the ABG changed the treatment or disposition in 2.5% of cases, whereas the PO_2 and PCO_2 results of the ABG assay changed the treatment or disposition of 1% of patients. There was good correlation between venous pH and arterial pH.

Conclusions.—ABG results rarely influence the decisions of emergency physicians in regard to diagnosis, treatment, or disposition in patients with suspected DKA. Venous pH findings correlated well and with enough precision with arterial pH to substitute for ABG analysis in these patients.

▶ So when does an emergency physician need an ABG? Not for managing DKA patients, according to this study. Provided that our patients are similar to those in the study hospital and that our decision-making procedures are similar, our own clinical gestalt (after exam, electrolytes, urinary ketones, and capillary blood glucose) is adequate to plan the care of these patients. And should we want to refine our DKA management plan, the ABG can be replaced by venous blood gas studies.

In 5 cases (2.5%), the pH value of the ABG (and this value would be shown on the venous blood gas reading, according to these authors and many others) changed management but not disposition, and in 1 of these 5 cases, the pH value changed management and disposition (changed to admission).

This study reminds us that ABG levels really offer us one value that no other noninvasive test can give: arterial oxygen partial pressure (PaO_2). In 1 case of 200 patients seen, the management of the patient changed based on the PaO_2. Pneumonia was suspected for a low PaO_2 value by ABG and antibiotics were started, but there was no definitive diagnosis of pneumonia in the patient (there were no fever, cough, or low pulse oximetry readings, and the chest radiograph did not show a pneumonic process).

In 1 case, the blood carbon dioxide partial pressure ($PaCO_2$), changed management, as it suggested that the patient had ventilatory failure and needed biphasic positive airway pressure. However, the authors note that they could have made this decision by clinical means alone without the use of the venous blood gas result.

What is also noteworthy about this study is that in the cause of transparency of research methods and data, the authors have made their decision-making data collection form available to subscribers of *Academic Emergency Medicine* by the Internet.

N. B. Handly, MD, MSc, MS

Syncope

Derivation of the San Francisco Syncope Rule to Predict Patients With Short-term Serious Outcomes

Quinn JV, Stiell IG, McDermott DA, et al (Univ of California, San Francisco; Univ of Ottawa, Ont, Canada)
Ann Emerg Med 43:224-232, 2004   2–12

Introduction.—More than 1 million patients are evaluated for syncope each year in the United States, and in most cases the cause is benign. The diagnostic workup and treatment are challenging, however, for a certain percentage of those coming to the ED will have a life-threatening or potentially life-threatening condition. The San Francisco Syncope Rule for predicting patients at risk for short-term serious outcomes was derived from a prospective cohort study.

Methods.—Patients included in the cohort were seen with acute syncope or near syncope at the ED of a large university teaching hospital. The attending physician made the final decision to enroll a patient, and the 7-day outcome was recorded at follow-up by a study nurse. For each patient, physicians completed a data form containing 50 potential predictor variables: 34 historical variables; 11 variables related to the physical examination; and 5 involving laboratory, radiographic, and ECG findings.

Results.—From July 2000 through February 2002, syncope accounted for 1.4% of 58,884 ED visits. The average patient age was 62 years, 59% were women, and 55% were admitted. Seventy-nine (11.5%) of the 684 patients evaluated by attending physicians had a serious outcome by day 7. A total of 26 of 50 potential predictor variables were associated with a serious outcome. Variables associated with organic heart disease and the use of anti-arrhythmic medications and diuretics were significantly associated with serious outcomes. The clinical decision rule derived from analyses includes an abnormal ECG (non–sinus rhythm or new changes compared with the previous ECG), a complaint of shortness of breath, a hematocrit of less than 30%, a triage systolic blood pressure of less than 90 mm Hg, and a history of congestive heart failure. Application of this rule to the study cohort would have yielded a sensitivity of 96.2% and a specificity of 61.9%.

Conclusion.—The San Francisco Syncope Rule can be used as a risk stratification tool to help physicians decide which patients require admission because of the possibility of a short-term serious outcome. When applied to the study cohort, the clinical decision rule would have decreased the admission rate by 10%.

▶ The decision-making process for disposition can be complex, depending on, in part, underlying disease, the need to manage severe symptoms such as pain or persistent vomiting, and reliability of outpatient follow-up. Perhaps a theme that would go through our heads is "What would happen if I sent him/her home?"

Quinn et al have developed a syncope rule to predict those patients in whom "bad things" would likely happen within 7 days from initial ED workup for syncope. While syncope is such a complex disease process and might have other severe consequences not included in this study, the CHESS (history of Congestive heart failure, low Hematocrit, Electrocardiographic changes, low Systolic blood pressure, Shortness of breath) rule for the indicators of the SF syncope rule predicts a set of serious outcomes of 96% sensitivity and 62% specificity.

One might wonder if this study could have been directed to describe those patients who would not have a serious outcome within 7 days, so that we might know who we can send home. Unfortunately, we have a problem, as the authors recognize: They may not have considered the complete spectrum of serious outcomes in their model. Additionally, what happens to patients who do not or cannot receive adequate follow-up beyond the 7 days time?

For the moment, we have a tool to define patients who need to be admitted. A refinement to this tool would help us distinguish those who need monitored beds from those who can be admitted to nonmonitored beds. This is a solid effort. The accompanying editorial[1] discusses how this study meets many quality criteria of decision rule creation and is a useful guide to the methodology of clinical decision-making rules.

N. B. Handly, MD, MSc, MS

Reference

1. Gallagher EJ: Shooting an elephant. *Ann Em Med* 43:233-237, 2004.

A Risk Score to Predict Arrhythmias in Patients With Unexplained Syncope
Sarasin FP, Hanusa BH, Perneger T, et al (Univ of Geneva; Univ of Pittsburgh, Pa)
Acad Emerg Med 10:1312-1317, 2003   2–13

Background.—The noninvasive testing currently recommended for evaluation of syncope in the ED includes a thorough clinical history, physical examination, and 12-lead ECG. These measures result in a diagnosis of syncope in approximately 50% of cases. One critical issue for the remaining patients with unexplained symptoms after such noninvasive testing is the identification of patients at risk for significant arrhythmias as the cause of syncope. In clinical practice, however, assessment of a patient's risk of significant arrhythmia is a difficult challenge. A risk score predictive of arrhythmias for patients with unexplained syncope after noninvasive testing in the ED was created and validated.

Methods.—One cohort of 175 Swiss patients with unexplained syncope was used to develop and cross-validate a risk score for this study; a second cohort of 269 similar American patients was used to validate the system. Arrhythmias as a cause of syncope were diagnosed by cardiac monitoring or electrophysiologic testing. Data from the patient's history and from 12-lead ECG analysis were used to identify predictors of arrhythmias. Logistic regression analysis was used to identify predictors for the risk-score system.

Results.—The prevalence of arrhythmia as a cause of syncope was 17% in the Swiss (derivation) cohort and 18% in the American (validation) cohort. The factors predictive of arrhythmias were abnormal ECG, a history of congestive heart failure, and age older than 65 years. The risk of arrhythmias in the derivation cohort ranged from 0% in patients with no risk factors to 6% for patients with 1 risk factor, 41% for patients with 2 risk factors, and 60% for patients with 3 risk factors. In the validation cohort, the risk of arrhythmias ranged from 2% with no risk factors to 17% with 1 risk factor, 35% with 2 risk factors, and 27% with 3 risk factors.

Conclusions.—A risk score for prediction of arrhythmias in patients with unexplained syncope was validated in this report. The risk score is based on clinical and ECG factors available in the ED and identifies patients at risk for arrhythmias.

▶ If our suspicions are the basis of our differential diagnoses, then what is the basis of our suspicions? Clearly, that is based on experience. Evidence-based experience we now recognize as the most valuable.

The authors developed an evidence-based system to identify if arrhythmia would be the cause for unexplained syncope. Getting the terms right is important. The authors divided the patients admitted to the ED with syncope into those whose cause was "easily identified" and those whose cause was "unexplained" after history, physical, and ECG. Previous studies have shown that about 50% of patients with syncope have an unexplained cause after this initial work-up.

The authors developed a risk score that would predict which of these unexplained syncope events would be the result of arrhythmias. Their technique was to use chart information from a hospital in Switzerland to derive the scoring system (logistic regression) and then to validate this system at a hospital in Pittsburgh.

They found 3 factors that describe the risk of final cause of arrhythmia: age greater than 65 years, history of congestive heart failure, and an abnormal ECG (atrial fibrillation, sinus pauses from 2 to 3 seconds, sinus bradycardia at rates of 25 to 45 beats/min, conduction disorders, evidence of old myocardial infarction, evidence of left ventricular hypertrophy, and multiple premature ventricular contractions).

The authors recognized an important weakness in their work. There was no objective method that defined arrhythmia (significant or otherwise) prior to the study. Thus, there is an unknown bias in the study. Yet it is interesting to note that both in the Swiss and Pittsburgh samples, the patients with final diagnosis of arrhythmia were of similar frequency (about 17% to 18%). Whether this reflects a training standardization internationally is unclear.

In the ED, we are challenged to direct our patients to the appropriate levels of care. Patients with the risks described in this study are likely those we already want to send to monitored beds; this evidence helps support our thinking. Further work might be done to find those patients who are safe to discharge home.

N. B. Handly, MD, MSc, MS

Electrical Cardioversion of Emergency Department Patients With Atrial Fibrillation
Burton JH, Vinson DR, Drummond K, et al (Maine Med Ctr, Portland, Ore)
Ann Emerg Med 44:20-30, 2004   2–14

Background.—Atrial fibrillation (AF) is the most common sustained cardiac arrhythmia and the most common arrhythmia in the ED. Electrical cardioversion of the ED patient with AF has not been well investigated. The outcomes and complications associated with ED electrical cardioversion in patients with AF were determined.

Methods.—A retrospective survey of health records was conducted to investigate a consecutive cohort of ED patients with AF who underwent electrical cardioversion in 4 EDs during 42 months. Medical records were reviewed by trained personnel for demographic characteristics, clinical descriptors, medical interventions, complications, and ED return visits within 7 days, and the data were analyzed using descriptive statistics. The study population included 388 patients, 20 to 93 years old (mean age, 61 years).

Results.—The duration of AF was less than 48 hours in 99% of the patients. Electrical cardioversion was successful in 332 (86%) of 388 patients. In 25 electrical cardioversion episodes, 28 complications occurred, including 22 attributable to procedural sedation and analgesia and 6 attributable to electrical cardioversion. Most of the patients (86%) were discharged to home from the ED, including 301 patients after successful electrical cardioversion and 32 after failed electrical cardioversion. Thirty-nine (10%) patients returned to the ED within 7 days, and 25 of these patients (including 6% of successful cardioversion patients) returned because of relapse of AF.

Conclusions.—This multicenter review of electrical cardioversion in ED patients found that selected ED patients with AF had high rates of electrical cardioversion success, infrequent hospital admission, and few immediate- and short-term complications.

▶ Selection of patients for ED cardioversion and for ED discharge still requires prospective investigation. The subset of patients with chest pain, shortness of breath, or hypotension presumably due to their tachyarrhythmia clearly need immediate electrical conversion but should be observed for a day or 2 after that. Patients with recurrent episodes should be converted with either drugs or electricity (although the evidence would favor use of electricity).

Based on the limited data provided by this study, these patients can be safely sent home with proper attention to adjustment of prophylactic antiarrhythmics and with awareness that almost 1 of 10 will return with a recurrence. New patients with AF may be appropriate candidates for ED cardioversion but should have a thorough evaluation of the cause of their arrhythmia, which, in most cases, means hospital admission.

As with so many other procedures, preparation is everything in electrical cardioversion. The key to a safe outcome is expert knowledge and skill in performing conscious sedation. Proper head positioning and immediately available equipment for ventilatory support is critical, as is experience and comfort with the sedative agent to be used. Half of the patients with a complication related to sedation in this study had oxygen desaturation, which may be partly preventable by preoxygenation and careful attention to marginal ventilatory effort.

W. P. Burdick, MD, MSEd

Initial Clinical Evaluation of Cardiac Systolic Murmurs in the ED by Noncardiologists

Reichlin S, Dieterle T, Camli C, et al (Univ Hosp Basel, Switzerland)
Am J Emerg Med 22:71-75, 2004   2–15

Background.—Cardiac systolic murmurs are common; they may be benign or may signal the presence of heart disease. Initial screening of patients with suspected heart murmurs is reliant on clinical methods, including history taking and cardiac auscultation. The goal of this clinical examination is not to arrive at a specific diagnosis but rather to identify patients in need of additional testing for detection or quantification of valvular heart disease. The accuracy of cardiac auscultation by cardiologists has been found to be high, but the clinical performance of noncardiologists performing auscultation has not been well defined. The sensitivity and specificity of the initial clinical evaluation in distinguishing innocent murmurs from valvular heart disease were measured, and the clinical predictors of the presence of valvular heart disease confirmed by echocardiography were determined.

Methods.—The initial clinical evaluation, including auscultation, was compared with findings on transthoracic echocardiography in 203 consecutive patients who were seen at a medical ED with a systolic murmur. Cardiac auscultation was performed independently in every patient by 3 physicians: a study physician, the ED physician, and the ED attending physician. Patients were enrolled in the study if 2 of the 3 physicians agreed that a systolic murmur was present.

Results.—Of the 203 patients, 132 (65%) had innocent murmurs and 71 patients (35%) had valvular heart disease. The sensitivity and specificity of the initial clinical routine evaluation in diagnosing echocardiographic valvular heart disease were 82% and 69%, respectively. Independent significant positive predictors of valvular heart disease were a systolic murmur with a grade greater than 2/6 and a pathologic ECG. Patients younger than

50 years with a systolic murmur graded 2/6 or less had innocent murmurs in 98% of cases.

Conclusion.—The initial clinical evaluation, including auscultation, by experienced ED physicians in internal medicine can accurately distinguish between innocent murmurs and valvular heart disease in patients with cardiac systolic murmurs.

▶ This study from Switzerland assesses the skill of ED physicians to distinguish "innocent" from valvular disease murmurs. The investigators used transthoracic echo for a gold standard. Overall, they found that senior ED physicians are able to diagnose valvular disease murmurs with a sensitivity of 82% and a specificity of 69%.

Whether these results can be applied everywhere is not clear. I would guess that training to recognize murmurs and their loudness varies from institution to institution. All the physicians in the study were internists; internal medicine residents were rotating through the medicine section of the ED. How would the performance of doctors trained in emergency medicine residencies compare?

The authors find that murmurs with loudness greater than 2/6 have an odds ratio of 8.3 of being valvular disease. The interobserver kappa was 0.55 for the 1/6 to 6/6 murmur loudness scale; this is only fair agreement. So from physician to physician, the problem is the assignment of loudness that would distinguish "innocent" from valvular disease murmurs. Perhaps one way to objectify loudness would be to use visual recording stethoscopes so that murmur loudness can be calibrated.

N. B. Handly, MD, MSc, MS

Vagal Response Varies With Valsalva Maneuver Technique: A Repeated-Measures Clinical Trial in Healthy Subjects

Wong LF, Taylor DM, Bailey M (Royal Melbourne Hosp, Parkville, Australia; Monash Univ, Melbourne, Victoria, Australia)
Ann Emerg Med 43:477-482, 2004   2–16

Background.—The Valsalva maneuver is the forced expiration against a closed glottis that is a safe, cost effective, and probably underused method for treating supraventricular tachyarrhythmias. Variable success rates of the Valsalva maneuver for the treatment of paroxysmal supraventricular tachycardia have been reported, and this variation may be the result of variations in performance techniques. The magnitude of the vagal reflexes initiated by 5 variations of the Valsalva maneuver technique was compared in an effort to determine which technique generates the greatest vagal response and to make recommendations for its use in clinical practice.

Methods.—A single-blind, repeated-measures, clinical trial was conducted among 65 subjects in sinus rhythm. The study subjects performed each Valsalva maneuver—supine, supine with epigastric pressure, supine with leg raise, semirecumbent position, and sitting position—5 times in random order. The means of the longest ECG R-R intervals during the relaxation phase and the postmaneuver pulse rates for each technique were compared. The mean differences between the premaneuver and postmaneuver R-R intervals for each technique were also compared.

Results.—The supine with epigastric pressure and supine techniques resulted in longer mean postmaneuver intervals than the leg raise, semirecumbent, and sitting position techniques, which equates to slower mean postmaneuver pulse rates for the supine with epigastric pressure and supine techniques than with the leg raise, semirecumbent, and sitting position techniques. The supine with epigastric pressure and supine technique also resulted in the greatest premaneuver versus postmaneuver differences.

Conclusions.—In a comparison of 5 variations of the Valsalva maneuver, the results demonstrated that the supine with epigastric pressure and supine Valsalva maneuver techniques generated stronger vagal responses than the other variations in healthy subjects in sinus rhythm, as measured by R-R intervals and pulse rates. However, the vagal responses of these 2 techniques were similar, and the addition of epigastric pressure may provide little advantage.

▶ If you must use the Valsalva technique, use it with the patient supine and epigastric pressure applied. Having said that, I'm not sure that Valsalva has a very important role in supraventricular tachycardia management anymore now that safe and effective adenosine is such a widely used tool. It may be used in the few minutes it takes to find and draw up the drug, but Valsalva is often neither easy nor comfortable for patients. The same could be said for carotid sinus massage, with the added caveat that this technique is not only uncomfortable but potentially dangerous.

W. P. Burdick, MD, MSEd

3 Respiratory Distress

Asthma

Levalbuterol Compared With Racemic Albuterol in the Treatment of Acute Asthma: Results of a Pilot Study
Nowak RM, Emerman CL, Schaefer K, et al (Henry Ford Health System, Detroit; Cleveland Clinic and MetroHealth Ctr, Ohio; Sepracor Inc, Marlborough, Mass; et al)
Am J Emerg Med 22:29-36, 2004   3–1

Background.—For acute asthma attacks, β2-agonists are a primary component of therapy. About one third of patients are not responsive to treatment with racemic albuterol and are admitted to hospital for an average stay of 3 to 4 days. It has been estimated that the financial impact of asthma in the United States is $11.3 billion, with hospital admissions accounting for most of these costs. Alternative approaches to improve clinical outcomes have been attempted but have had little effect in reducing admission rates. Racemic albuterol is composed of equal amounts of (R)-albuterol (also known as levalbuterol) and (S)-albuterol, and it has been shown that these 2 enantiomers have different pharmacologic properties.

Levalbuterol produces both bronchodilatory and bronchoprotective effects; (S)-albuterol has no bronchodilator activity but is not inert. The most effective dose of levalbuterol for treatment of acute bronchospasm was investigated, and the efficacy of levalbuterol was compared with that of racemic albuterol.

Methods.—In this prospective, open-label, nonrandomized pilot study, patients with acute asthma (those with forced expiratory volume in 1 second [FEV_1] of 20% to 55% of predicted) were sequentially enrolled into cohorts of 12 to 14 patients and received 0.63, 1.25, 2.5, 3.75, or 5.0 mg levalbuterol or 2.5 or 5.0 mg racemic albuterol every 20 minutes for 60 minutes.

Results.—After the initial dose, FEV_1 changes were 56% for 1.25-mg levalbuterol and 6% and 14% for 2.5 and 5 mg-racemic albuterol, respectively (Fig 1). After 3 doses, FEV_1 changes were 74%, 39%, and 37% for 1.25-mg levalbuterol, 2.5-mg racemic albuterol, and 0.63-mg levalbuterol, respectively. Doses of levalbuterol greater than 1.25 mg did not provide further improvement in bronchodilation. Baseline plasma (S)-albuterol levels were found to be negatively correlated with baseline FEV_1 and percent change in

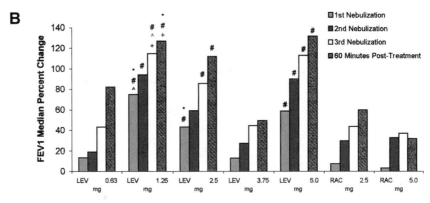

*p<0.05 vs. RAC 2.5 mg; #p<0.05 vs. RAC 5.0 mg; ^p<0.05 vs. LEV 0.63 mg; +p<0.05 vs LEV 3.75 mg

FIGURE 1.—Forced expiratory volume in 1 second (FEV_1) median percentage change from bseline. B, Data for patients with baseline FEV 35% of predicted normal. *Abbreviations: LEV*, Levalbuterol; *RAC*, racemic albuterol. (Courtesy of Nowak RM, Emerman CL, Schaefer K, et al: Levalbuterol compared with racemic albuterol in the treatment of acute asthma: Results of a pilot study. *Am J Emerg Med* 22:29-36, 2004.)

FEV_1. Levalbuterol at a dose of 1.25 mg provided effective bronchodilation that was greater than that of both racemic albuterol doses.

Conclusion.—The negative correlation between (S)-albuterol levels and FEV_1 may suggest a deleterious effect of (S)-albuterol. These findings support the need for larger comparative studies of levalbuterol in comparison with racemic albuterol in the treatment of acute asthma.

Comparison of Racemic Albuterol and Levalbuterol for Treatment of Acute Asthma

Carl JC, Myers TR, Kirchner HL, et al (Case Western Reserve Univ, Cleveland, Ohio)

J Pediatr 143:731-736, 2003   3–2

Background.—Racemic albuterol is the β_2-selective agonist most commonly used for the treatment of acute asthma. However, the (R)-enantiomer levalbuterol has far more potent β_2-receptor binding activity than does the (S)-enantiomer. Levalbuterol was compared with racemic albuterol for the treatment of acute asthma in children.

Methods.—This randomized controlled trial included 482 patients treated in the ED and in the inpatient asthma care unit of an urban children's hospital. These patients accounted for a total of 547 enrollments. The patients' mean age was 7 years; most were African American boys with moderate to severe chronic asthma. The children received either 2.5 mg nebulized racemic albuterol or 1.25 mg levalbuterol, given every 20 minutes to a maximum of 6 doses.

Findings.—The hospitalization rate, the main study outcome, was 36% in patients receiving levalbuterol versus 45% in those receiving racemic albuterol (Figure). The relative risk of admission in the racemic albuterol

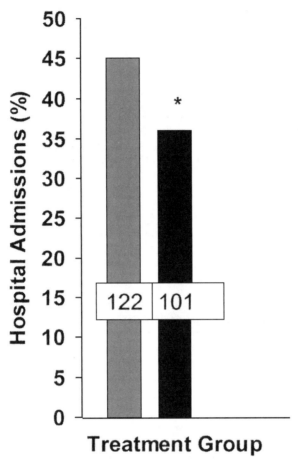

FIGURE.—Hospital admissions in each treatment group, shown as percentage of total in each group. *Figures on the bars* are numbers of patients. * $P = .02$ compared with racemic albuterol; *black bar*, levalbuterol; *shaded bar*, racemic albuterol. (Reprinted by permission of the publisher from Carl JC, Myers TR, Kirchner HL, et al: Comparison of racemic albuterol and levalbuterol for treatment of acute asthma. *J Pediatr* 143:731-736, 2003. Copyright 2003 by Elsevier.)

group was 1.25 (95% CI, 1.01-1.57). The number needed to treat with levalbuterol to prevent 1 hospital admission was 10.6. No significant difference was found between groups in length of hospital stay (about 45 hours in the levalbuterol group vs 50 hours in the racemic albuterol group). The use of albuterol before the patients went to the ED was associated with a 40% increase in the hospitalization rate. No significant adverse events occurred in either group.

Conclusions.—For children receiving emergency treatment for acute asthma, levalbuterol is associated with a significant reduction in hospitalization rate compared with racemic albuterol. The savings achieved by reducing asthma admissions are likely to offset the additional cost of levalbuterol. However, levalbuterol does not seem to reduce the hospital length of stay.

▶ Is a component of our standard therapy with racemic albuterol making patients worse? Racemic albuterol is a mixture of (R)-albuterol (levalbuterol) and (S)-albuterol. It is the latter component that has been implicated by in vitro studies as a possible cause of airway hyperreactivity and bronchoconstriction. It also promotes eosinophil recruitment and activation and increases the production of histamine and immunoglobulin 4, all of which work against the beneficial effects of levalbuterol. Clinical trials are beginning to demonstrate the significance of these in vitro findings at the bedside.

Data from both studies (Abstracts 3–1 and 3–2) look convincing. Levalbuterol has a significantly greater effect on forced expiratory volume in 1 second than racemic albuterol, particularly in those with the worst lung function. In addition, Carl et al (Abstract 3–2) were able to demonstrate a 20% drop in admissions with the isomeric form of albuterol. Given the wide use of this drug for a very prevalent condition, levalbuterol seems to be destined to be a clear replacement for racemic albuterol.

W. P. Burdick, MD, MSEd

Near-Fatal Asthma Related to Menstruation
Martinez-Moragón, E, for the Spanish High Risk Asthma Research Group (Hosp de Sagunto, Valencia, Spain; et al)
J Allergy Clin Immunol 113:242-244, 2004   3–3

Background.—Menstruation has been reported to be a possible trigger of near-fatal asthma (NFA) episodes. However, the evidence of this correlation remains weak. The role of menstruation as a contributor to the development of NFA episodes in women of reproductive age was further investigated.

Methods.—Forty-four women with NFA were included in the multicenter trial. Patients and clinical data were obtained. Spirometric and allergy studies were also performed when the patients were in stable condition. An NFA episode was defined as a severe exacerbation with 1 or more of these events: respiratory arrest, need for mechanical ventilation, $PaCO_2$ exceeding 50 mm Hg, and pH of less than 7.30.

Findings.—Significantly more NFA episodes occurred on the first day of menstruation than on the remaining days. Twenty-five percent of women experiencing NFA episodes had these exacerbations on the first day of their menstrual cycle. In addition, patients seeking care on the first day of menstruation used more inhaled salbutamol as rescue medication.

Conclusions.—In women with unstable asthma, menstruation may be a contributing factor to the development of NFA episodes. Self-management plans of asthmatic women of reproductive age should include systematic recording of asthma symptoms and pulmonary function during the perimenstrual phase.

▶ Martinez-Moragón et al suggest that menstruation was not the isolated trigger of NFA in these patients but served as a contributing factor in patients whose asthma was already unstable and severe. While they may be right, it is important to be aware that their findings contrast with those previously reported by Mitchell and others.[1]

R. K. Cydulka, MD, MS

Reference

1. Mitchell I, Tough SC, Semple LK, et al: Near-fatal asthma: A population-based study of risk factors. *Chest* 121:1407-1413, 2002.

Use of Endoscopic Fibrinogen–Thrombin in the Treatment of Severe Hemoptysis

de Garcia J, de la Rosa D, Catalán E, et al (Hospital Universitari Vall d'Hebron, Barcelona)
Respir Med 97:790-795, 2003   3–4

Background.—The mortality rate of severe hemoptysis is reported to range from 7% to 10%. Asphyxia and intractable hypoxemia caused by the inundation of blood within the alveoli are the most frequent causes of death. Maintenance of airway patency and control of bleeding are the primary immediate goals in the treatment of severe hemoptysis because of its unpredictable course. Bronchial artery embolization (BAE) is the treatment of choice for most patients with severe hemoptysis. However, this procedure may be unavailable and may even fail or be contraindicated in 4% to 13% of patients. The efficacy of fibrinogen-thrombin (FT) instilled endoscopically as a treatment for patients with massive hemoptysis in whom BAE is contraindicated was evaluated.

Methods.—A prospective clinical study was performed from August 1993 to February 1996 in which FT instillation by fiberoptic bronchoscopy was performed in all patients with severe hemoptysis in whom BAE could not be performed. Patients were followed up until June 2001.

Results.—Of the 101 patients with hemoptysis greater than 150 mL/12 h, 11 (11%) underwent FT instillation. In a mean of 39.4 months of follow-up, early relapse of severe hemoptysis occurred in 2 patients (18%), and a long-time relapse occurred in 1 patient. The mean duration of the procedure was 3 minutes, and no attributable complications were observed in any of the patients.

Conclusions.—Topical treatment with FT should be considered in the initial endoscopic evaluation of patients with severe hemoptysis while awaiting BAE or surgery. FT instillation should also be considered in patients in whom BAE has proved ineffective or is contraindicated.

▶ These authors report their experience with endoscopically applied FT in treating severe hemoptysis. Their patient population included 11 who were either unable to undergo the standard interventional radiologic technique of BAE (either the service was not available at that time or was deemed contraindicated due to patient overanticoagulation) or in those in whom BAE had failed. They were followed up for 72 months with contact every 6 months.

Their approach included use of cold normal saline, 1:20,000 epinephrine in cold normal saline, and collapse of the bleeding bronchial orifice with suction prior to application of FT solution. The region was dried with a flow of oxygen. Four of the 11 had hemoptysis that required embolization or surgery after endoscopy, while 2 had minor hemoptysis that did not require further treatment. We cannot use these figures to approximate our "all comers" population; however, there is no question that this technique can be a successful temporization technique in the ED setting.

Addition of bronchoscopy to the ED armamentarium is worth considering. Costs will include training, equipment purchase, and maintenance (including sterilization). However, the skills to use the scope have value in airway and esophageal problems that often cannot wait for attention from consultants.

N. B. Handly, MD, MSc, MS

Tracheal and Lung Sounds Repeatability in Normal Adults
Sánchez I, Vizcaya C (Catholic Univ of Chile)
Respir Med 97:1257-1260, 2003   3–5

Introduction.—Acoustical signals from the respiratory system are historically evaluated only by clinical auscultation. Lung and tracheal sounds have been the focus of extensive research during the past 2 decades. Photopneumography is a procedure for identifying and analyzing respiratory sounds measured by sensors positioned on the trachea and chest wall. This technique permits objective information and the ability to save and compare respiratory sounds that cannot be obtained via classic auscultation. Tracheal and lung sounds were characterized in young adults. The temporal intrasubject variability in these measurements was examined.

Methods.—Tracheal and lung sounds were evaluated in 7 and 10 adults, respectively. Acoustic measurements for tracheal sounds were performed at 5 different time points during 1 month. Lung sounds were evaluated on 7 occasions during a year. Contact sensors placed on the suprasternal notch and posterior right lower lobe were used for sound recording. Participants breathed through a pneumotachograph at flows of 0.9 to 1.1 L/s. Signals were low-pass filtered and amplified. Fourier analysis was used to assess sounds within a target flow range. Determined were the frequencies below which 25%, 50%, 75%, and 99% of the spectral power between 100 and 2000 Hz was contained.

Results.—There were no differences between the measurements obtained on different days comparing each participant (P = nonsignificant). The spectral pattern of tracheal and lung sounds was stable with low intrasubject variability (Fig 2).

Conclusion.—The spectral pattern of tracheal and lung sounds is stable and demonstrates low intrasubject variability.

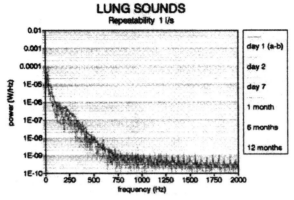

FIGURE 2.—Lung sound reproducibility in 1 selected normal subject breathing at 1 L/s ± 10% on 7 occasions during a 1-year period. Note that variation is small, and the slope of the curve is stable, with most of signals below 600 Hz.(Reprinted from *Respiratory Medicine* courtesy of Sánchez I, Vizcaya C: Tracheal and lung sounds repeatability in normal adults. *Respir Med* 97:1257-1260, 2003, by permission of the publisher W B Saunders Company Limited, London.)

▶ First the phonoechocardiogram, now the phonopneumogram. This is an interesting tool that may have utility in teaching lung auscultation to students and residents. Seeing a graphic image of the "shape" of a heart murmur has helped many students train their ears. I suspect this would also be the case for learning to identify adventitious lung sounds. This study also demonstrates that lung sounds for an individual do not vary significantly over time but that there is about a 20% variation in the quality of breath sounds across individuals.

W. P. Burdick, MD, MSEd

Congestive Heart Failure

Noninvasive Ventilation in Cardiogenic Pulmonary Edema: A Multicenter Randomized Trial
Nava S, Carbone G, DiBattista N, et al (Istituto Scientifico di Pavia, Italy; Gradenigo Hosp, Turin, Italy; S Orsola Hosp, Bologna, Italy; et al)
Am J Respir Crit Care Med 168:1432-1437, 2003   3–6

Background.—The rationale for the use of continuous positive airway pressure in patients with acute pulmonary edema is based on the fact that it may limit the decline in functional residual capacity, improve respiratory mechanics and oxygenation, and decrease left ventricular afterload. However, the best therapy for treatment of an episode of acute respiratory failure due to cardiogenic pulmonary edema is controversial. Studies of the use of noninvasive pressure support ventilation (NPSV) in cardiogenic pulmonary edema have been performed in the ICU when overt respiratory failure is already present and in small groups of patients. NPSV was compared with conventional oxygen therapy in the treatment of acute cardiogenic pulmonary edema.

Methods.—This multicenter study was conducted in EDs and included 130 patients with acute respiratory failure who were randomly assigned to receive medical therapy plus oxygen (65 patients) or NPSV (65 patients). The main outcome measure was the need for intubation. Secondary outcomes were in-hospital mortality and changes in some physiologic variables.

Results.—Partial pressure of arterial oxygen/fraction of inspired oxygen (PaO_2/FIO_2), respiratory rate, and dyspnea were improved significantly faster with NPSV. Intubation rate, hospital mortality, and duration of hospital stay were similar in the 2 groups. In the subgroup of patients with hypercapnia, NPSV provided improvement in partial pressure of arterial carbon dioxide ($PaCO_2$) significantly faster and reduced the intubation rate in comparison with medical therapy (2 of 33 patients vs 9 of 31). Adverse events, including myocardial infarction, were evenly distributed between the 2 groups.

Conclusion.—The early use of NPSV during acute respiratory failure accelerates the improvement of PaO_2/FIO_2, $PaCO_2$, dyspnea, and respiratory rate but does not affect the overall clinical outcome. However, NPSV does reduce the intubation rate in the subgroup of patients with hypercapnia.

▶ Nava and colleagues report that NPSV improves oxygenation, respiratory rate, and dyspnea faster than standard treatment in patients presenting to the ED with cardiac pulmonary edema but doesn't prevent intubation. In addition, his data suggest that NPSV may be more effective in preventing intubation in hypercapnic patients. However, more investigative work needs to be done in this area as CO_2 level was not a significant predictor variable for intubation when entered into a logistic regression model. Many emergency physicians have been using NPSV when treating cardiogenic pulmonary edema for a long time so it's nice to see that our positive anecdotal experience (ie, patients feel better faster) is being borne out. The flip side is that our negative anecdotal experience is also being borne out: Some patients need to be intubated and nothing we can do will save them from that unpleasant (but lifesaving) experience.

R. K. Cydulka, MD, MS

Focused Training of Emergency Medicine Residents in Goal-directed Echocardiography: A Prospective Study
Jones AE, Tayal VS, Kline JA (Carolinas Med Ctr, Charlotte, NC)
Acad Emerg Med 10:1054-1058, 2003   3–7

Background.—Previous studies have shown the utility and reliability of focused US when used by emergency physicians for various clinical situations in the ED. Focused echocardiography by emergency physicians has been proposed as a method of rapidly diagnosing the presence of pericardial tamponade in hemodynamically unstable patients and the presence or absence of cardiac contraction during cardiac arrest resuscitation. There is continuing debate as to whether emergency physicians should perform and interpret echocardiograms and what training should be required to define competency. Whether a focused transthoracic echocardiography (TTE) training course would improve the accuracy of completion and interpretation of a goal-directed TTE by emergency medicine residents was determined.

Methods.—This prospective, observational, education study was designed to evaluate the change in physician performance on pretraining and posttraining examinations testing competency in goal-directed TTE defined by 5 criteria, including image orientation, anatomy identification, chamber size grading, ventricular function estimation, and pericardial effusion identification. The study group was composed of emergency medicine residents with 10 to 20 hours of noncardiac US didactics and 20 to more than 150 proctored noncardiac US examinations. All the study subjects underwent 5 hours of focused echocardiography didactics and 1 hour of proctored practical echocardiography training designed and implemented by an emergency physician US director and a cardiologist. Before beginning the course, study participants completed a written 23-question test on these concepts and performed a TTE on a healthy subject, testing 16 elements that define a properly performed examination. After the training course, study participants completed both examinations.

Results.—A total of 21 ED residents underwent the standardized testing and training. The mean correct score on the precourse written examination was 54%, and the postcourse mean correct score on the examination was 76%. The percentage correct on the precourse practical examination was 56% compared with 94% on the postcourse practical examination.

Conclusion.—A focused 6-hour echocardiography training course significantly improved emergency medicine residents' percentage scores on both written and practical examinations testing essential components necessary for correct performance and interpretation of focused TTE.

Accuracy of Emergency Physician Assessment of Left Ventricular Ejection Fraction and Central Venous Pressure Using Echocardiography
Randazzo MR, Snoey ER, Levitt MA, et al (Alameda County Med Ctr, Oakland, Calif)
Acad Emerg Med 10:973-977, 2003   3–8

Introduction.—Emergency physicians (EPs) routinely manage critically ill patients with an indeterminate or changing hemodynamic status. ED bedside echocardiography may provide useful information concerning cardiac function and volume status. The accuracy of EP performance of echocardiography in the evaluation of left ventricular ejection fraction (LVEF) and central venous pressure (CVP) was examined in a cross-sectional observational trial at an urban teaching ED.

Methods.—A convenience sample of patients seen in the ED between September 2000 and February 2001 was evaluated. Level III–credentialed EP sonographers who had undergone a 3-hour instructional session in limited echocardiography, focusing on LVEF and CVP measurement, performed echocardiograms. Vital signs and indications for echocardiography were recorded on a data sheet. The LVEF was expressed as an absolute percentage and was rated as poor (<30%), moderate (30%-55%), or normal (>55%). CVP was categorized as low (<5 cm), moderate (5-10 cm), or high (>10 cm). Formal echocardiograms were performed within a 4-hour window on all patients and were interpreted by a staff cardiologist.

Results.—A total of 115 patients were evaluated for LVEF; complete data for CVP were available in 94 patients. The indications for echocardiography were chest pain (45.1%), congestive heart failure (38.1%), dyspnea (5.7%), and endocarditis (10.6%). Results demonstrated a LVEF correlation of $r^2 = 0.712$, with 86.1% overall agreement. Subgroup analysis showed the highest agreement (92.3%) between EP and formal echocardiograms within the normal LVEF category, 70.4% agreement in the poor LVEF category, and 47.8% in the moderate LVEF category. CVP measurements demonstrated a 70.2% overall raw agreement between EP and formal echocardiograms. Subgroup analysis showed the highest agreement (83.3%) within the high CVP category, 66.6% in the moderate, and 20% in the low categories.

Conclusion.—Experienced EP sonographers with a small amount of focused additional instruction in limited bedside echocardiography can accurately evaluate LVEF in the ED.

▶ Cardiac US has been adopted by EPs to answer specific questions about pericardial effusions/tamponade and wall motion. Our experience with cardiac US has grown, and we are seeing the benefit of completing additional studies to assess LVEF and CVP. Assumptions have been made about how much and what kind of training is required to be proficient at cardiac scanning.

The first work (Abstract 3–7) reviews the results of a training program to improve results by emergency residents on a written and practical skills tests for cardiac US. Validation is important because we want to know a study tells us something about the real world performance. Jones et al (Abstract 3–7) admit that their tests were not validated. However, they were able to show that significant improvements in knowledge and practical skills can occur after 6 hours of training (including 1 hour of practical training). We do not know if more or less hours would give equivalent or proportional improvements or whether the ratio of didactic versus practical training could be optimized. It would be useful to give these tests to cardiologists trained in echocardiography to see where a criterion standard level of performance might lie.

Randazzo et al (Abstract 3–8) designed their study to test accuracy of EM-completed echocardiograms compared to echocardiograms performed by cardiology staff. This provides a validation step in their work that the Jones et al article lacks. A 3-hour training course on echocardiology was used to prepare the test subjects for measuring LVEF and CVP. The test subjects had already completed general emergency medicine US training. After this course, the test subjects were able to make US measurements that compared well with the cardiologists'.

EPs can learn and use echocardiography to diagnose and stratify patients with brief training programs. These are useful tools for us. How about adding a stress echo course so that we can complete our workup of patients who are at low risk (enzyme negative throughout stays in a chest pain unit)?

N. B. Handly, MD, MSc, MS

Science or Fiction: Use of Nesiritide as a First-Line Agent?
Noviasky JA, Kelberman M, Whalen KM, et al (St Elizabeth Med Ctr, Utica, NY; Mohawk Valley Heart inst, Utica, NY; St Joseph's Hosp, Syracuse, NY; et al)
Pharmacotherapy 23:1081-1083, 2003   3–9

Background.—Nesiritide is a recombinant form of human B-type natriuretic peptide recently approved for the treatment of acute decompensated chronic heart failure (CHF) in the United States. Many reviews of this agent suggest it is appropriate as first-line therapy for symptomatic patients with this condition. However, the current authors disagree with the use of nesiritide as a first-line agent in such patients. The safety, efficacy, and cost of this agent were discussed.

Discussion.—The Vasodilation in the Management of Acute CHF (VMAC) trial demonstrated that patients given nesiritide had fewer adverse events than those given nitroglycerin. Twenty percent of nitroglycerin recipients had frequent headache compared with 8% of nesiritide recipients. However, there was a 60% relative-risk increase in patient dropout because of adverse effects from nesiritide compared with nitroglycerin.

Data from the VMAC trial also showed a trend toward reduced survival with nesiritide. At 90 days, mortality in the nesiritide and nitroglycerin groups was 19% and 13%, respectively. In patients with right-heart catheters, nesiritide and nitroglycerin significantly reduced pulmonary capillary wedge pressure (PCWP) compared with placebo. When nitroglycerin was infused at a greater concentration, the PCWP declined by 5 mm Hg at 1 hour and 7 mm Hg at 3 hours. This effect appeared consistent with that of nesiritide at similar periods, with reductions of 5.5 and 5.8 mm Hg at 1 and 3 hours, respectively. The dyspnea rating at 3, 6, and 24 hours did not differ significantly between groups.

In general, nesiritide requires less dosage titration than nitroglycerin. However, this factor alone does not compensate for the initial expense of the agent. Nesiritide is about 40 times more expensive than standard agents such as nitroglycerin.

Conclusions.—For these reasons, nesiritide should not be used as first-line therapy in patients with acute decompensated CHF. A more appropriate approach would be to administer nitroglycerin and IV diuretics at 2 or more times the usual daily diuretic dose before using nesiritide.

▶ With the use of published data from the VMAC trial[1] and additional unpublished data provided to the Food and Drug Administration from the VMAC trial, Noviasky and colleagues reframe the outcomes of the VMAC study. The authors present a cogent argument that nitroglycerin and furosemide may be preferred over nesiritide for the treatment of acute decompensated CHF.

Clearly, more data are needed, as well as a trial of appropriately dosed nitro-glycerin and lasix versus nesiritide.

R. K. Cydulka, MD, MS

Reference

1. Publication Committee for the VMAC Investigators (Vasodilatation in the Man-agement of Acute CHF): Intravenous nesiritide vs nitroglycerin for treatment of decompensated congestive heart failure: A randomized controlled trial. *JAMA* 287:1531-1540, 2002.

Pulmonary Embolism

D-Dimer for the Exclusion of Acute Venous Thrombosis and Pulmonary Embolism: A Systematic Review
Stein PD, Hull RD, Patel KC, et al (Saint Joseph Mercy-Oakland, Pontiac, Mich; Wayne State Univ, Detroit; Univ of Calgary, Alta, Canada; et al)
Ann Intern Med 140:589-602, 2004   3–10

Background.—Tests for D-dimer to exclude venous thromboembolic dis-ease have been available since the 1980s, but despite an extensive body of literature, the diagnostic role of D-dimer for the evaluation of deep venous thrombosis (DVT) or pulmonary embolism (PE) has not been clarified. This uncertainty is a reflection of multiple D-dimer assays and concerns regarding differing sensitivities and variability. A systematic review investigated trials that assessed sensitivity, specificity, likelihood ratios, and variability among D-dimer assays.

Methods.—A search was conducted of the PubMed and EMBASE data-bases from 1983 to 2003 and from 1988 to 2003, respectively, for relevant studies in all languages. Prospective studies were selected if they compared D-dimer with a reference standard. Studies of high methodologic quality were included in the primary analyses, whereas additional weaker studies were included in sensitivity analysis. Data on study-level factors were col-lected by 2 authors. These data included the D-dimer assay used, the cutoff value, and whether patients had suspected DVT or PE.

Results.—For DVT, the enzyme-linked immunosorbent assay (ELISA) and quantitative rapid ELISA dominated the rank order for these values, with sensitivities of 0.96 and 0.96 and negative likelihood ratio of 0.2 and 0.09, respectively. For PE, the ELISA and quantitative rapid ELISA also dominated the rank order for these values. The ELISA and quantitative rapid ELISA have negative likelihood ratios that provide a high certainty for exclusion of DVT or PE. The positive likelihood values, which are in the gen-eral range of 1.5 to 2.5, did not greatly increase the certainty of diagnosis. These findings were not affected by sensitivity analyses (Fig 2). A limitation to this study is that, although many studies evaluated multiple D-dimer as-says, the findings are based largely on indirect comparisons of test perfor-mance characteristics across studies.

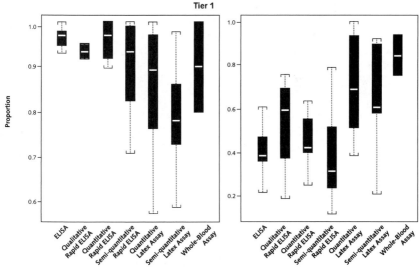

FIGURE 2.—Boxplots of findings for sensitivity and specificity among D-dimer assays for patients with suspected DVT. *Top* and *bottom* of each box represent upper and lower quartiles of values for sample; *white bars* represent medians. Bars extend above and below each box to maximal and minimal values in sample or, if there are extreme data points, to limits based on interquartile range, defined as distance from lower quartile to upper quartile. Outliers beyond these limits are plotted separately. *Quantitative latex assay*, Quantitative latex agglutination assay; *semiquantitative latex assay*, semiquantitative latex agglutination assay; *whole-blood assay*, whole-blood agglutination assay. (Courtesy of Stein PD, Hull RD, Patel KC, et al: D-Dimer for the exclusion of acute venous thrombosis and pulmonary embolism: A systematic review. *Ann Intern Med* 140:589-602, 2004.)

Conclusions.—This analysis of D-dimer assay trials found that the ELISAs generally dominate the comparative ranking among the D-dimer assays for sensitivity and negative likelihood ratio. For exclusion of PE and DVT, a negative result on quantitative rapid ELISA is as diagnostically useful as a normal lung scan or negative duplex US finding.

▶ By using an ELISA, and particularly the quantitative rapid ELISA D-dimer assay, the clinician can count on a negative result to convincingly rule out DVT and to a lesser extent, PE. Significantly less consistent and less sensitive are the semiquantitative rapid ELISA, the latex assays, and whole-blood assays. It is worth finding out what test your laboratory is using.

W. P. Burdick, MD, MSEd

Diagnosing Pulmonary Embolism in Outpatients With Clinical Assessment, D-Dimer Measurement, Venous Ultrasound, and Helical Computed Tomography: A Multicenter Management Study

Perrier A, Roy P-M, Aujesky D, et al (Geneva Univ; Angers Univ, France; Univ Hosp, Lausanne, Switzerland)

Am J Med 116:291-299, 2004　　　　　　　　　　　　　　　　　3–11

Background.—There has been extensive research in recent years into the development of noninvasive and cost-effective diagnostic strategies for pulmonary embolism. A diagnostic strategy for pulmonary embolism was evaluated that combined clinical assessment, plasma D-dimer measurement, lower limb venous US, and helical CT.

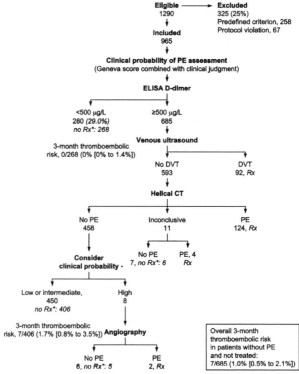

FIGURE.—Flow chart summarizing the diagnostic process in the study. Several patients who were categorized as not having pulmonary embolism by the study criteria were anticoagulated during follow-up for reasons other than venous thromboembolism. The number of patients who were not anticoagulated at any time during follow-up is indicated in the Figure under the caption "no Rx." Those numbers were used to calculate the 3-month thromboembolic risk. Ranges in square brackets indicate 95% CIs. *Abbreviations: DVT,* Deep vein thrombosis; *ELISA,* enzyme-linked immunosorbent assay; *PE,* pulmonary embolism; *Rx,* treatment. (Reprinted from Perrier A, Roy P-M, Aujesky D, et al: Diagnosing pulmonary embolism in outpatients with clinical assessment, D-dimer measurement, venous ultrasound, and helical computed tomography: A multicenter management study. *Am J Med* 116:291-299, 2004. Copyright 2004 with permission from Excerpta Medica Inc.)

Methods.—The study was conducted among 965 consecutive patients with clinically suspected pulmonary embolism who were seen at the EDs of 3 general and teaching hospitals. All patients underwent sequential noninvasive testing. The clinical probability was assessed by a prediction rule combined with implicit judgment. All patients were followed up for 3 months.

Results.—A normal D-dimer level (<500 µg/L by a rapid enzyme-linked immunosorbent assay) excluded venous thromboembolism in 280 patients (29%), and finding a deep vein thrombosis by US established the diagnosis in 92 patients (9.5%). Helical CT was required in only 593 patients (61%) and showed pulmonary embolism in 124 patients (12.8%). Pulmonary embolism was considered to be excluded in the 450 patients (46.6%) with negative US and CT scan findings and a low to intermediate clinical probability. The 8 patients with negative US and CT scan findings despite a high clinical probability were then evaluated with pulmonary angiography. Helical CT was inconclusive in 11 patients. The overall prevalence of pulmonary embolism was 23%. Patients classified as not having pulmonary embolism did not receive anticoagulation therapy during follow-up and had a 3-month thromboembolic risk of 1.0% (Figure).

Conclusions.—This study described a noninvasive diagnostic strategy that combined clinical assessment, D-dimer measurement, US, and helical CT. This approach provided a diagnosis in 99% of outpatients suspected of having pulmonary embolism and appeared to be safe, provided that CT was combined with US to exclude the disease.

▶ The authors present a very logical flow chart for the diagnosis of a pulmonary embolus that combines the use of D-dimer measurement, Doppler US, and helical CT. This approach still missed about 1% of patients with pulmonary emboli, but it represents a significant improvement in our diagnostic ability.

W. P. Burdick, MD, MSEd

Efficacy of Alteplase Thrombolysis for ED Treatment of Pulmonary Embolism With Shock
Le Conte P, Huchet L, Trewick D, et al (Univ Hosp, Nantes, France)
Am J Emerg Med 21:438-440, 2003   3–12

Background.—Massive pulmonary embolism (MPE) is rarely encountered in the ED. Immediate treatment is essential to avoid death at an early stage in patients seen with MPE. Clinical suspicion is often very high in MPE, with sudden onset of acute dyspnea, chest pain, or syncope. Physical examination is often poor or nonspecific, and chest x-ray films often provide no help in the diagnosis. A confirmatory procedure following the guidelines of the European Society of Cardiology is necessary. The management of MPE is based on symptomatic treatment and thrombolysis in the absence of complications.

The efficacy of thrombolysis versus heparin in the treatment of MPE has not been formally demonstrated in large, prospective randomized studies,

but thrombolysis is likely effective in reducing early mortality. The efficacy and tolerability of thrombolysis using 0.6 mg/kg of Alteplase (Boehringer Ingelheim, Germany) in patients with MPE was assessed.

Methods.—A retrospective review was conducted of 21 patients seen with a massive pulmonary embolism confirmed by either scintigraphy or spiral CT. The patients were treated on the basis of a standard rationale followed by thrombolysis with 0.6 mg/kg Alteplase over 15 minutes. The main outcome measures were hospital mortality, vital signs before and 2 hours after thrombolysis, and incidence of hemorrhagic events.

Results.—There were 5 patient deaths (23.8%); 4 of these deaths occurred during the first 4 hours after hospital admission. Systolic and diastolic blood pressure were significantly improved 2 hours after the beginning of thrombolysis. There were 5 minor hemorrhagic events.

Conclusion.—A bolus treatment with Alteplase is potentially effective and well tolerated in patients with pulmonary embolism and shock.

▶ Since there was no control group, all we can take away from this study is that Alteplase does not appear to hurt people, and even that conclusion would be premature, based on the small sample size. The slightly lower mortality compared with historical controls is not very meaningful since acuity and co-morbidities of the 2 samples may have differed substantially.

The first premise of any study using thrombolytics is rapid diagnosis. In this retrospective study, patients were assessed within 1 hour using ventilation-perfusion scans or spiral CT. While this study does not signal a change in practice, EDs need to be developing rapid diagnosis protocols in anticipation of effective thrombolytics.

W. P. Burdick, MD, MSEd

4   Chest Pain

Transfer for Primary Angioplasty Versus Immediate Thrombolysis in Acute Myocardial Infarction: A Meta-analysis
Dalby M, Bouzamondo A, Lechat P, et al (Pitie-Salpetriere Univ Hosp, Paris)
Circulation 108:1809-1814, 2003   4-1

Background.—Percutaneous intracoronary intervention (PCI) has been found to be superior to thrombolysis in the treatment of acute myocardial infarction (AMI). However, as only a minority of patients with AMI come directly to centers that provide PCI, the real choice for these patients is immediate treatment with thrombolyis or transfer and delayed treatment with PCI. Of these 2 options, the 1 that is more preferable for patients experiencing an AMI was assessed by a meta-analysis.

Study Design.—A comprehensive literature and major cardiac conference review from 1985 to September 2002 found 6 randomized trials (3750 patients) comparing the outcomes of primary transfer PCI to those of local thrombolysis for patients with AMI. Transfer time was always under 3 hours. The primary end point was the 30-day combined criteria (CC) of death, reinfarction, or stroke. Individual end points were also evaluated separately. Relative risk was used to evaluate the treatment effect.

Findings.—The CC was significantly reduced in the group of patients with AMI transferred to other institutions for PCI compared with the group receiving immediate on-site thrombolysis. This was also true for each end point considered separately. A trend was also observed toward a reduction in the all-cause mortality rate.

Conclusions.—This meta-analysis indicates that the prognosis of patients with AMI is more improved after percutaneous coronary intervention than after thrombolysis, even if patients have to be transferred to receive delayed PCI. To optimize treatment for patients with AMI, health-care systems must organize rapid transfer networks.

▶ If transport can be accomplished within 2 hours, the meta-analysis evidence presented in this article clearly indicates that it is better to use angioplasty than thrombolysis, even if it means transporting the patient to another hospital. The difference in the composite end point, which included reinfarction, stroke, and mortality rate, was dramatic—6.7% for percutaneous coronary intervention versus 13.5% for thrombolysis.

W. P. Burdick, MD, MSEd

Insurance Status and the Treatment of Myocardial Infarction at Academic Centers

Hiestand BC, Prall DM, Lindsell CJ, et al (Ohio State Univ, Columbus; Univ of Cincinnati, Ohio; Univ of Pennsylvania, Philadelphia; et al)
Acad Emerg Med 11:343-348, 2004   4–2

Background.—Disparities in the treatment of patients with acute coronary syndromes on the basis of race and sex have been documented in many studies. However, other causes may be responsible for these treatment disparities. Whether insurance status affects the quality of care in patients with acute myocardial infarction (AMI) coming to academic health centers was determined.

Methods.—The database used in this study was the Internet Tracking Registry for Acute Coronary Syndromes (i*trACS), a prospective multicenter registry of patients with chest pain coming to the ED who receive an ECG (n = 17,737). A subset of patients who were diagnosed as having AMI were selected from the database (n = 936). These patients were classified as having either ST-segment elevation MI (n = 178) or non–ST-segment elevation MI (n = 758). Insurance status, age, race, and sex were extracted as predictor variables, and the influence of these variables on treatment modality was investigated using logistic regression, adjusted for clustering within sites.

Results.—The odds of a self-paying patient with ST-segment elevation MI receiving fibrinolytics were 3.23 times higher than for other patients. Patients with Medicare coverage were less likely to receive fibrinolytics, and a tendency was noted for these patients to undergo percutaneous coronary intervention less often. The odds of a privately insured patient receiving coronary artery bypass grafting or percutaneous coronary intervention were higher than for other patients.

Conclusions.—Insurance coverage affects the treatment of patients with AMI; self-paying patients are more likely to receive invasive treatments.

▶ Emergency medicine physicians often act as patient advocates. If the best therapy is not being offered to one of our patients because of their insurance status, then it is important for us to go to bat for them and push for it. Remembering our obligation as patient advocates will help in the short run, but until we create systems for universal health care, there will be discrepancies in access to state-of-the-art medical care. We need to resist thinking that our current system is the way it has to be.

W. P. Burdick, MD, MSEd

Socioeconomic Status, Service Patterns, and Perceptions of Care Among Survivors of Acute Myocardial Infarction in Canada

Alter DA, for the SESAMI Study Group (Univ of Toronto)
JAMA 291:1100-1107, 2004   4–3

Introduction.—No investigation has formally examined how service patterns and perceptions of care vary across socioeconomic strata in Canada for an acute life-threatening illness. Patients with acute myocardial infarction (AMI) from various socioeconomic backgrounds were evaluated to determine how they perceive their care in Canada's universal health care system and to correlate patients' backgrounds and perceptions with actual care received.

Methods.—Data were obtained from the Socioeconomic Status and Acute Myocardial Infarction study, an ongoing prospective observational cohort investigation of patients hospitalized with AMI throughout Ontario, Canada. A total of 2256 patients discharged from 53 hospitals across Ontario between December 1999 and June 2002 were contacted 30 days after AMI. The primary outcome measures were postdischarge use of cardiac specialty services; satisfaction with care; willingness to pay directly for quicker service or more choice; and mortality rate according to income and education, adjusted for age, sex, ethnicity, clinical factors, on-site angiography capacity at the admitting hospital, and rural-urban residence.

Results.—Compared with patients in lower socioeconomic strata, more affluent or better-educated patients were more likely to undergo coronary angiography (67.8% vs 52.8%; $P < .001$), receive cardiac rehabilitation (43.9% vs 25.6%; $P < .001$), or be followed up by a cardiologist (56.7% vs 47.8%; $P < .001$). Socioeconomic differences in cardiac care persisted after adjusting for confounders. Despite receiving more specialized services, patients with higher socioeconomic status were more likely to be dissatisfied with their access to specialty care (adjusted risk ratio, 2.02; 95% confidence interval, 1.20-3.32) and favor out-of-pocket payments for more rapid access to a wider choice of treatment options (30% vs 15% for patients with household incomes of Can $60,000 or higher vs less than Can $30,000, respectively; $P < .001$). After adjusting for baseline characteristics, socioeconomic status was not significantly linked with death at 1 year after hospitalization for AMI.

Conclusion.—Compared with persons with lower incomes or less education, upper-middle-class Canadians gain preferential access to services with the publicly funded health care system; they are more likely to favor supplemental coverage or direct purchase of services.

▶ In the Canadian universal health care system, one cannot purchase any additional or parallel insurance. The socioeconomic "elite" who must remain within the system are thought to provide a level of expectation and influence that elevates the service for all the public. It is not clear, however, whether these higher expectations are always medically appropriate.

In this study of care and satisfaction among survivors of AMI, the authors found that those of higher education are more likely to receive cardiologic specialty care (including catheterization, rehab, or post-AMI follow-up by a cardiologist). Since there were no system-wide, described indications for these interventions, it is still not clear whether the increased use of these interventions was appropriate or not. A closer review of the patient records in this sample after deciding indications for use of cardiac interventions would help answer the question of appropriateness of these actions. It is also important to consider whether the less-educated population was receiving adequate care—we have no information to determine the level of care by this study. Again, by deciding a set of indications for procedures before re-examining the data, it would be possible to answer this question. However, whether the expectations of the elite drive adequate care of the "non-elite" would not be clear without changing the study further (such as letting the "elite" drop out of the system, at least temporarily).

Additionally, while these patients received more care, it was found that those who had completed more education were less satisfied with the care delivered (significantly more were extremely dissatisfied with their overall care and access to specialists, and significantly fewer thought that the procedural wait time was extremely short). The higher educated and higher income elite were more willing to pay for additional choices in care (which seems to follow a pattern observed in other countries with a universal insurance scheme but did not prevent purchasing extra insurance outside the national scheme).

It is unlikely that these results are biased by self-reporting of care delivered. The study authors did review charts for a substantial number of these patients to verify the extent of care. It is suggested that the current insurance scheme in Canada might need to be rethought in light of these results. The lesson for all of us is that equal care is difficult to deliver—we are subject to a number of forces, including our patients' education and experience.

N. B. Handly, MD, MSc, MS

Women's Early Warning Symptoms of Acute Myocardial Infarction
McSweeney JC, Cody M, O'Sullivan P, et al (Univ of Arkansas, Little Rock; East Carolina Univ, Greenville, NC; Univ of Kentucky, Lexington; et al)
Circulation 108:2619-2623, 2003   4–4

Background.—The diagnosis of coronary heart disease (CHD) in women is challenging, and few studies have focused on the scope of women's prodromal and acute symptoms of CHD. Little is known about early warning or prodromal CHD symptoms in women before acute myocardial infarction (AMI). The prodromal and AMI symptoms in women are described.

Methods.—The study participants included 515 women diagnosed with AMI from 5 sites. The McSweeney Acute and Prodromal Myocardial Infarction Symptom Survey was used to survey them for 4 to 6 months after discharge, asking about symptoms, comorbidities, and demographic characteristics.

Results.—The women were predominantly white (93%), high school educated (54.8%), and older, with mean age of 66 ± 12 years. Prodromal symptoms were reported by 95% of those surveyed. The most frequent prodromal symptoms experienced more than 1 month before AMI were unusual fatigue (70.7%), sleep disturbance (47.8%), and shortness of breath (42.1%). Only 29.7% reported chest discomfort, which is a hallmark symptom in men. The most common acute symptoms were shortness of breath (57.9%), weakness (54.8%), and fatigue (42.9%). Acute chest pain was absent in 43% of respondents. Women had more acute than prodromal symptoms. The average prodromal score, symptom weighted by frequency and intensity, was 58.5 ± 52.7, whereas the average acute score, symptom weighted by intensity, was 16.5 ± 12.1. These 2 scores were correlated. Women with more prodromal symptoms had more acute symptoms. After controlling for risk factors, prodromal scores accounted for 33.2% of acute symptoms.

Conclusions.—Most women have prodromal symptoms before AMI. However, it is unknown whether prodromal symptoms are predictive of future events.

▶ This is a story about careful listening and open-ended questions. As the authors point out, "Failure by clinicians to assess for and differentiate between chest pain and sensations may be a significant contributing factor in the chest pain controversy." If one just asks about chest pain, one will get answers about only chest pain and miss out on the range of symptoms that may be prodromes to myocardial events. Recognizing that these very nonspecific symptoms may be indications of myocardial ischemia is the other part of the equation.

The general principle is to begin an interview with an open mind, and open-ended questions, and not ask direct questions that will only (no surprise) give answers to the questions you have already thought of. "Tell me the story of what brings you here today," and "were you perfectly well before that?" are among the most productive inquiries in my armamentarium. The smartest doctors can't possibly think of the panoply of symptoms a patient might have, and if the patient is trying to be cooperative, they will answer those questions asked of them and no more. The open-ended approach, which takes no more time when you factor in the reduction of unnecessary tests and repeat assessment when everything comes back "negative," is one that often takes a great deal of convincing before clinicians are willing to use it but yields the best patient care in the end.

W. P. Burdick, MD, MSEd

Mortality Benefit of Immediate Revascularization of Acute ST-Segment Elevation Myocardial Infarction in Patients With Contraindications to Thrombolytic Therapy: A Propensity Analysis

Grzybowski M, Clements EA, Parsons L, et al (Wayne State Univ, Detroit; Spectrum-Health Hosp, Grand Rapids, Mich; Ovation Research Group, Chicago; et al)
JAMA 290:1891-1898, 2003   4–5

Background.—Thrombolytic therapy is the most widely used method for management of patients with acute ST-segment elevation myocardial infarction (STEMI). However, there are no definitive recommendations for management of these patients who have contraindications to thrombolytic therapy. There is some evidence that percutaneous coronary intervention may be more effective than thrombolytic therapy, but it is not clear that immediate mechanical reperfusion (IMR) in these patients can improve outcome. Whether IMR, which was defined as percutaneous coronary intervention or coronary artery bypass surgery, is associated with improved mortality rate in patients with STEMI who are eligible for IMR but have contraindications to thrombolytic therapy was evaluated.

Methods.—The National Registry of Myocardial Infarction 2, 3, and 4 enrolled 1,799,704 patients with acute myocardial infarction from June 1994 to January 2003. A total of 19,917 patients with acute STEMI were eligible for IMR but had thrombolytic contraindications. Patients transferred to or from other facilities, those who received intracoronary thrombolytics, and those who did not receive medications within 24 hours of arrival were excluded. The main outcome measure was in-hospital death.

Results.—Of the 19,917 patients included in the study, 4705 patients (23.6%) received IMR and 5173 patients (25.9%) died. In-hospital mortality rates in the IMR and non-IMR treated groups in the unadjusted analysis were 11.1% (521 of 4705 patients), and 30.6% (652 of 15,212 patients), respectively, for a risk reduction of 63.7%. Additional analysis with a propensity matching score to reduce the effects of bias found that 3905 patients who received IMR continued to have a lower risk for in-hospital death than 3905 matched patients (10.9% vs 20.1%, respectively), for a risk reduction of 45.8%. A significant treatment effect was found to persist after application of a second logistic model to the matched group to adjust for residual differences.

Conclusions.—Immediate mechanical reperfusion was found to be associated with a reduced risk of in-hospital death after appropriate adjustments in this population. Of the patients in this study who were eligible for IMR, 76.4% did not receive it. It would appear from these findings that the use of IMR in patients with STEMI and the contraindications to thrombolytic therapy should be strongly considered.

▶ As soon as contraindications to thrombolytic therapy are identified, prompt movement to mechanical revascularization is clearly indicated. The mortality rate of patients who received this intervention was less than half of those who did not in this large multicenter trial. For emergency physicians, this means clearly identified referral patterns and protocols to expedite decision making and rapid movement of the patient to the catheterization lab or the operating room.

The type of analysis used in this study is a method that determines the "propensity" for a subject to be included in the treatment group instead of the control group. Theoretically, if there is no propensity to treatment, then there is no bias in assignment to treatment in the study. Since random assignment was not used in this study, a possibility exists that there was bias in the decision to send certain patients and not others to treatment. A propensity score considers all the known patient characteristics and collapses them into a single predictor variable that can then be used to assess and adjust for bias by matching control and treatment subjects. As with any nonrandomly assigned subjects, however, there may be unknown variables that are potentially important that would not be taken into account.

W. P. Burdick, MD, MSEd

Acute Myocardial Infarction: Contrast-Enhanced Multi–Detector Row CT in a Porcine Model
Hoffmann U, Millea R, Enzweiler C, et al (Harvard Med School, Boston)
Radiology 231:697-701, 2004   4–6

Background.—Earlier studies have demonstrated the feasibility of conventional CT for infarct imaging in animal models. The role of contrast material–enhanced retrospectively ECG-gated multi–detector row CT for the detection of acute myocardial infarction was assessed in a porcine model of total coronary occlusion.

Methods.—Seven Yorkshire farm pigs were studied. Contrast-enhanced retrospectively ECG-gated multi–detector row CT was performed 3 hours after total occlusion of the distal left anterior descending artery (5 pigs) or the second diagonal branch (2 pigs). Reformatted short-axis end-systolic and end-diastolic CT data sets were assessed for myocardial perfusion deficits, coronary occlusion, and abnormal myocardial wall motion. Perfusion deficits were compared with microsphere-determined blood flow and triphenyltetrazolium chloride–stained tissue samples for infarct assessment by using Bland-Altman analysis and analysis of variance.

Results.—The study was completed by 5 animals. One animal died, and one data set had nondiagnostic image quality. Myocardial perfusion deficits, occlusion of the left anterior descending or second diagonal branch, and akinesis of the infarcted segment were identified in all 5 animals that completed the study. The CT end-diastolic and end-systolic volume of perfusion deficit was similar to that of infarcted tissue at triphenyltetrazolium chloride staining. Infarcted myocardium at CT demonstrated a reduction of 76.1% in microsphere-determined blood flow and a significant reduction of myocardial CT attenuation in comparison with normal myocardium (Fig 2). Myo-

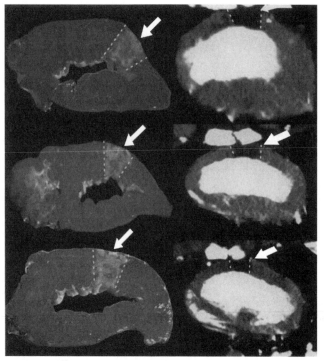

FIGURE 2.—**Right,** Three consecutive multi–detector row CT images of an acute transmural infarct in short-axis orientation. The infarct can be visually detected by low CT tissue attenuation due to lack of contrast enhancement (*arrows*). **Left,** Corresponding triphenyltetrazolium chloride (TTC)-stained specimen (short-axis orientation). The infarct is displayed as a region of unstained myocardium (*arrow*). (Courtesy of Hoffman U, Millea R, Enzweiler C, et al: Acute myocardial infarction: Contrast-enhanced multi–detector row CT in a porcine model. *Radiology* 231:697-701, 2004. Copyright Radiological Society of North America.)

cardial wall motion analysis showed absence of systolic wall thickening in infarcted myocardium.

Conclusions.—These findings demonstrate the feasibility of multi–detector row CT with retrospective ECG gating for detection and further characterization of acute myocardial infarction in a porcine model of complete coronary occlusion.

▶ It's coming: a patient with a suspected myocardial infarction and a nondiagnostic ECG is whisked to CT for a definitive diagnosis. This porcine model demonstrating the utility of CT for diagnosis brings us one step closer to the use of CT to diagnose myocardial infarction. Just as we have learned with CT diagnosis of appendicitis, it won't be right 100% of the time, but it will reduce the group of "undecideds" considerably.

W. P. Burdick, MD, MSEd

The Prognostic Value of High-Sensitive C-Reactive Protein and Cardiac Troponin T in Young and Middle-Aged Patients With Chest Pain Without ECG Changes
Blum A, Safori G, Hous N, et al (Poria Hosp, Lower Galilee, Israel)
Eur J Intern Med 14:310-314, 2003   4–7

Introduction.—There is growing evidence concerning the prognostic importance of inflammatory markers in angina pectoris. The independent value of high-sensitivity C-reactive protein (hsCRP), cardiac troponin T (cTnT), or their combination has yet to be determined in young patients with angina pectoris without ECG changes. The 6-month prognostic value of serum hsCRP and cTnT was evaluated in young and middle-aged patients admitted to the hospital with chest pain without ECG changes.

Methods.—Forty young or middle-aged patients (45 ± 10 years old; 2 women, 38 men) with new onset angina pectoris with no ECG changes or CPK-MB elevation were prospectively evaluated between June 2000 and June 2001. Blood was obtained at admission, separated, and serum was frozen at $-80°C$ for 1 year until thawed and evaluated as 1 batch to measure hsCRP and cTnT levels. Patients were monitored clinically for 6 months.

Results.—The strongest independent marker of an adverse outcome was the hsCRP level at the time of admission (sensitivity 66.7%; specificity 94.1%); cTnT level added somewhat to specificity (97.1%). It did not add to the sensitivity seen at the hsCRP level.

Conclusion.—The hsCRP level at admission may be an independent prognostic marker in young and middle-aged patients with angina pectoris without ECG changes and without CPK-MB elevation.

▶ How many times have you heard the cardiologists complain about your decision to admit a young patient who turns out to have normal ECGs, negative cardiac enzymes, and a negative stress test? What if you could show that these patients were at increased risk of a cardiac event in 6 months?

Drs Blum et al monitored 40 such patients for 6 months (these patients had normal ECGs, negative cardiac enzymes, and negative exercise stress and thallium tests). These patients were stratified by hsCRP levels. Outcomes measured were recurrent chest pain with rehospitalization, angiography, myocardial infarction, coronary artery bypass grafting, and cardiac sudden death. At a cutoff of 15 mg/dL, hsCRP can predict a 6-month adverse outcome with a sensitivity of 66.7% and specificity of 94.1%. The cTnT level contributed little additionally to the sensitivity and specificity to detect these 6-month outcomes. The authors acknowledge that these results are based on a small sample of 40 patients.

Would an elevated hsCRP level help justify your admission decision? Probably not yet, as the method needs further validation. However, if hsCRP is to be used as a marker of future risk, what kind of monitoring will be necessary for these patients? How will we know when an "event" is likely to occur? Will we need to use monitoring equipment such as event monitors for these patients?

N. B. Handly, MD, MSc, MS

Predictors of Major Bleeding in Acute Coronary Syndromes: The Global Registry of Acute Coronary Events (GRACE)
Moscucci M, for the GRACE Investigators (Univ of Michigan, Ann Arbor; et al)
Eur Heart J 24:1815-1823, 2003   4–8

Introduction.—The outcome of patients with acute coronary syndrome has improved with recent advances in therapy, but the complication of major bleeding remains a significant risk. Data from the prospective, multicenter Global Registry of Acute Coronary Events (GRACE) were used to develop a prediction rule for identifying patients at higher risk of major bleeding.

Methods.—Bleeding status was known for 24,045 patients with ACS enrolled in GRACE between April 1999 and September 2002. Cases were categorized as ST segment elevation myocardial infarction (STEMI), non–ST segment elevation myocardial infarction (NSTEMI), unstable angina, and other cardiac/noncardiac diagnoses.

Results.—Major bleeding developed in 933 (3.9%) patients in the study group. Patients with this complication were significantly older and had lower mean arterial pressure and a lower body mass index. Other baseline clinical characteristics associated with an increased risk of major bleeding were female sex, peripheral vascular disease, renal insufficiency, and a history of bleeding. Patients with unstable angina were less likely to have major bleeding than were patients with STEMI or NSTEMI (2.3% vs 4.8% and 4.9%, respectively). The associations between major bleeding and advanced age, female sex, a history of bleeding, and renal insufficiency remained significant after adjustment for drug interventions and invasive diagnostic and therapeutic procedures.

Conclusion.—Major bleeding, a relatively frequent noncardiac complication in patients hospitalized for acute coronary syndrome, is significantly associated with an increased risk of hospital death (odds ratio, 1.64). Gastrointestinal bleeding accounted for 31.5% of major bleeding complications and vascular access site bleeds for 23.8%. Patients at increased risk for major bleeding can be identified by baseline demographic and clinical characteristics.

Creatinine Clearance and Adverse Hospital Outcomes in Patients With Acute Coronary Syndromes: Findings From the Global Registry of Acute Coronary Events (GRACE)

Santopinto JJ, Fox KAA, Goldberg RJ, et al (Hosp Municipal de Bahia Blanca, Argentina)

Heart 89:1003-1008, 2003   4–9

Introduction.—Mild renal impairment is known to be associated with an increased risk of coronary artery disease and stroke, but the prognostic significance of creatinine clearance in patients hospitalized with acute coronary syndrome (ACS) is unknown. Data from the Global Registry of Acute Cardiac Events (GRACE) were examined to determine whether creatinine clearance at admission is an independent predictor of hospital mortality and adverse outcomes in patients with ACS.

Methods.—The study sample of 11,774 patients with ACS and available renal function data was divided into 3 groups according to creatinine clearance rates: greater than 60 mL/min (normal or minimally impaired renal function; 7591 patients); 30 to 60 mL/min (moderate renal dysfunction; 3397 patients); and less than 30 mL/min (severe renal dysfunction, 786 patients). Patients were also categorized as having ST segment elevation myocardial infarction (STEMI) or non-ST segment elevation myocardial infarction/unstable angina (NSTEMI/UA). In-hospital outcomes were compared according to renal function, demographic and clinical characteristics, and medication use.

Results.—Compared with patients whose renal function was normal or near normal, those with moderate or severe renal dysfunction were older, more likely to be women, and to have more comorbidities on admission. There was an association between worsening renal dysfunction and both the frequency of ECG changes and the risk of major bleeding. In patients with STEMI, ECG changes were seen less often as renal impairment increased. Patients with moderate or severe renal dysfunction were more likely to have received drugs to treat or prevent renal and atherosclerotic disease before hospital admission, but they were less likely to receive such agents during acute hospitalization. Patients with moderate renal dysfunction were twice as likely to die, and those with severe renal dysfunction were 4 times more likely to die, than patients with normal or near normal renal function. This elevated risk remained after adjustment for other variables.

Conclusion.—Creatinine clearance is an important independent predictor of hospital death and major bleeding episodes in patients with ACS. Even moderate renal insufficiency significantly increases these risks.

▶ These studies (Abstracts 4–8 and 4–9) both use the GRACE data to analyze hospital process and outcome. Patients were entered into the registry based on admission criteria (rather than discharge diagnosis) and followed up in a prospective observation mode. The intention of the designers of this registry was to minimize selection bias by having standardized yet broad inclusion criteria for entry in to the study. Additionally, this study is multicenter and multinational. It was planned that this study sample would better represent the "all comers" (to the ER) population than have some previous studies that used criteria for inclusions based on events after admission to the ER.

The article by Moscucci et al (Abstract 4–8) used logistic regression to show that increasing age, female gender, history of bleeding, or renal insufficiency are independent risk factors in patients' major bleeding. They then found that major bleeding was an independent risk factor for mortality.

The article by Santopinto et al (Abstract 4–9) reports the role of creatinine clearance, which was estimated from serum creatinine clearance, as a risk of major bleeding, stroke, acute myocardial infarction, and mortality.

There was an interrelationship of these determinants: females tended to be older and with worsening renal function in the patients in GRACE.

Abnormal renal function was a common risk in each of these 2 studies. While more could be done to create an inclusion criteria for "all patients suspected of acute cardiac syndrome" in future studies, it is worthwhile to closely watch the patients with poor renal function to avert possible bleeding episodes and death.

N. B. Handly, MD, MSc, MS

Lack of Utility of Telemetry Monitoring for Identification of Cardiac Death and Life-Threatening Dysrhythmias in Low-Risk Patients With Chest Pain
Hollander JE, Sites FD, Pollack CV Jr, et al (Univ of Pennsylvania, Philadelphia)
Ann Emerg Med 43:71-76, 2004   4–10

Background.—Identification of high-risk patients with chest pain on presentation to the ED has improved in the past 2 decades; however, the rapid and accurate identification of low-risk patients continues to be problematic. Clinical and computer algorithms can successfully stratify patients by risk, but they are not able to identify a group of patients as low risk so that they could not be safely and immediately released from the ED. As a result, liberal admission policies have remained the standard approach, and low-risk patients with chest pain are often admitted to monitored beds. However, the use of telemetry beds in these patients is not evidence based. The hypothesis was tested that monitoring admitted low-risk patients with chest pain for dysrhythmia is low yield, and that fewer than 1% of such patients would have life-threatening dysrhythmias requiring treatment.

Methods.—A prospective cohort study was conducted of ED patients with chest pain with a Goldman risk score of less than 8%, a normal initial creatine kinase-MB level, and a negative troponin I level admitted to non-ICU monitored beds. The main outcome measure was cardiovascular death and life-threatening ventricular dysrhythmia during telemetry.

Results.—A total of 3681 patients with chest pain presented to the ED, 1750 of whom were admitted to non-ICU monitored beds. Of these patients, 1029 had a Goldman risk score of less than 8%, a troponin I level of less than 0.3 ng/mL, and a creatine kinase-MB level of less than 5 ng/mL, which accounted for 59% of all chest pain telemetry admissions. There were no patients who sustained ventricular tachycardia/ventricular fibrillation requiring treatment on the telemetry service during hospitalization. There were 2 deaths, but neither was from cardiovascular causes or was preventable by monitoring.

Conclusions.—These findings do not support the routine use of telemetry monitoring for low-risk patients with chest pain. However, admission of these patients to nonmonitored beds may help reduce crowding in the ED without increasing the risk of adverse events caused by dysrhythmia in patients with a Goldman risk of less than 8%, an initial troponin I level of less than 0.3 ng/mL, and a creatine kinase-MB level of less than 5 ng/mL.

▶ When I was a resident, I had an attending physician who made a point of adding the letter "D" to the "ABC" of emergency medicine. That "D" stood for "disposition." Good patient care, improved ED throughput, and reduced ED crowding require our moving patients to their best disposition as efficiently as possible.

Which patients with potential cardiac problems can be sent home and which can be sent to unmonitored beds? Hollander et al question whether telemetry admission is necessary for patients at low risk for lethal dysrhythmias. There is no evidence to base the admission of all patients to telemetry settings. We assume that the risk of lethal dysrhythmia guides us in our current admission plan strategy.

The authors followed the hospital course of patients who did not rule in for acute myocardial infarction and had a Goldman risk of less than 8% after ED work-up. The primary outcomes were in hospital cardiac death and life-threatening dysrhythmias. They hypothesized that these patients could have been safely managed in a nonmonitored bed. None of the 1029 patients included in the study had cardiac death or sustained ventricular tachycardia or ventricular fibrillation. However, 136 were eventually diagnosed with acute myocardial infarction or unstable angina, and about 250 required procedures of catheterization or coronary artery bypass grafting—so that about 25% of these "low-risk" patients in this group would require an increase in intensity of observation and care (possibly requiring a transfer to a coronary care unit bed during the acute phase). They did not follow up with these patients after hospital discharge.

The use of this stratification rule might make better use of scarce hospital resources by sending these patients to an unmonitored bed from the ED. It is presumed that the patients requiring increased intervention during the hospital stay would all be recognized by serial ECGs and cardiac enzyme studies, clinical exam, or pain. Further work is needed to identify criteria that might be used to decide which patients would be at low enough risk that they could be sent home.

N. B. Handly, MD, MSc, MS

Predictors of Delay in Presentation to the ED in Patients With Suspected Acute Coronary Syndromes

Grossman SA, Brown DFM, Chang Y, et al (Harvard Med School, Boston)
Am J Emerg Med 21:425-428, 2003   4–11

Background.—The morbidity and mortality rates of acute coronary syndromes are correlated with the extent of myocardial damage. Most deaths from cardiac arrest occur outside the hospital in patients who have not received medical attention. There is increasing evidence that the benefits of myocardial-preserving therapies, such as thrombolytics and primary angioplasty, are directly related to the duration of ischemia. However, delays in seeking medical attention for patients with acute coronary syndromes will prevent the early application of life-saving treatment, diminishing efficacy. Previous studies have suggested that there is a median 3-hour delay between the onset of symptoms and arrival in the ED in patients with a typical presentation of acute myocardial infarction. The delay (lag time) from symptom onset to ED arrival was measured in patients with suspected acute coronary syndromes, and the lag times among predetermined subgroups of patients stratified by age, sex, and typical versus atypical presentation were compared.

Methods.—A prospective observational study was conducted at an urban ED to measure lag time among adults who presented within 48 hours of onset with symptoms suggestive of acute coronary syndrome. Univariate and multiple regression analyses were performed by using 5 predictors, including age, sex, and symptoms at presentation and 2 different outcomes (acute myocardial infarction and acute coronary syndrome).

Results.—A total of 374 patients were enrolled in the study, with a mean age of 63 years (38% of patients were aged 70 years or older). Nearly three quarters (73%) of all patients with suspected acute coronary syndrome presented with chest pain; 27% presented with atypical symptoms. The overall mean lag time was 8.7 hours. In subgroup analysis, patients aged 70 years or older were more likely to have lag times greater than 12 hours (29% vs 19%); those without chest pain had longer mean lag times (11.6 hours vs 7.6 hours).

Conclusions.—The delay from onset of symptoms suspicious of acute coronary syndromes to arrival in the ED is an average of 9 hours. The delay in ED presentation appeared to be group specific, and advanced age and patients with atypical symptoms are predictive of longer lag times. These findings are contrary to the previously published data and may change the current view of the prevention of acute coronary syndromes and the management of these patients.

▶ This study presents a disturbing pattern of longer delays in arrival at the ED for patients with symptoms suggestive of acute coronary syndromes than previously reported. The authors find delays on average of 8 hours; if the patient is older or has atypical symptoms, the delay can be longer than 12 hours.

What could make this sample group different from previous studies that showed less delay is that the attending physician made a subjective decision of inclusion into the study; however, without any standardized protocol, the attending physician still has final responsibility for the care of his or her patients.

Apparently, our public awareness campaigns have not been effective in reaching the public. We emergency physicians need to join with other health practitioners to develop better systems for educating our patients. This may include involving family members and other support groups besides directly addressing the patients at risk.

N. B. Handly, MD, MSc, MS

Incomplete Data Reporting in Studies of Emergency Department Patients With Potential Acute Coronary Syndromes Using Troponins
Glavan B, Shewakramani S, Hollander JE (Univ of Pennsylvania, Pa)
Acad Emerg Med 10:943-948, 2003   4–12

Background.—The care of patients who arrive at the ED with potential acute coronary syndromes is a continuing challenge because significant amounts of time and resources are devoted to the care of these patients. Several strategies to aid in the risk stratification of ED patients with potential acute coronary syndromes have been developed; however, none of these tools has achieved widespread acceptance. One possible explanation for the slow incorporation of these risk stratification tools is the difficulty in comparing their utility across multiple studies. A multidisciplinary panel has been organized by the Emergency Medicine Cardiac Research and Education Group to develop standardized reporting criteria for risk stratification studies of ED patients with potential acute coronary syndromes. The need for such criteria was assessed by reviewing published studies. The goal was to determine whether these core criteria are currently being reported.

Methods.—A systematic review of the MEDLINE database was used to identify studies published from 2000 to 2001 in 8 journals representing emergency medicine, cardiology, and general medicine that evaluated the cardiac troponins for risk stratification of ED patients with chest pain. Each study was independently analyzed by 2 raters with a structured tool. The presence or absence of 47 core criteria in 8 major reporting categories, which were determined by expert consensus, was abstracted from the articles. Discrepancies between the 2 raters were resolved by consensus. The data from this study were presented as percent frequency of occurrence with 95% confidence intervals.

Results.—A total of 22 articles were included in the review. The was a median of 7.5 initial discrepancies per article between the 2 reviewers, but the reviewers achieved consensus on all articles.

Conclusions.—This literature review found that many of the 47 items considered core criteria by the expert committee engaged in formulating risk stratification guidelines for patients with possible acute coronary syndrome were not often reported in major cardiology and emergency medicine journals. There is a need for standardized reporting guidelines because important information is not currently being reported.

▶ The Utstein templates were designed to standardize language and better describe patient care activities. These templates would help standardize the studies and reports generated about them. At present, the emergency medicine cardiac research and education group has identified a number of criteria that should be part of emergency medicine acute coronary syndrome/troponin studies and should be reported in each publication.

The authors found a significant variability in reporting of the results of acute coronary syndrome/troponin papers from 2000 to 2001. This means that many papers could not be compared. Consider some of those missing elements: time from onset to presentation was stated in only half of the 22 papers reviewed; risk factors were stated typically in fewer than half of the papers; and reference levels for cardiac marker studies were presented in approximately 60% of these papers.

Standardization makes it possible to compares studies at different sites and times, which would make it possible to know if results can be generalized for most practices. We would do well to design our studies and papers with a set of standards such as proposed by the Emergency Medicine Cardiac Research and Education Group; and as readers of publications, we should be mindful of how well any study abides by them.

N. B. Handly, MD, MSc, MS

Spontaneous Coronary Artery Dissection Causing Acute Coronary Syndrome: An Early Diagnosis Implies a Good Prognosis
Roig S, Gómez JA, Fiol M, et al (Hosp Son Dureta, Palma de Mallorca, Spain; Hosp Bellvitge, Barcelona; Hosp Sant Pau, Barcelona)
Am J Emerg Med 21:549-551, 2003   4–13

Background.—Spontaneous coronary artery dissection (SCAD) is a rare cause of acute ischemic heart disease. It occurs most frequently but not exclusively in healthy young women with no associated heart disease, particularly in late pregnancy and the early postpartum period. The incidence, cause, and pathogenesis of SCAD have not been clearly discerned. The prognosis for most patient with SCAD is poor, and morbidity and mortality rates are high. A series of SCAD cases with a good outcome and an early diagnosis and aggressive treatment, including percutaneous angioplasty and stent implantation and cardiac surgery, are described.

Methods.—A retrospective study of patients with SCAD was conducted in 3 coronary care units in third-level university hospitals to investigate the demographic characteristics, clinical settings, treatments, and in-hospital course. The diagnosis of SCAD was made by coronary angiography in 5 women and 2 men aged 28 to 64 years.

Results.—Oral contraceptives were used by 2 patients, with 1 taking them during the postpartum period. The most frequent clinical presentation of SCAD was an acute anterior wall myocardial infarction, which occurred in 4 to 7 days. The left anterior descending artery was involved in 6 cases. An urgent coronary angiogram was performed in all patients. Definitive treatment included percutaneous angioplasty and stent implantation in 3 cases, coronary artery bypass in 2 cases, and cardiac transplantation in 1 case. One patient was treated medically. There were no in-hospital deaths.

Conclusions.—SCAD is an unusual cause of acute coronary syndrome that should be included in the differential diagnosis of acute myocardial infarction, particularly when it affects young, healthy women. The prognosis of these patients could be improved by an early clinical suspicion and diagnosis with urgent coronary angiography and aggressive treatment, including percutaneous angioplasty with stent implantation and cardiac surgery.

▶ This is a report of 7 lucky individuals whose artery dissection was found and treated successfully. They were lucky because many patients with SCAD die suddenly. We do not know the frequency of SCAD in the general or acute coronary syndrome (ACS)–specific population. This report suggests that women in third trimester pregnancy or the postpartum period may be at greater risk due to the hormonal changes of pregnancy. Connective tissue disorders, such as Marfan syndrome, were not found in this case series. This is not to say that connective tissue disorders are not risks for SCAD, as these patients may be more likely to die suddenly and would not be caught in time with a presentation of ACS.

Clearly, we have to respond rapidly to manage our ACS patients. All these patients presented with ACS recognized by the physicians as either unstable angina or acute myocardial infarction. However, we are often confronted by atypical chest pains—where we have a model of low risk of ACS in our heads. Low-risk patients—the pregnant or postpartum women in this report—with chest pain need to be stratified quickly to distinguish the pain of ACS from noncardiac causes.

N. B. Handly, MD, MSc, MS

Disagreement in the Interpretation of Electrocardiographic ST Segment Elevation: A Source of Error for Emergency Physicians?
Erling BF, Perron AD, Brady WJ (Univ of Virginia, Charlottesville)
Am J Emerg Med 22:65-70, 2004   4–14

Background.—Evaluating an ECG is a subjective, complex process that carries the potential for interobserver disagreement. The extent of disagreement among emergency physicians (EPs) in the interpretation of ECG ST-segment elevation (STE) was investigated.

Methods.—Attending EPs retrospectively analyzed STE and waveform morphology on the ECGs of 599 patients. ECGs interpreted with discrepancy were analyzed to determine the patterns of disagreement.

Findings.—Overall, 35.2% of the patients had STE determined by at least 1 attending EP, 19% by 1 EP, 10% by 2 EPs, and 71% by 3 EPs. Discrepancy in interpretation occurred in 28.9% of the ECGs. The mean STE was 1.31 mm per lead for ECGs with disagreement and 2.93 mm per lead for those with agreement. Agreement on STE was more likely when ECGs had reciprocal S depression. Discrepant interpretations of ST-segment morphology occurred on 8.2% of the ECGs, with STE determined by at least 2 EPs.

Conclusions.—Discrepancy on interpretations of ECG STE among EPs is common. Disagreement is related to the amount of STE present on the ECG. ECG patterns underlying interpretive disagreement on STE may be a predictable source of error in emergency medicine.

▶ Let the ECG reader beware! Erling and colleagues have identified the following ECG STE patterns that are particularly troublesome, at least for emergency physicians:

1. Acute myocardial infarction with atypical or concave ST-segment morphology
2. Left ventricular hypertrophy
3. Bundle branch blocks
4. Benign early repolarization
5. Pericarditis
6. Left ventricular aneurysm.

Particular attention should be paid when STE is less than 2 mm or when STE is noted in the inferior leads.

R. K. Cydulka, MD, MS

Prognostic Value of Myeloperoxidase in Patients With Chest Pain
Brennan M-L, Penn MS, Van Lente F, et al (Cleveland Clinic Found, Ohio)
N Engl J Med 349:1595-1604, 2003   4–15

Background.—The leukocyte enzyme myeloperoxidase has been linked to both inflammation and cardiovascular disease. Whether plasma levels of myeloperoxidase might be a marker of major adverse cardiovascular events (MACEs) was investigated.

Methods.—The subjects were 604 patients (58.6% men; mean age, about 62 years) seen in the ED with chest pain. Plasma levels of myeloperoxidase, troponin T (TnT), and C-reactive protein (CRP) were measured at baseline. Patients were followed up for 6 months to determine MACEs (myocardial infarction [MI], reinfarction, need for revascularization, death).

Results.—Of the 148 patients, 23.5% had MI, 37.6% had suspected coronary syndrome, 17.1% had unstable angina, and 21.5% had noncardiac chest pain. Plasma myeloperoxidase levels correlated significantly but weakly with TnT and CRP levels. The incidence of MI increased significantly as the baseline myeloperoxidase level increased (13.9% in lowest myeloperoxidase quartile vs 38.4% in highest quartile), even in patients whose baseline TnT level was less than 0.1 ng/mL.

The baseline myeloperoxidase level was a significant predictor of a MACE at 30 days (unadjusted odds ratio [OR], 4.7; highest vs lowest quartiles) and at 6 months (unadjusted OR, 4.7; highest vs lowest quartiles). The baseline myeloperoxidase level remained a significant predictor of 30-day and 6-month MACEs, even after data adjustment for age, sex, CRP level, hyperlipidemia, revascularization, MI, and acute coronary syndrome.

In particular, in patients whose TnT levels were persistently less than 0.1 ng/mL, an increasing baseline myeloperoxidase level was significantly associated with MACEs at 30 days (adjusted ORs, 2.2, 4.2, and 4.1, for the second, third, and fourth quartiles vs the first quartile) and at 6 months (adjusted ORs, 1.9, 4.4, and 3.9 for the second, third, and fourth quartiles vs the first quartile).

Conclusion.—The baseline plasma myeloperoxidase level is a significant and independent predictor of a MACE at 30 days and 6 months, even in patients with negative TnT levels.

▶ The search for cardiac markers or predictors of adverse outcomes in acute coronary syndrome continues. Brennan and colleagues report that a single initial measurement of plasma myeloperoxidase independently predicts an early risk of MI and a risk of major cardiac events within 30 to 60 days of presentation to an ED with chest pain. Although the data support myeloperoxidase as a more sensitive measure than the others, its receiver operating characteristic curves are nothing to write home about. It is neither sensitive nor specific, nor does it boast a good positive or negative prediction value. Clearly, more work needs to be done to determine how or whether myeloperoxidase can be combined with other markers to identify high-risk patients with chest pain in the ED.

By the way, why weren't any emergency physicians listed as investigators in this study of 604 sequential patients presenting to the ED with chest pain?

R. K. Cydulka, MD, MS

5 Abdominal Pain

Magnetic Resonance Cholangiopancreatography: A Meta-analysis of Test Performance in Suspected Biliary Disease
Romagnuolo J, Bardou M, Rahme E, et al (Univ of Calgary, Alta, Canada; McGill Univ, Montreal, Quebec, Canada)
Ann Intern Med 139:547-557, 2003   5–1

Background.—MR cholangiopancreatography (MRCP) is a noninvasive method for imaging the biliary tree. A meta-analysis was performed to evaluate MRCP retrospectively as a method for the diagnosis of biliary disease and obstruction.

Study Design.—A MEDLINE search was performed for articles published between January 1987 and March 2003 in English and French that allowed construction of 2 × 2 contingency tables of MRCP compared with a gold standard for presence, level, or cause of biliary obstruction. Two independent observers graded study quality. The overall sensitivity, specificity, and positive and negative predictive values were calculated. The results were summarized as a quantitative receiver-operating characteristic (ROC) curve (Fig 3).

Findings.—The meta-analysis included 67 studies with 4711 patients. MRCP had a 95% overall pooled sensitivity and 97% overall pooled specificity. It was less sensitive for stones (92%) and malignant conditions (88%) than for obstruction. Diagnostic performance was higher in larger studies,

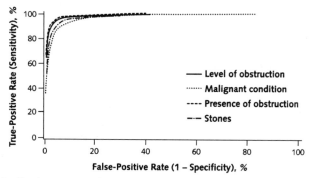

FIGURE 3.—Receiver-operating characteristic curves for magnetic resonance cholangiopancreatography targeted at each of 4 imaging end points. (Courtesy of Romagnuolo J, Bardou M, Rahme E, et al: Magnetic resonance cholangiopancreatography: A meta-analysis of test performance in suspected biliary disease *Ann Intern Med* 139:547-557, 2003.)

those lacking consecutive enrollment, and those that did not use a gold standard comparison of all patients.

Conclusions.—MRCP is an effective, noninvasive procedure for the diagnosis of biliary obstruction but is not as accurate at differentiating benign from malignant causes of obstruction. Its exact role in the diagnosis of biliary disease remains to be elucidated.

▶ As MRI becomes more effective in diagnosing entities previously requiring invasive procedures performed by specialty consultants, it is more likely that emergency physicians will be ordering it for their patients. We need to learn the benefits and limitations of this newly available modality. It appears that MRI is very useful for assessing obstruction and stones but somewhat less useful for finding malignancy.

Over time, I can see MRI as the test that follows abdominal US (done either at the bedside or in the US suite) when the US appears to be negative, or there are technical difficulties in patients with high pretest probability of disease.

W. P. Burdick, MD, MSEd

Value of Helical Computed Tomography in the Management of Upper Esophageal Foreign Bodies
De Lucas EM, Sádaba P, García-Barón PL, et al (Hosp Universitario Marqués de Valdecilla, Cantabria, Spain)
Acta Radiol 45:369-374, 2004   5–2

Background.—Because barium swallow studies can impede subsequent esophagoscopy, many patients with suspected esophageal foreign bodies (FBs) whose plain films are negative are sent directly for esophagoscopy. Yet even endoscopic esophagoscopy is an invasive procedure, and a noninvasive method for evaluating these patients is desirable. The utility of helical CT in the diagnosis of upper esophageal FBs was investigated.

Methods.—Thirty-six patients (10 men and 26 women; mean age, 70 years) with a history of fish or chicken bone impaction were studied. Results of oral examination and indirect laryngoscopy were negative in each case. All patients underwent a barium swallow study with 4 radiographs, and unenhanced helical CT of the neck. Patients with positive findings in either study underwent esophagoscopy, and all patients were monitored for 72 hours.

Results.—Both helical CT and barium swallow studies were normal in 20 patients, and all 20 had satisfactory clinical outcomes. Both CT and barium study results were positive for an FB in the cervical esophagus in 12 patients, and the FB was confirmed by esophagoscopy. Of the remaining 4 patients, CT detected an impacted fish bone in 1 patient and an esophageal perforation caused by a fish bone in a second patient. In both cases, barium study did not detect these anomalies, but they were confirmed at esophagoscopy. Of the remaining 2 patients, CT indicated FBs that were not found by barium study or esophagoscopy.

Conclusion.—Helical CT of the neck was 100% sensitive in diagnosing upper esophageal FBs in these patients. Helical CT is noninvasive, and results are quickly available. It is recommended that helical CT should be the first choice for evaluating suspected upper esophageal FBs that would not be expected to be visible on plain radiographs.

▶ Advances in helical CT will continue to change the way we practice medicine. This is a beautiful demonstration of the power of this imaging modality, as it clearly demonstrates the presence and location of a fish bone in the esophagus. In this study, the FB was visible on plain film. In other circumstances where there is an unconfirmed suspicion of a foreign body in the esophagus (or elsewhere), helical CT may spare the patient from undergoing endoscopy by ruling it out noninvasively.

W. P. Burdick, MD, MSEd

Decline in Admission Rates for Acute Appendicitis in England
Kang JY, Hoare J, Majeed A, et al (Univ College, London; Hammersmith Hosp, London)
Br J Surg 90:1586-1592, 2003   5–3

Background.—The use of laparoscopy, ultrasonography, and CT scanning has been described for the evaluation of acute abdominal pain in an attempt to reduce the number of negative appendectomies and the incidence of surgery, even if the incidence of acute appendicitis were to remain constant. Time trends in hospital admissions for acute appendicitis were determined in England between 1989 and 1990 and between 1999 and 2000, and in population mortality rates for appendicitis from 1979 to 1999.

Methods.—Hospital episode statistics for admission were obtained from England's Department of Health, and mortality data were obtained from the Office for National Statistics.

Results.—From 1989 to 1990 and 1999 to 2000, age-standardized hospital admission rates for acute appendicitis decreased by 12.5% in male patients and by 18.8% in female patients. The proportions of admissions that resulted in surgery remained stable. Admission rates for nonspecific mesenteric lymphadenitis declined, but admission rates for abdominal pain increased between 1989 and 1990 and between 1995 and 1996 (Fig 1), during which time the International Classification of Diseases codes changed. Admission rates for abdominal pain decreased between 1995 and 1996 and between 1999 and 2000. Analysis of age-specific admission rates for acute appendicitis and abdominal pain from 1989 to 1990 and from 1995 to 1996 showed the decline in acute appendicitis was not attributable to a change in diagnostic practice. The mortality rates for acute appendicitis were stable throughout the study period.

FIGURE 1

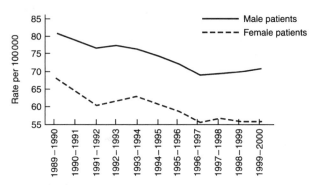

a Acute appendicitis

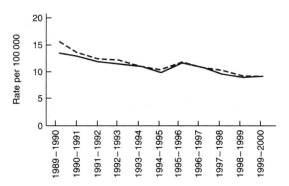

b Unspecified appendicitis

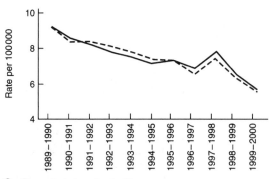

c Mesenteric lymphadenitis

(Continued)

FIGURE 1 (cont.)

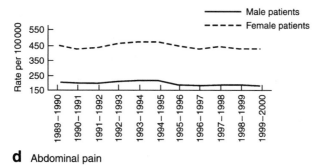

d Abdominal pain

FIGURE 1.—Age-standardized hospital admission rates by diagnosis. a, Acute appendicitis; b, unspecified appendicitis; c, mesenteric lymphadenitis; d, abdominal pain. (Courtesy of Kang JY, Hoare J, Majeed A, et al: Decline in admission rates for acute appendicitis in England. *Br J Surg* 90:1586-1592, 2003. Reprinted by permission of Blackwell Publishing.)

Conclusion.—There was a decline in admission rates for acute appendicitis in England during the study period that could not be explained by changes in the International Classification of Diseases.

▶ Why should the incidence of appendicitis vary over time and from one region or socioeconomic class to another? Apparently, the frequency of appendicitis increased at the end of the 19th century and beginning of the 20th century until it peaked in the 1930s and has been declining ever since. Various theories have been advanced to explain the change, including fiber ingestion, antibiotic use, and living standards, but none has held up and the trends remain a mystery. In the meantime, expect to see fewer cases of appendicitis over the coming years.

W. P. Burdick, MD, MSEd

Meta-analysis of the Clinical and Laboratory Diagnosis of Appendicitis
Andersson REB (County Hosp Ryhov, Jönköping, Sweden)
Br J Surg 91:28-37, 2004   5–4

Background.—Authorities disagree on the relevance of certain components of the clinical diagnosis of appendicitis. The diagnostic value of disease history, clinical findings, and laboratory test results in patients with suspected appendicitis was retrospectively investigated.

Methods.—A literature search of all published studies on the clinical and laboratory diagnosis of appendicitis in patients hospitalized with suspected disease yielded 24 studies. A total of 28 diagnostic variables were reported. Meta-analyses of receiver-operator characteristic (ROC) areas and positive and negative likelihood ratios were generated.

Findings.—The best discriminators of appendicitis were inflammatory response variables, including granulocyte count, proportion of polymorphonuclear blood cells, white blood cell count, and C-reactive protein con-

TABLE 5.—Discriminatory and Predictive Power of Combinations of Variables

| | Reference | ROC Area | Likelihood Ratio | | |
			All Variables Absent	At Least One Variable Present	All Variables Present
Guarding or rebound and WBC count $\geq 10.0 \times 10^9$/L	49	0.84 (0.80, 0.88)	0.14 (0.08, 0.24)	0.94 (0.72, 1.22)	11.34 (6.65, 19.56)
WBC > 10.0×10^9/L and CRP > 8 mg/L	57	0.96 (0.92, 1.00)	0.03 (0.00, 0.14)	0.53 (0.20, 1.37)	23.32 (6.87, 84.79)*
WBC > 10.0×10^9/L and CRP > 12 mg/L	32	0.85 (0.80, 0.90)	0.05 (0.01, 0.18)	1.07 (0.75, 1.47)	8.22 (4.73, 14.38)
WBC > 12.0×10^9/L and CRP > 6 mg/L	52	0.74 (0.66, 0.87)	0.06 (0.01, 0.33)	2.00 (1.45, 3.09)	—
WBC > 10.0×10^9/L CRP > 8 mg/L and IL-6 > 60 ng/L	57	0.87 (0.80, 0.94)	0.03 (0.01, 0.16)*	2.06 (1.35, 3.25)	16.96 (3.08, 98.66)
WBC > 9.0×10^9/L and proportion of PMN cells > 75%	55	0.66 (0.59, 0.73)	0.17 (0.07, 0.42)	1.54 (1.32, 1.79)	—
WBC > 10×10^9/L proportion of PMN cells > 70% and CRP > 12 mg/L	32	0.79 (0.74, 0.84)	0.03 (0.01, 0.16)	1.57 (1.28, 1.91)	20.85 (5.47, 80.27)
WBC > 9.0×10^9/L proportion of PMN cells > 75% and CRP > 6 mg/L	55	0.65 (0.58, 0.72)	0.05 (0.01, 0.28)*	1.44 (1.29, 1.63)	—
WBC > 9.0×10^9/L proportion of PMN cells > 75%, manual bands > 5% and CRP > 6 mg/L	55	0.65 (0.58, 0.72)	0.05 (0.01, 0.29)*	1.43 (1.28, 1.62)	—

Note: Values in parentheses are 95% confidence intervals.
*One case was added to an empty cell for the calculations, giving underestimated ROC area and likelihood ratios.
Abbreviations: ROC, Receiver-operating characteristic; WBC, white blood cell count; CRP, C-reactive protein; IL, interleukin; PMN, polymorphonuclear.
(Courtesy of Andersson REB: Meta-analysis of the clinical and laboratory diagnosis of appendicitis. Br J Surg 91:28-37, 2004. Reprinted by permission of Blackwell Publishing.)

centration; descriptors of peritoneal irritation, including rebound and percussion tenderness, guarding, and rigidity; and migration of pain. The ROC areas of these factors ranged from 0.78 to 0.68. Inflammatory variables had a particularly strong discriminatory power for perforated appendicitis, with ROC areas ranging from 0.85 to 0.87. When 2 or more inflammatory variables were increased, appendicitis was likely. When all inflammatory variables were normal, appendicitis was unlikely.

Conclusion.—Individually, all clinical and laboratory variables are weak indicators of appendicitis. However, in combination they have a high discriminatory power. (Table 5). The most important diagnostic information is obtained from laboratory assessment of the inflammatory response, clinical descriptors of peritoneal irritation, and a history of migration of pain.

▶ Andersson's meta-analysis flies in the face of the emergency medicine conventional wisdom and suggests that laboratory markers of inflammation are helpful in making the diagnosis of appendicitis. However, this is only true when they are combined with signs of peritoneal irritation and a history of pain migration. Busting another long-held belief, Andersson also notes that the rectal examination adds no discriminatory or predictive power when evaluating a patient with possible appendicitis. In spite of these findings, I suspect the following 2 statements are true. (1) In some EDs, it's probably faster and cheaper to get the CT scan than it is to wait for the results of multiple blood tests. (2) In many EDs, the surgeons won't operate until they see the scan. My advice is to evaluate the literature yourself and decide what will result in the most efficient and medically sound care in your setting.

R. K. Cydulka, MD, MS

The Ability of Traditional Vital Signs and Shock Index to Identify Ruptured Ectopic Pregnancy

Birkhahn RH, Gaeta TJ, Van Deusen SK, et al (New York Methodist Hosp, Brooklyn)
Am J Obstet Gynecol 189:1293-1296, 2003   5–5

Background.—Of women seeking ED care in the first trimester of pregnancy, 10% to 15% are found to have ectopic pregnancies (EP). A tool to quickly and accurately identify women with ruptured EP would help clinicians make better treatment decisions. A shock index (SI), which has proved useful for identifying hemorrhage in trauma patients, may be a more sensitive, specific indicator of ruptured EP than heart rate (HR) or systolic blood pressure (SBP). Correlations between vital signs and hemoperitoneum were determined.

Methods and Findings.—This retrospective case-control study included 52 patients. Initial HR, SBP, and HR plus SBP were correlated with respect to the quantity of hemoperitoneum. Predictive values were then determined. Twenty-five women studied had ruptured pregnancies, and 27 had unruptured EP. Correlation coefficients were 0.50 for HR, -0.34 for SBP, and 0.69 for HR plus SBP. The sensitivity for HR was 28%; for SBP, 36%; and for HR plus SBP, 72%. The specificities were 96%, 96%, and 67%, respectively. Abnormal SI better predicted rupture than HR or SPB alone. In addition, SI was more strongly associated with degree of hemoperitoneum.

Conclusions.—Normal vital signs alone poorly predict the presence or ruptured EP. HR plus SBP best correlates with the quantity of intraperitoneal hemorrhage. Prospective research is now needed to determine a value for SI with enhanced clinical use for detecting ruptured EP.

▶ The bottom line on this study is that the SI can serve as a triage tool for initiating resuscitation but little else. Clinical suspicion and early US are really the keys to rapid diagnosis and treatment of this potentially lethal condition.

R. K. Cydulka, MD, MS

Sonographic Comparison of the Tubal Ring of Ectopic Pregnancy With the Corpus Luteum

Stein MW, Ricci ZJ, Novak L, et al (Albert Einstein College of Medicine, Bronx, NY)

J Ultrasound Med 23:57-62, 2004   5–6

Background.—The tubal ring is well known as a sonographic sign of ectopic pregnancy. However, a dilemma arises in the case of a pregnant patient without a sonographically visible intrauterine pregnancy when a thick-walled adnexal cystic structure is present without clear depiction of a separate ovary. Is this finding indicative of an ectopic pregnancy or a corpus luteum within the ovary, splaying the normal ovarian tissue around it? The utility of various sonographic features were compared in differentiating between the tubal ring of ectopic pregnancy and the corpus luteum.

Methods.—A retrospective review of first-trimester transvaginal sonograms demonstrated a cystic adnexal structure in 79 women. Each of these structures was evaluated for 6 specific sonographic characteristics: echogenicity of its wall compared with that of the ovary and endometrium; wall thickness in 2 planes; color Doppler flow distribution and percentage of wall circumference; and internal texture.

Results.—Ectopic pregnancies were present in 41 of 79 (52%) women, and 38 women (48%) had corpora lutea. In the ectopic pregnancies, 11 of 35 (32%) ectopic walls were more echogenic than the endometrium, compared with none of the corpora lutea. A cyst wall less echogenic than the endometrium was more likely in corpora lutea (84% vs 31%). More than twice as many ectopic rinds were more echogenic than ovarian tissue compared with corpora lutea (76% vs 34%). The only predictive internal texture feature was a clear pattern, which was more common in the corpora lutea. No significant difference in mural flow distribution or extent was observed between the 2 groups.

Conclusion.—The relative echogenicity of the rind of an adnexal cystic mass compared with that of the endometrium and that of the ovarian parenchyma is valuable in distinguishing between an ectopic pregnancy and a corpus luteum. In addition, the presence of an anechoic cyst fluid is a useful feature to consider in clinically ambiguous cases because this finding favors the diagnosis of a corpus luteum. The pattern and degree of Doppler wall vascularity did not aid the differentiation of these entities.

▶ This article provides some insight into the potential difficulty of differentiating the tubal ring of an ectopic pregnancy from a corpus luteum cyst even by experienced radiologists, an important consideration as ectopic pregancies become more comfortable with bedside US and seek to rule in an ectopic pregnancy in the absence of an intrauterine pregnancy. There have been a number of methods proposed to differentiate corpus luteum cyst from tubal ring in the presence of a thick-walled adnexal cystic structure without a clearly seen ovary, but none have been shown to be completely reliable in excluding or definitively diagnosing ectopic pregnancies.

Of note, in addition to examining characteristics of tubal rings, the authors also note that complex free fluid was present in significantly more patients with ectopic pregnancies than corpus luteum cysts. Sickler et al have previously shown that the presence of echogenic free fluid is 100% sensitive and 95% specific in the detection hemoperitoneum in patients with suspected ectopic pregnancies.[1] Evaluation for the presence and nature of free fluid in the cul-de-sac should be routinely done by emergency physicians evaluating patients with suspected ectopic pregnancies.

S. L. Werner, MD

Reference

1. Sickler GK, Chen PC, Dubinsky TJ, et al: Free echogenic pelvic fluid: Correlation with hemoperitoneum. *J Ultrasound Med* 17:431-435, 1998.

Performance of a New, Rapid Assay for Detection of *Trichomonas vaginalis*
Kurth A, Whittington WLH, Golden MR, et al (Univ of Washington, Seattle; Univ of Alabama, Birmingham)
J Clin Microbiol 42:2940-2943, 2004   5–7

Background.—Current screening tests for *Trichomonas vaginalis* tend to have low sensitivity, to be expensive, or to require a long time before rendering results. A new point-of-care assay for rapidly detecting trichomoniasis was evaluated.

Methods.—Participants were 936 women attending sexually transmitted disease clinics in Seattle (n = 497) or Birmingham, Alabama (n = 439). After a vaginal swab was collected for wet preparation microscopy, 2 additional swabs were collected. One specimen was submitted for culture, while the other specimen was studied via the XenoStrip-Tv (Xenotope Diagnostics, Inc, San Antonio, Tex). The assay is designed as a point-of-care test, but assays were performed in a single laboratory to ensure uniform testing conditions. With the assay, specimens were mixed for 1 minute in a microfuge tube containing the sample buffer; then the specimen solution was expressed from the swab. The XenoStrip-Tv test strip was placed in the expressed specimen solution, and results were read at 10 minutes (and, for negative specimens, again at 20 minutes).

Results.—Culture results were positive in 8.7% of the Seattle cohort and in 21.0% of the Birmingham cohort. Compared with culture, the assay had a sensitivity of 76.7% in Seattle and 79.4% in Birmingham; corresponding specificity values were 99.8% and 97.1%. The assay had a positive predictive value of 97.1% in Seattle and 87.9% in Birmingham; corresponding negative predictive values were 97.8% and 94.7%. Performance of the rapid assay did not vary according to vaginal symptoms or other vaginal or cervical syndromes or infection. Assay sensitivity did, however, vary according to the time when cultures first became positive: for every additional 1-day delay until *T vaginalis* was first detected in culture, the sensitivity of the assay decreased by 71%. Compared with wet preparation results, the rapid assay was significantly more sensitive in detecting *T vaginalis* infection (78.5% vs 72.4%), but significantly less specific (98.6% vs 100%).

Conclusion.—The XenoStrip-Tv test is a simple-to-use, point-of-care assay for rapidly identifying *T vaginalis* infection in areas with a moderate to high prevalence of trichomoniasis.

▶ This one looks like a winner—a cheap quick test for a highly contagious sexually transmitted infection. Although its sensitivity is only around 77%, it is better that microscopic examination of a wet prep sample. Waiting for culture results is not practical since follow-up and return for treatment is never easy with ED patients. The authors do not mention the price, but the benefits are potentially substantial.

W. P. Burdick, MD, MSEd

The Significance of Measuring the Time Course of Serum Malondialdehyde Concentration in Patients With Torsion of the Testis
Kehinde EO, Mojiminiyi OA, Mahmoud AH, et al (Kuwait Univ)
J Urol 169:2177-2180, 2003   5–8

Background.—Testicular torsion is a urologic emergency that affects approximately 1 in 158 men before age 25 years. Ideally, the prompt release of testicular torsion should result in the restoration of testicular endocrine and exocrine function. However, despite restoration of endocrine and exocrine function in the affected testicle, spermatogenesis is often impaired in both the affected and contralateral side. The postulated mechanisms resulting in testicular malfunction after ipsilateral testicular torsion include sympathetic orchiopathy, autoimmune mechanism, and ischemia-reperfusion injury. There is an urgent need to identify methods for limiting the damage to a torsed testis and to decrease the testicular atrophy rate below the current level of approximately 40%. The time course of malondialdehyde, a measure of free radical damage, in patients undergoing standard surgical treatment for testicular torsion was determined.

Methods.—This prospective study included patients with testicular torsion. Blood samples were obtained after administration of general anesthesia but before surgical incision and at 10 minutes, 30 minutes, and 24 hours after detorsion. Orchiopexy was performed in patients with viable testes (group 1), and orchiectomy was performed in patients with nonviable testes (group 2). Similar blood samples were obtained from control patients, including patients younger than 40 years who were undergoing other surgical procedures involving manipulation of the testes. The level of malondialdehyde in each serum sample was determined by thiobarbituric acid reaction.

Results.—A total of 65 patients were included in the study, including 56 patients with testicular torsion and 9 control patients. Of the 56 patients with testicular torsion, 11 (19.6%) with testicular torsion underwent ipsilateral orchiectomy and contralateral orchiopexy. The remaining 45 patients (80.4%) underwent bilateral orchiopexy. However, serum malondialdehyde was estimated in only 34 of the 56 patients with torsion. The mean malondialdehyde levels at 0, 10, and 30 minutes, 24 hours, and at 3 and 6 months were 3.3, 3.69, 3.69, 2.9, 2.65, and 2.39 nmol/mL in the 24 patients in group 1; 3.53, 4.56, 3.87, 2.87, 2.82, and 2.64 nmol/mL in the 10 patients in group 2; and 3.6, 3.08, 3.18, 2.95, 2.88, and 2.65 nmol/mL in the control group, respectively. The highest level of serum malondialdehyde occurred at 10 minutes after detorsion in groups 1 and 2. A statistically significant difference in malondialdehyde was noted between groups 1 and 2 compared with the control group at 10 minutes. Serum malondialdehyde returned to baseline levels at 24 hours in all patients.

Conclusions.—Testicular torsion and its treatment with detorsion is an example of ischemia-reperfusion injury. This produces measurable changes in malondialdehyde in human beings. Serum malondialdehyde could be used to determine the extent of injury in patients with testicular torsion.

▶ There are several explanations of injury to the testes after torsion/detorsion (T/D). In T/D patients, testicular spermatogenesis is found to be an average of 36% of expected values, suggesting that the contralateral side is also harmed in the process. The proposed disease mechanisms include orchiopathy (that there was some underlying yet unrecognized disease state of the testes that was present prior to T/D); an autoimmune disorder (that some set of normally unexposed self-antigens are presented to the immune system, which leads to damage to both ipsilateral and contralateral testes); and an ischemia-reperfusion injury (dependent on release of free radicals that then cause damage to testicular tissue).

The authors chose to measure serum malondialdehyde levels as a marker of free radical levels associated with possible ischemia-reperfusion injury in testicular T/D. They had 3 patient groups to follow: (1) those with torsion without testicular necrosis, (2) those with torsion in whom the surgeons believed the testis was unviable (treated with orchiectomy), and (3) a group of control patients without torsion who were having procedures involving testicular manipulation (such as correcting hydrocele and orchiopexy).

The authors found that malondialdehyde levels increased 10 minutes after detorsion with even greater elevation after detorsion of nonviable testes. The authors suggest that these results are most consistent with ischemia/reperfusion injury. As the testis is detorsed, free radicals are released into the blood. However, there is an elevated level of malondialdehyde in all the patients after general anesthesia. What role does exposure to anesthesia have in measurable malondialdehyde? Does this mean that there is a time and duration of exposure to the free radicals that are important to defining injury conditions? More work is needed to prove that ischemia/reperfusion is responsible for ipsilateral and contralateral testicular injury.

If ischemia/reperfusion is clearly a factor in testicular injury, then not only do we have to make the diagnosis quickly, but we must provide treatments such as hyperbaric oxygen or antioxidants to limit the damage. Stay tuned.

N. B. Handly, MD, MSc, MS

Korean Hand Acupressure for Motion Sickness in Prehospital Trauma Care: A Prospective, Randomized, Double-blinded Trial in a Geriatric Population

Bertalanffy P, Hoerauf K, Fleischhackl R, et al (Univ Hosp of Vienna; Vienna Red Cross)
Anesth Analg 98:220-223, 2004   5–9

Background.—Motion sickness can increase the discomfort experienced by patients being transported by ambulance. The Korean hand acupressure point K-K9 can produce an antiemetic effect. A prospective, randomized, double-blind study was conducted to investigate the utility of Korean acupressure in reducing motion sickness for older patients during ambulance rides.

Study Design.—The study group consisted of 100 patients at least 60 years of age with a history of motion sickness or postoperative nausea and vomiting and an estimated ambulance ride of more than 20 minutes. Baseline demographic and hemodynamic variables were assessed. Patients were queried about nausea and other symptoms not directly related to nausea. Skin sensors were placed to determine vasodilation status. Patients were then randomly assigned to either K-K9 stimulation or sham stimulation (Fig 1). The patient was then transported by ambulance. At the hospital, all variables were reanalyzed. The patient's overall satisfaction with care was also evaluated.

Findings.—At hospital arrival, nausea scores were significantly lower in the Korean acupressure group than in the sham acupressure group. Significantly more patients were vasodilated in the sham acupressure group. Heart rate was significantly higher in the sham group. Overall patient satisfaction was significantly higher in the Korean acupressure group. Neither group had a significant blood pressure change.

Conclusion.—Korean hand acupressure at the K-K9 point was associated with reduced motion sickness and sympathetic activity and increased patient

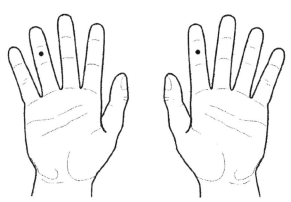

FIGURE 1.—The K-K9 point (**left**) and the sham point (**right**). (Courtesy of Bertalanffy P, Hoerauf K, Fleischhackl R, et al: Korean hand acupressure for motion sickness in prehospital trauma care: A prospective, randomized, double-blinded trial in a geriatric population. *Anesth Analg* 98:220-223, 2004.)

satisfaction. This technique is both easy and inexpensive and could enhance the quality of care for patients during ambulance transport.

▶ Motion sickness is a common problem among both patients and providers in the prehospital environment. Many of the commonly used medications available to treat or prevent the symptoms associated with motion sickness have undesirable side effects, including somnolence and dystonic reactions. This prospective, randomized, double-blinded study provides solid evidence of the efficacy of a simple, nonpharmaceutical alternative medicine approach to treating motion sickness. The K-K9 acupressure point has previously been shown useful in postoperative nausea, but this is the first study of a nonpharmaceutical approach to motion sickness.

While the study was limited to patients over 65 with minor trauma, the technique may be useful in a broader range of patients, and even for prehospital providers susceptible to motion sickness. (I think I will try it on my next rough aeromedical transport.) As some forms of alternative or complementary medicine gain acceptance in the medical community, this study should lead us to consider their evaluation and potential use in the prehospital environment as well.

S. L. Werner, MD

6 Acute Neuropsychiatric Problems

A Prospective, Double-blind, Randomized Trial of Midazolam Versus Haloperidol Versus Lorazepam in the Chemical Restraint of Violent and Severely Agitated Patients
Nobay F, Simon BC, Levitt MA, et al (Univ of California, San Francisco; Alameda County Med Ctr, Highland Campus, Oakland, Calif)
Acad Emerg Med 11:744-749, 2004   6–1

Background.—Violent and severely agitated patients are a common and serious problem in most major EDs. Physical restraints are often necessary for these patients, and some may require augmentation of their restraints by chemical sedation. The safety, efficacy, and expediency of chemical restraints have been documented in several studies, and butyrophenones (haloperidol and droperidol) have emerged as leaders in the area of chemical restraint. In recent years, benzodiazepines, such as lorazepam, have been added to the list of safe and effective options for chemical restraint. Whether midazolam is superior to lorazepam or haloperidol in the management of violent or severely agitated patients in the ED was determined. Superiority would be indicated by a significantly shorter time to sedation and a shorter time to arousal.

Methods.—This randomized, prospective, double-blind study was performed in an urban county teaching ED among a convenience sample of 111 violent and severely agitated patients. The patients were randomly assigned to receive IM midazolam (5 mg), lorazepam (2 mg), or haloperidol (5 mg). The mean ($\pm$SD) age of the patients was 40.7 ($\pm$13) years.

Results.—The mean ($\pm$SD) time to sedation was 18.3 ($\pm$14) minutes for patients receiving midazolam, 28.3 ($\pm$25) minutes for patients receiving haloperidol, and 32.2 ($\pm$20) minutes for those receiving lorazepam. The mean time to arousal was 81.9 minutes for midazolam, 126.5 minutes for haloperidol, and 217.2 minutes for lorazepam. There were no significant differences among the 3 drugs in terms of changes in systolic and diastolic blood pressure, heart rate, respiratory rate, and oxygen saturation.

Conclusions.—Midazolam has a significantly shorter time to onset of sedation and a more rapid time to arousal than lorazepam or haloperidol. However, the efficacy of the 3 drugs was similar.

▶ The striking finding in the results is the wide range of pharmacokinetics of identical drug and drug dose manifested by the patients in this study. Although the mean onset for haloperidol was 28.3 minutes, the range was 3.3 to 53.3 minutes. The range for midazolam was 4.3 to 32.3 minutes. The take-home message for me is this: if you can possibly get an IV catheter into the patient and deliver the medication IV, do it that way and achieve a much faster, more predictable onset.

I agree with the authors that the shorter duration of action makes midazolam preferable for an agitated patient. It is also nice to avoid the potential complication of a dystonic reaction occasionally seen with haloperidol. In patients who are frankly psychotic and would benefit from an antipsychotic medication, however, haloperidol would remain my choice.

W. P. Burdick, MD, MSEd

Xanthochromia Is Not Pathognomonic for Subarachnoid Hemorrhage
Graves P, Sidman R (Rhode Island Hosp, Providence)
Acad Emerg Med 11:131-135, 2004   6–2

Introduction.—Most patients with subarachnoid hemorrhage (SAH) can be diagnosed with CT, but a lumbar puncture (LP) is required to exclude SAH. The presence of CSF xanthochromia within several hours of symptom onset suggests SAH and is considered to distinguish SAH from a traumatic spinal tap. An in vitro observational study examined the hypothesis that xanthochromia, the yellow discoloration of CSF caused by hemoglobin catabolism, may be seen as well in traumatic LP.

Methods.—A model of traumatic LP was developed by adding whole blood to pigment-free CSF to obtain red blood cell (RBC) concentrations of 0, 5000, 10,000, 20,000, 30,000, and 40,000 RBC/μL. Samples were centrifuged and the supernatant analyzed by spectrophotometry, measuring absorbance from 400 to 700 nm immediately and at hourly intervals after the initial mixing of RBC and CSF. Xanthochromia was considered present on the basis of values obtained in previous studies. Before this study, additional experiments were conducted to ensure that its methods did not cause xanthochromia.

Results.—Xanthochromia was detected immediately in samples with at least 30,000 RBC/μL, at 1 hour in samples with 20,000 RBC/μL, and within 2 hours in samples with 10,000 RBC/μL or less. Four hours elapsed before all samples containing 5000 RBC/μL became positive. No spectrophotometric evidence of xanthochromia was noted in CSF controls (Fig 1).

Conclusion.—In this model, CSF xanthochromia could be seen within 2 hours after traumatic LP and even sooner in samples with greater than 10,000 RBC/μL. Clinicians should be aware that xanthochromia unrelated

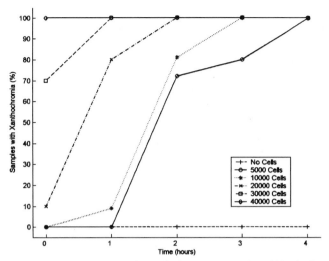

FIGURE 1.—Percent of samples positive for xanthochromia over time by red blood cell concentration. (Courtesy of Graves P, Sidman R: Xanthochromia is not pathognomonic for subarachnoid hemorrhage. *Acad Emerg Med* 11:131-135, 2004.)

to SAH may be detected in traumatic LPs with a high RBC count. When the time between sample acquisition and analysis is delayed or the CSF RBC count is elevated above 10,000 RBC/µL, xanthochromia should not be relied on to confirm a diagnosis of SAH.

▶ "If there is xanthochromia present, it must be a subarachanoid hemorrhage" is a bromide that has existed for a long time. Never say never in medicine, and the authors show us why. Even samples with 5000 cells showed a significant level of xanthochromia at 2 hours. I know your lab never tests samples that long after they have been obtained, but it sometimes happens around my shop, and it is quite useful to be aware of these data.

W. P. Burdick, MD, MSEd

▶ Graves and Sidman use a clever model to demonstrate that CSF xanthochromia may be noted very quickly in traumatic LPs containing 10,000 RBC/µL or more. Although they would like us to use these data to prevent unnecessary testing and admission for CT-negative patients in whom a subarachnoid hemorrhage is being considered, I'm not sure many emergency physicians will have the nerve to discharge a patient with a severe headache/suspected subarachnoid hemorrhage and xanthochromic spinal fluid even if the tap was traumatic! The consequences for a mistake on this one are too great.

R. K. Cydulka, MD, MS

The Relationship of Intraocular Pressure to Intracranial Pressure

Lashutka MK, Chandra A, Murray HN, et al (Ohio State Univ, Columbus)

Ann Emerg Med 43:585-591, 2004   6–3

Background.—Increased intracranial pressure (ICP) presents a difficult management challenge in the critical care and ED setting. In these patients, brain herniation and death can be prevented by early detection of intracranial hypertension and resulting timely medical and neurosurgical intervention. However, the detection of increased ICP in the ED can be problematic. A noninvasive method for detection of increased ICP in the ED would facilitate early medical intervention and possibly improve outcomes. The hypothesis that an increase in ICP could be detectable by an increase in intraocular pressure using noninvasive existing technology, such as a handheld tonometer, was tested.

Methods.—This prospective observational pilot study was conducted at a community hospital among patients with an invasive ICP monitor. The study included 27 patients, and 76 individual measurements were performed. Patients were excluded if they had known glaucoma or had sufficient ocular or facial trauma that precluded determination of intraocular pressure. Simultaneous measurements of intracranial or intraocular pressure were recorded.

Results.—All of the patients with an abnormal ICP had an abnormal intraocular pressure, and all patients with a normal ICP had a normal intraocular pressure.

Conclusion.—Abnormal intraocular pressure, as measured with the handheld tonometer, was found to be an excellent indicator of abnormal ICP in patients with known intracranial disease.

▶ This pilot study on a convenience sample of patients at high risk for elevated ICP may offer the possibility of a noninvasive assessment of the presence of elevated ICP. While the authors reference evidence for reliability of the measurements from their handheld tonometer, it would have been useful for them to report these data for the present study. My experience with these devices is that they tend to be very unreliable, undermining their utility for predicting elevated ICP. Assuming a reliable device is in use, I can imagine using this type when information to decide whether to institute ICP-lowering interventions in the ED in those marginal cases that are not suitable for surgical intervention is available and where a direct ICP monitor is anticipated but is not yet in place.

W. P. Burdick, MD, MSEd

Neuroprotective Effects of (S)-*N*-[4-[4-[(3,4-Dihydro-6-hydroxy-2,5,7,8-tetramethyl-2*H*-1-benzopyran-2-yl)carbonyl]-1-piperazinyl]phenyl]-2-thiophenecarboximid-amide (BN 80933), an Inhibitor of Neuronal Nitric-Oxide Synthase and an Antioxidant, in Model of Transient Focal Cerebral Ischemia in Mice
Ding-Zhou L, Marchand-Verrecchia C, Palmier B, et al (Université René Descartes, Paris; Institut Henri Beaufour, Les Ulis, France)
J Pharmacol Exp Ther 306:588-594, 2003   6–4

Background.—Both nitric oxide and reactive oxygen species have been implicated in neuronal death due to cerebral ischemia in experimental studies in mice. These species can act independently or in concert by forming the highly reactive oxidant peroxynitrite. Nitric oxide synthase inhibitors and scavengers of reactive oxygen species have therefore been proposed as strategies for neuroprotection in stroke.

Results of a previous study showed that a combined treatment associating an nitric oxide synthase inhibitor and an antioxidant/superoxide anion scavenger provides a synergistic neuroprotective effect in transient focal ischemia in rats. This finding resulted in the development of a new therapeutic concept that combines activities inhibiting neuronal nitric oxide synthase and lipid peroxidation in one molecule.

BN80933 is a representative of this novel class of agent that was shown to significantly reduce infarct volume and to improve neurologic signs in transient focal ischemia in rats. The purpose of this study was to confirm these findings in mice and to further study the effects of BN 80933 on inflammatory response, including blood-brain barrier disruption, brain edema, and neutrophil infiltration after transient middle cerebral artery occlusion (MCAO).

Methods.—BN 80933 was dissolved in 5% glucose and injected into the tail vein (10 mL/kg) of mice in whom focal cerebral ischemia was induced by MCAO.

Results.—IV administration of BN 80933 at 3 and 10 mg/kg 3 hours after transient MCAO resulted in significant reduction (26% to 36%) of the infarct volume evaluated at 24 and 48 hours after the ischemia. The neurologic score was also improved. In addition, BN 80933 at both dosages provided a 42% to 75% reduction in the extravasation of Evans blue in brain parenchyma observed 24 hours after ischemia. This reduction in blood-brain barrier disruption was associated with decreased brain edema as demonstrated by a 37% reduction in brain water content induced by BN 80933 at 3 mg/kg 24 hours after MCAO. Neutrophil infiltration in brain parenchyma, which was evaluated by the myeloperoxidase activity, was also reduced by 45% to 56% in animals treated with BN 80933 at 3 and 10 mg/kg.

Conclusion.—These findings provided evidence of the protective capacity of a novel compound, BN 80933, against brain ischemic injury and confirmation that BN 80933 is a promising new agent for the treatment of stroke.

▶ BN 80933—not a catchy name for new stroke treatment drug but a heck of a lot easier than its chemical name. Inhibiting nitric oxide production as well as inhibiting reactive oxygen molecules seems to dramatically reduce infarct size and improve neurologic function in this mouse model. If reductions in the range of 30% for infarct size are confirmed in other studies, "BN 80933, stat" may come rolling off our tongues in the near future.

W. P. Burdick, MD, MSEd

Intraarterial Thrombolytic Therapy Within 3 Hours of the Onset of Stroke
Bourekas EC, Slivka AP, Shah R, et al (Ohio State Univ, Columbus)
Neurosurgery 54:39-46, 2004   6–5

Background.—It has been shown by the National Institute of Neurological Disorders and Stroke (NINDS) Recombinant Tissue Plasminogen Activator Stroke Study Group that IV administration of recombinant tissue plasminogen activator (rt-PA) given within 3 hours of onset of ischemic stroke can improve the clinical outcome. Intraarterial (IA) thrombolysis has been shown to offer advantages to IV thrombolysis, but no previous reports have been published of experience with IA therapy within 3 hours of the onset of symptoms. The first retrospective analysis of a 2-institution experience with IA thrombolysis given within 3 hours of stroke onset was described.

Methods.—The study group included 36 patients with angiographically demonstrated occlusions who were treated with urokinase or rt-PA within 3 hours of the onset of stroke. Outcome measures included the percentage of patients with no or minimal neurologic disability at 30 to 90 days as measured by the modified Rankin Scale, percentage recanalization, incidence of symptomatic intracranial hemorrhage, and mortality rate. The results were compared with those of the NINDS rt-PA study.

Results.—The median admission National Institutes of Health Stroke Scale score was 14. Fifty percent of the treated patients had a modified Rankin Scale score of 0 or 1, which was indicative of little or no disability at 1 to 3 months, compared with 39% of treated patients in the NINDS trial. The incidence of recanalization was 75%. The incidence of symptomatic intracranial hemorrhage was 11%, compared with 6.4% with IV rt-PA in the NINDS trial, and the mortality rate was 22%, compared with 17% with IV rt-PA in the NINDS trial.

Conclusions.—IA thrombolysis administered within 3 hours of stroke onset is a feasible and viable alternative to IV rt-PA on the basis of improved clinical outcomes, high percentage of recanalization, and comparable mortality rate, despite the increased incidence of symptomatic intracranial hemorrhage observed in this study. It remains to be determined whether IA thrombolysis is superior to IV therapy.

▶ For decades, we have watched stroke patients through the course of their illness, hoping that they recover. Thrombolytic therapy has offered hope of treatment but at the cost of making matters worse by precipitating an intracerebral hemorrhage. This risk is made even more serious by the fact that some of the patients treated with lytic therapy may not actually have an IA thrombus causing the neurologic deficit. As the authors point out, IA lytic therapy is appealing because it allows confirmation of the diagnosis, focused treatment, and direct evidence for success. In fact, when the catheter is in place, it may be better to perform angioplasty, as the studies have shown for myocardial infarction.

Unfortunately, as with cardiac catheterization, this procedure requires an on-call team that can immediately respond to the need for neurovascular catheterization. If that can be accomplished within the narrow window that ischemic brain tissue needs to stay alive, then we may be closer to the dream of effective stroke therapy.

W. P. Burdick, MD, MSEd

Telemedicine in Emergency Evaluation of Acute Stroke: Interrater Agreement in Remote Video Examination With a Novel Multimedia System
Handschu R, Littmann R, Reulbach U, et al (Friedrich Alexander Universitaet, Erlangen-Nuremberg, Germany)
Stroke 34:2842-2846, 2003   6–6

Background.—A number of therapeutic strategies have been shown to be effective in the treatment of acute stroke, leading to shortened time windows for intervention. The systemic administration of recombinant tissue plasminogen activator (tPA) has been shown to cause a significant reduction in mortality rate compared with placebo when administered within 180 minutes after the onset of symptoms. However, tPA may also cause severe intracerebral hemorrhage, and in daily practice crucial factors influence the risk-to-benefit ratio and may increase mortality rate. Rapid, careful evaluation of patients is mandatory in acute stroke care, but this requires an experienced stroke neurologist. The development of telemedicine technology may provide new opportunities to bring this expertise quickly to more patients. Whether remote video examination is feasible and reliable when used for emergency stroke care using the National Institutes of Health Stroke Scale (NIHSS) was tested.

Methods.—A novel multimedia telesupport system for transfer of real-time video sequences and audio data was used. The remote examiner was able to direct the set-top camera and zoom from distant overview to close-ups with the personal computer in his or her office. Acute stroke patients admitted to the study facility's stroke unit were examined on admission in the ED. Standardized examinations were performed by using the NIHSS (German version) by telemedicine and compared with bedside application.

Results.—A total of 41 patients were examined. The average total examination time was 11.4 minutes, with a range of 8 to 18 minutes. None of the examinations had to be stopped or interrupted for technical reasons, although in 2 sessions the examination process was affected by minor problems with brightness and audio quality.

Conclusions.—The results of this study support the feasibility and reliability of remote examination of acute stroke patients in the ED. Some minor problems, such as brightness, optimal camera position, and audio quality, need to be solved for more widespread application of this technology.

▶ There is pressure to create special stroke centers because some of the skills needed to use tools (eg, tPA, interventional radiologic techniques) require a level of practice that comes from frequent experience.

Telemedicine may be a way to provide the experience of specially trained physicians to hospitals at some distance and reduce the pressure to create these special skills centers. This study reports the experience with telemedicine to perform a neurologic exam in the acute stroke setting. The authors compared 2 expert physicians performing the NIHSS exams: 1 in the presence of the patient (P) and the other "connected" to the patient by multimedia equipment and the internet (C).

The κ coefficient, a measure of agreement of the 2 physicians, indicated that there was good agreement between physicians P and C. However, how well physician C can replace physician P requires more than measures of agreement. It is important to show that there are no systemic biases (such as observing consistently less or greater NIHSS scores that might lead to inappropriate decisions to use tPA).

There are some parts of the exam that require the intervention of physician P, so at the moment it is necessary to have someone able to understand the examination well enough to be the hands of the remote physician C for parts of the neurologic exam. Whether tools will be available to perform procedures remotely in the future is unclear. That will require real-time connections between the expert and patient sites.

Stay tuned.

N. B. Handly, MD, MSc, MS

Magnetic Resonance Imaging as a Diagnostic Adjunct to Wernicke Encephalopathy in the ED

Chung SP, Kim SW, Yoo IS, et al (Chungnam Natl Univ, Daejeon, South Korea; Gachon Med School, Incheon, South Korea)

Am J Emerg Med 21:497-502, 2003   6–7

Background.—Wernicke's encephalopathy (WE) is an uncommon neurologic emergency that is a result of thiamine deficiency. The prevalence of WE has been reported to range from 0.8% to 2.8%; however, the true prevalence is believed to be higher because only 20% of WE patients are clinically diagnosed before autopsy. The utility of MRI for the evaluation of patients with suspected WE was illustrated.

Case 1.—Man, 39, was brought to the ED with a 3-day history of confused mental state. He had undergone low anterior resection for rectal cancer 14 months earlier, followed by several admissions for chemotherapy and management of intestinal obstruction. His body weight had declined by approximately 20 kg because of poor oral intake. He was alert and cooperative but disoriented on examination. Eye movement was limited and not conjugated. Cerebellar movement was ataxic. After normal findings on CT, MRI was performed. Findings on MRI included hyperintense areas in the bilateral medial thalami and the periaqueductal region of the midbrain.

Case 2.—Woman, 46, was transferred to the ED for mental status change. She had ingested more than 50 tablets of Dapsone 5 days earlier and was admitted to another facility for gastric lavage and methylene blue therapy. Her blood pressure was 110/70 mm Hg on examination at the ED, and her heart rate was 103 beats/min. The patient was drowsy and disoriented, and cyanosis was observed on her whole body. The initial met-hemoglobin (MetHb) level was 47%. The MetHb level decreased after methylene blue administration, but mental confusion and ataxia were present. MRI showed a hyperintense lesion around the third ventricle, the mammillary bodies, and the periaqueductal area.

Case 3.—Man, 50, with a history of chronic alcoholism was brought to the ED with mental status change of 1 day's duration. He had eaten almost nothing for 1 week because of malaise. His blood pressure was 210/120 mm Hg, and his heart rate was 108 beats/min. The patient was drowsy and uncooperative. His pupils were isochoric, with prompt light reflex and without any limitation of the eye movement. Tremors were noted in both hands. CT findings were nonspecific. Diffusion-weighted MRI was performed and showed high signal intensity in the bilateral medial thalami and posterior tip of the putamen.

Case 4.—Woman, 71, with an unremarkable medical history was brought to the ED with mental deterioration for a duration of 30 minutes. Her vision had been blurred all day, and she had not been able to read letters for 8 hours before her presentation. The woman first visited a private hospital, where her mental status decreased while she awaited examination. On examination at the study ED, her blood pressure was 90/60 mm Hg and her heart rate was 100 beats/min. The patient was drowsy and dysarthric but oriented, and her eye movement was not limited. She had no visual field defect and her motor and sensory functions were normal. Cerebellar function was ataxic. Diffusion-weighted imaging showed high signal intensity in the bilateral thalami. The patient was admitted to the neurology department with a diagnosis of bilateral lacunar infarction of thalami.

Conclusions.—The diagnosis of WE has been based for the most part on history and clinical symptoms. These case studies support the usefulness of MRI as a diagnostic adjunct in patients with suspected WE.

▶ WE (a triad of oculomotor dysfunction, ataxia, and confabulation) is caused by a thiamine deficiency that results from poor intake, poor absorption, or body weight loss. We often think of the chronic alcoholic at risk for WE. The authors call our attention to the problem of diagnosing WE and how MR may be useful. They note that WE is predominantly diagnosed clinically or at autopsy. Our clinical evaluation may be limited in the ED among patients with other medical illnesses, with decreased level of consciousness, or if our suspicions are low and thus we could use some help.

In their presentation of 4 cases, the authors suggest that MRI may be helpful in diagnosing WE. It is notable that no gold standard for WE was identified for the purposes of this study, although MR changes noted in 3 of the patients were typical of WE. There was no report of improvement in condition with thiamine administration for these 3 patients, which is central to the diagnosis of WE.

While it is great to be reminded of the pathophysiology of WE, I doubt very much that they have proved that MRI is going to play a role in ED diagnosis of WE based on this study. The sensitivity and specificity cited for the study is about 50%; we might as well flip a coin to make the diagnosis—it is cheaper than the MRI! Then again, thiamine is cheap and easy to give to our patients without the coin flip.

The case of the patient who overdosed on Dapsone is interesting. While we do not know if she had WE, the authors call attention to the possibility that the Dapsone ingestion or methylene blue treatment may be the cause of a WE-like syndrome.

N. B. Handly, MD, MSc, MS

Migraine Preventive Medication Reduces Resource Utilization
Siberstein SD, Winner PK, Chmiel JJ (Thomas Jefferson College of Medicine, Philadelphia; Abbott Labs, Abbott Park, Ill)
Headache 43:171-178, 2003   6–8

Background.—It has been estimated that approximately 18 million women and 5.6 million men have severe migraine; of these, an estimated 8.7 million women and 2.6 million men are moderately or severely disabled as a result of their migraines. However, it is estimated that only 48% of patients with migraines are identified and that only 41% of those identified are treated with prescription medication. Consensus guidelines from the US Headache Consortium and the American Academy of Neurology have recommended migraine preventive medication for patients with severe symptoms and those for whom the condition significantly interferes with their daily routine or in whom acute therapy is contraindicated or ineffective. However, the effects of preventive migraine therapy on the use of medical and pharmaceutical resources has not been extensively studied. Whether long-term resource utilization is reduced by the addition of a preventive medication to a migraine management regimen that already includes acute medication was investigated.

Methods.—A retrospective analysis was conducted of resource utilization data in a large claims database to evaluate the effect of new evidence-based guidelines for the treatment of migraine on medical and pharmaceutical resources.

Results.—The addition of a preventive medication to a migraine management regimen resulted in a reduction in the use of other migraine medications. The number of visits to physician offices and emergency departments was also reduced. Finally, the use of both acute and preventive medications was associated with lower utilization of CT and MRI scans.

Conclusion.—These findings support the effectiveness of migraine preventive drug therapy in reducing consumption of resources when migraine-preventive medications are added to a regimen that comprises only an acute medication.

▶ By using a retrospective analysis of a claims database, the authors compare resource utilization for migraine sufferers based on their use of preventive medications. (Preventive medications with "high" efficacy include amitriptyline, divalproex sodium, propranolol, and timolol.) The medication used for acute management was sumatriptan.

Resource utilization included the amount of acute medication prescribed, cost of this medication, primary physician and emergency department (ED) visits, and cranial imaging (CT and MRI) studies. By using historic controls in the periods before preventive medication and after beginning use of preventive medication, the prescriptions and cost of sumatriptan decreased. The prescription of sumatriptan was a proxy for sumatriptan use because no direct measure of use was available in the claims database.

The problem with the study is that there is no way to remove the effect of the intervention of the doctor who prescribes preventive medication to control resource use. There is likely to be an improved patient-physician relationship when the physician is managing the headache in a preventive mode. Fewer ED visits and imaging studies may reflect better contact with the physician caring for the headaches and a patient's better understanding of the disease (including better recognition of triggers and symptoms to decrease the need for acute medication and ED intervention).

Because emergency physicians often do not have good historic information about the patient who arrives in the ED, there may be no way to reduce the number of CT studies among those who have come to us. Note that for the patients in this study there was clearly a decrease in CT imaging studies regardless of the use of preventive medications. MRI occurred at greater frequency in study patients given preventive medications—again this may reflect a bias of the physicians using preventive medications to use MR or CT more frequently at the beginning of the workup of patients being prescribed preventive medications.

It is not clear whether we in the ED should be prescribing preventive medications. We should be aware that preventive medications are a part of migraine management. Directing our headache patients to primary care physicians or neurologists who manage migraines could well reduce ED visits by these patients. The authors acknowledge that if regional practice patterns vary, these results may not be applicable outside of the Midwest, where 75% of the patients in this claims database reside. In our hospital, MCP in Philadelphia, sumatriptan use is not common (anecdotally) and not part of our routine acute therapeutics bag of tricks (which typically includes narcotics, nonsteroidal anti-inflammatories, and antiemetics).

N. B. Handly, MD, MSc, MS

Cost-Effectiveness of Oral Phenytoin, Intravenous Phenytoin, and Intravenous Fosphenytoin in the Emergency Department
Rudis MI, Touchette DR, Swadron SP, et al (Univ of Southern California, Los Angeles; Oregon State Univ, Portland)
Ann Emerg Med 43:386-397, 2004   6–9

Introduction.—Patients who come to the ED with seizures often receive an oral or IV loading dose of phenytoin. The cost-effectiveness of 3 methods of loading phenytoin in the ED was examined in terms of cost per adverse event and cost per hour of ED time saved.

Methods.—Data were obtained from a prospective, randomized clinical trial that compared oral phenytoin, IV phenytoin, and IV fosphenytoin in 45 patients admitted to the ED after seizure. Eligible patients had been receiving maintenance phenytoin for an existing seizure disorder and had a serum phenytoin concentration of less than 5 µg/mL at admission. Patients were observed for 24 hours after the study medication was administered. Oral phenytoin was given in increments of 400 mg every 2 hours until a dose of 20 mg/kg was reached. Dosing for the IV routes was 18 mg/kg for phenytoin and 18 mg/kg phenytoin equivalent for fosphenytoin. The calculated costs included the cost of drugs, supplies, and personnel.

Results.—When labor costs were not included, oral phenytoin cost $2.83 per patient, IV phenytoin cost $23.48 per patient, and IV fosphenytoin cost $176.79 per patient. When the costs of labor and adverse events management were included, per patient costs of the 3 options were, respectively, $40.06, $84.31, and $238.67.

The mean numbers of adverse events per patient were 1.06 for oral phenytoin, 1.93 for IV phenytoin, and 2.13 for IV fosphenytoin. The mean times to safe ED discharge were, respectively, 6.4 hours, 1.6 hours, and 1.3 hours. Thus, oral phenytoin was most effective in terms of lowest cost and number of adverse events. But with an additional $20.65 in cost of the drug, IV phenytoin resulted in a much faster discharge with only a small increase in adverse events. The far greater cost of IV fosphenytoin offered no important advantage over IV phenytoin in terms of fewer adverse events or faster discharge.

Conclusion.—Oral phenytoin is the least costly method for loading phenytoin in the ED. Faster discharge can be achieved with IV phenytoin, but the cost of IV fosphenytoin does not appear to be justified in any setting.

▶ I have lots of issues with this article, but I'll limit myself to two. Let's start with the simpler one. I disagree with Rudis' cost analysis of keeping a patient in the ED 6.4 hours versus less than 2 hours. During the 4-plus hours that Rudis and colleagues propose that a patient occupy a bed and monitor getting loaded with oral dilantin, I can use the bed for 2 additional fairly sick patients. That means 2 fewer angry, anxious patients in the waiting room, 2 fewer embarrassed patients in hallway beds, and 3 additional satisfied patients (including my patient with seizures who leaves after 1.7 hours instead of 6.4 hours).

My second issue is that I'm not sure which patients Rudis and colleagues are trying to address in this study. If it's patients who are still actively seizing in the ED, an IV benzodiazepine is the treatment of choice. If it's a patient with a known seizure disorder and a subtherapeutic phenytoin level who had a seizure before arrival in the ED, suspect that by reloading the patient we are simply preventing more seizures for today but doing nothing to address the underlying reason that the phenytoin level is low to begin with, ie, noncompliance versus drug interaction versus absorption issues. Unfortunately, that seems to be the nature of the beast with many "acute exacerbations" of chronic diseases that we treat.

Although as an epidemiologist it pains me to discuss anecdotal experience, I feel I must. My experience with oral phenytoin loading has been abysmal. Patients either have another seizure during the loading process or—worse yet—have another seizure while in the waiting area. Call me old-fashioned or just plain cautious, but for alert patients who complain of a breakthrough seizure before arrival in the ED, have a subtherapeutic phenytoin level, and no one precipitating etiology, I'm going to stick with good old IV phenytoin and then address the real issue: Why is the level low and how can we work together to fix it on a daily basis?

R. K. Cydulka, MD, MS

7 Infections and Immunologic Disorders

Bacteremic Elder Emergency Department Patients: Procalcitonin and White Count
Caterino JM, Scheatzle MD, Forbes ML, et al (Allegheny Gen Hosp, Pittsburgh, Pa)
Acad Emerg Med 11:393-396, 2004   7–1

Background.—It is quite common for elderly patients to be seen in the ED without common signs and symptoms of bacterial infection. As a result, emergency physicians correctly predict bacteremia in less than two thirds of elderly patients, and this diagnosis requires the results of blood cultures that are not available for 24 to 48 hours. Medical decision making for these patients could be greatly improved by the development of an accurate, readily available test for bacteremia. Serum procalcitonin (PCT) and white blood cell (WBC) count for the detection of bacteremia in elderly patients was assessed.

Methods.—This prospective observational study was conducted among ED patients aged 65 years and older in whom blood cultures were drawn. The setting was an urban, tertiary care, academic ED. Serum for PCT and WBC count was obtained at the time of the ED visit. Receiver-operating characteristic curves, proportions, and likelihood ratios were calculated.

Results.—The entry criteria were met by 108 patients, of whom 14 had bacteremia. In comparing bacteremic patients with all others, PCT greater than 0.2 ng/mL was 93% sensitive and 38% specific, with a negative likelihood ratio of 0.18. Abnormal WBC count was 64% sensitive and 54% specific, with a negative likelihood ratio (LR[−]) of 0.78. The presence of either abnormal WBC count or left shift was 93% sensitive but 11% specific, with an LR(−) of 0.64. When considering only bacteremic patients versus noninfected patients, PCT at a cutoff of 0.2 ng/mL had an LR(−) of 0.12. The area under a receiver-operating characteristic curve was significantly greater for PCT than for an abnormal WBC count.

Conclusion.—A PCT level of 0.2 ng/mL is sensitive for bacteremia and is moderately helpful in excluding the diagnosis. WBC count with or without left shift performed poorly in this study in the diagnosis of bacteremia.

▶ I think I'll wait for a study with more power before I add PCT to the already long list of unhelpful laboratory tests ordered on sick elders who present to the ED for evaluation.

R. K. Cydulka, MD, MS

"Drink Plenty of Fluids": A Systematic Review of Evidence for This Recommendation in Acute Respiratory Infections
Guppy MPB, Mickan SM, Del Mar CB (Univ of Queensland, Australia)
BMJ 328:499-500, 2004   7–2

Introduction.—Physicians often recommend that patients with respiratory infections drink extra fluids. Theoretically, this advice is given to replace fluid losses from fever and respiratory tract evaporation, to correct dehydration from decreased intake, and to reduce the viscosity of mucous. Theoretical reasons also exist for not increasing fluid intake. Increased antidiuretic hormone secretion has been reported in patients (both children and adults) with lower respiratory tract infections. Taking extra fluids while antidiuretic hormone secretion is increased may produce hyponatremia and fluid overload. Fluid restriction may be appropriate management to prevent hyponatremia. To determine whether the recommendation of increased fluids for respiratory infections is beneficial or harmful, a retrospective review was performed.

Methods.—The study considered the following 3 questions: (1) Does recommending increased fluid intake for acute respiratory infections influence duration and severity of symptoms? (2) Are there adverse effects linked to these recommendations? and (3) Are any benefits or harm associated with the site (upper or lower respiratory tract) or severity of illness? A conventional search of the Cochrane Central Register of Controlled Trials, MEDLINE, Embase, and Current Contents was performed. References of relevant papers were reviewed, and experts in the field were contacted.

Results.—No randomized controlled trials were identified that compared increased or restricted fluid regimens in patients with respiratory infections. Two prospective prevalence trials reported hyponatremia at rates of 31% and 45% for children with moderate to severe pneumonia. None of these children demonstrated clinical signs of dehydration. Symptoms linked with hyponatremia were not reported. The deaths of 4 children with a serum sodium level less than 125 mmol/L were reported in 1 trial. Several case series in which hyponatremia developed in patients with respiratory infections (some were symptomatic) were reported; all were successfully treated with fluid restriction.

Conclusion.—Increased fluid consumption in patients with respiratory infections may cause harm. No randomized controlled trials have been reported that provide definitive evidence regarding recommendations to increase fluids, particularly, in patients with lower respiratory tract infections.

▶ In the presence of a respiratory infection, it is possible that there may be either an increase in insensate losses, leading to hypovolemia, or an increased release of antidiuretic hormone triggered by the changes in the lung, leading to increased fluid retention.

This is a quick study that looks a bit more closely at the old doctors' suggestion (in our best Dr Welby manner) of "drinking more fluids" in the presence of many infections. While there were few studies, there were 3 studies of infants that suggested that hyponatremia was an important risk with lower respiratory tract infections; thus, antidiuretic hormone release may dominate in the very young. There is not enough known to identify whether there was any increase of water versus milk consumption in these children.

Clearly, more needs to be done, but, until then, we need to consider that not every old saw has been well tested and proven useful (and not harmful).

N. B. Handly, MD, MSc, MS

Antibiotic Use for Emergency Department Patients With Acute Diarrhea: Prescribing Practices, Patient Expectations, and Patient Satisfaction
Karras DJ, for the EMERGEncy ID NET Study Group (Temple Univ, Philadelphia; et al)
Ann Emerg Med 42:835-842, 2003   7–3

Background.—The inappropriate use of antibiotics by physicians has been well documented. The factors that emergency physicians consider when prescribing antibiotics to patients with diarrhea were explored. Patient expectations, physician-perceived expectations, and patient satisfaction were analyzed.

Methods.—Ten academic EDs enrolled a total of 104 patients in the prospective observational cohort study. Adult patients and the parents or guardians of children enrolled were asked about their treatment expectations before they saw the physician. Satisfaction with medical care at discharge was also documented. Physicians were asked about what influenced their management decisions and their perceptions of patients' expectations.

Findings.—Twenty-five percent of the patients received antibiotics. Physicians were more likely to prescribe antibiotic therapy when patients had signs or symptoms suggesting bacterial enteritis, the unadjusted odds ratio being 2.5. Physicians were also more likely to prescribe antibiotics when they thought patients expected them to, with an unadjusted odds ratio of 2.3. However, physicians correctly identified these expectations in only 33% of instances. All patients receiving antibiotic therapy reported being satisfied with care, compared with 90% of those not receiving antibiotic therapy.

Conclusions.—Physicians in academic EDs prescribe antibiotic therapy to about 1 in 4 patients with acute diarrhea. Emergency physicians are more likely to prescribe antibiotics when the patient has signs or symptoms suggesting bacterial enteritis and when physicians believe that patients expect such treatment. However, physicians' perceptions of patient expectations tend to be inaccurate. Patient satisfaction correlates weakly with antibiotic prescription.

▶ The good news is that emergency physicians prescribe antibiotics less frequently and for more clinically valid reasons for acute diarrhea than we do for many other conditions, such as upper respiratory infection, presenting to the ED. It would have been interesting to have obtained stool cultures on all patients to see how good emergency physicians are at differentiating bacterial diarrhea from viral diarrhea.

R. K. Cydulka, MD, MS

Low Risk of Infection in Selected Human Bites Treated Without Antibiotics
Broder J, Jerrard D, Olshaker J, et al (Univ of Maryland, Baltimore)
Am J Emerg Med 22:10-13, 2004   7–4

Background.—The effects of antibiotics on infection rates in persons with low-risk human bites have not been studied prospectively. In the current prospective, controlled trial, rates of wound infections of patients with low-risk human bite wounds given antibiotics or placebo were compared. It was hypothesized that antibiotic treatment would not influence infection rates for such wounds.

Methods and Findings.—One hundred twenty-seven patients with low-risk human bites treated at 1 ED during a 2-year period were included in the study. Low-risk bites were defined as bites penetrating only the epidermis and not involving the hands, feet, skin, overlying joints, or cartilaginous structures. All study subjects were 18 years or older, and none were immunocompromised. Patients with puncture wounds, allergy to penicillin or related compound, or bites greater than 24 hours old were excluded. By random assignment, the study subjects received a cephalexin/penicillin combination or placebo. Infection developed in 1.6% of placebo recipients and in none of the antibiotic recipients.

Conclusions.—Antibiotic treatment may be unnecessary in some patients with low-risk human bites. In this series, infection rates appeared to be comparable in the group given antibiotic treatment and the group given placebo.

▶ Although I agree with Broder and colleagues' conclusions, this study is woefully underpowered. Achieving adequate power to prove that selected superficial human bites don't need antibiotics could be achieved with a nicely designed, simple multicenter trial using one of the already existing large emergency medicine networks. If the results of such a trial were similar to that of

Broder et al, the standard of care for selected human bites would be changed and a great deal of unnecessary antibiotic use could be discontinued.

R. K. Cydulka, MD, MS

A Prospective, Randomized Pilot Evaluation of Topical Triple Antibiotic Versus Mupirocin for the Prevention of Uncomplicated Soft Tissue Wound Infection

Hood R, Shermock KM, Emerman C (Cleveland Clinic Found, Ohio)

Am J Emerg Med 22:1-3, 2004   7–5

Background.—Soft tissue wounds are commonly treated in the ED. Many such injuries respond well to appropriate cleansing and debridement. However, the rate of wound infection after ED treatment reportedly ranges from 4.5% to 6.3%. The efficacies of triple antibiotic ointment (TAO) (a combination of neomycin sulfate, bacitracin zinc, and polymixin B sulfate) and mupirocin ointment (pseudomonic acid A) as prophylaxis for wound infections have been studied separately. The relative safety and efficacy of TAO and mupirocin for preventing uncomplicated soft tissue wound infections were compared.

Methods.—Ninety-nine patients were enrolled in and completed the randomized, prospective, interventional study. All patients met study criteria and were required to make 1 follow-up visit to the ED. Patients were assigned to TAO or mupirocin ointment after standard wound care and suturing.

Findings.—The 2 treatment groups were similar in self-reported rates of compliance with wound care and dressing changes. Signs of infections were observed in 12% of mupirocin recipients and in 6.1% of TAO recipients. Infection occurred in 4% and 0%, respectively. These differences, however, were not statistically significant. No serious adverse effects occurred in either group.

Conclusions.—This pilot study showed a similar rate of wound infection and adverse effects in patients treated with TAO and patients treated with mupirocin ointments. A larger equivalency trial is now needed to confirm these findings.

▶ Although I agree with the conclusion, there are so many methodological problems with this study that I don't know where to start.

Definition of the main inclusion criteria, ie, "uncomplicated soft tissue wound," would have been a nice touch. Second, it's unclear to me how one can study outcomes of wound care without standardization of initial wound care because this contributes more to outcome than does choice of topical antibiotic at discharge.[1] Third, Hood and colleagues' superficial description of the types of wounds entered into the study leaves me to wonder how many of these wounds needed antibiotic ointment at all. Fourth, were the wound evaluators, ie, the physicians overseeing the trained research nurses, trained? There is no mention of training in the article. Was there good agreement between these groups? I hope the methodologic flaws are corrected before the investigators attempt a larger trial.

R. K. Cydulka, MD, MS

Reference

1. Singer AJ, Hollander JE, Quinn JV: Current concepts: Evaluation and management of traumatic lacerations. *N Engl J Med* 337:1142-1148, 1997.

Severe Acute Respiratory Syndrome: Radiographic Appearances and Pattern of Progression in 138 Patients
Wong KT, Antonio GE, Hui DSC, et al (Chinese Univ of Hong Kong)
Radiology 228:401-406, 2003   7–6

Background.—More than 200 confirmed cases of severe acute respiratory syndrome (SARS) have been treated at the authors' institution since the initial outbreak in March 2003. The radiographic appearances and pattern of progression in 138 of these cases were reviewed.

Methods and Findings.—Chest radiographs obtained at presentation and during treatment from 72 women and 66 men were included in the study. Patients' ages ranged from 20 to 83 years. Seventy-eight percent of the patients had abnormal findings on their initial chest radiographs, which showed air-space opacity. The lower lung zone was involved in 64.8%, and the right lung was involved in 75.9%. Seventy-five percent had peripheral lung involvement. Involvement was more often unifocal (in 54.6% of patients) than multifocal or bilateral. None of the patients had cavitation, lymphadenopathy, or pleural effusion. Four patterns of radiographic progression were identified. Type 1, seen in 70.3% of the patients, was characterized by initial radiographic deterioration to peak level followed by radiographic improvement. Type 2, seen in 17.4%, consisted of fluctuating radiographic changes. Type 3, in 7.3%, was characterized by a static radiographic appearance, and type 4, in 5.1%, was characterized by progressive radiographic deterioration. In 74.6%, the initial focal air-space progressed to unilateral multifocal or bilateral involvement during treatment.

Conclusions.—Imaging plays an important role in diagnosing SARS and in monitoring patients' response to treatment. The most distinctive radiographic features in patients with SARS are predominant peripheral location, common progression pattern from unilateral focal air-space opacity to unilateral multifocal or bilateral involvement during treatment, and lack of cavitation, lymphadenopathy, and pleural effusion.

▶ Let's face it, you are not going to diagnose SARS by a chest radiograph. Enough variation in appearance of the radiographs was noted by these authors that the patterns they have described will not be sensitive or specific enough to make the diagnosis. SARS is going to be diagnosed by exposure history, fever, and a pattern of symptoms.

It is interesting that the "radiographic abnormalities" of infection are categorized by 4 temporal patterns; the one that is associated with a progressive worsening to an acute respiratory distress syndrome–like pattern progresses often to death. Twenty percent of patients had no abnormalities on the chest radiograph. What patient and treatment factors influence the other 3 patterns might be helpful in making treatment plans.

N. B. Handly, MD, MSc, MS

Predictive Model of Diagnosing Probable Cases of Severe Acute Respiratory Syndrome in Febrile Patients With Exposure Risk
Chen S-Y, Su C-P, Ma MH-M, et al (Natl Taiwan Univ, Taipei)
Ann Emerg Med 43:1-5, 2004   7–7

Background.—Severe acute respiratory syndrome (SARS) has rapidly become a worldwide threat to public health. After the first report of a SARS case in March 2003, the overwhelming numbers of patients who returned from affected areas or who had close contact with them and presented to hospital EDs seeking to rule out the possibility of having contracted SARS made it imperative to identify patients with a high probability of having SARS by simple clinical characteristics. The clinical characteristics of SARS were identified and a scoring system for early diagnosis was developed.

Methods.—Detailed clinical data were collected and assessed for all patients who were seen at the ED of the study institution with a temperature higher than 38.0°C (100.3°F) documented at home or at the ED. Exposure to SARS within 14 days was assessed. A diagnosis of probable SARS was made according to the definition of the Centers for Disease Control and Prevention. The scoring system was developed on the basis of items with significant differences among symptoms, signs, and laboratory tests on presentation between SARS and non-SARS groups.

Results.—Seventy patients were enrolled, 8 of whom were diagnosed as probably having SARS. None of the initially discharged patients or their relatives had SARS develop. Compared with the non-SARS group, the patients with SARS were younger, had a higher percentage of fever for more than 5 days, and had myalgia and diarrhea. The SARS group also had less occurrence of cough before or during fever and had lower absolute lymphocyte and platelet counts compared with the non-SARS group. A 4-item symptom score on the basis of presence of cough before or concomitant with fever, myalgia, diarrhea, and rhinorrhea or sore throat was found to detect SARS with 100% sensitivity and 75.9% specificity. A 6-item clinical score based on lymphopenia, thrombocytopenia, and the 4 symptom items had a sensitivity of 100% and specificity of 86.3% for the detection of SARS.

Conclusions.—A predictive model for the diagnosis of probable SARS was developed on the basis of certain symptoms and laboratory tests that are indicative of higher risk of febrile probable SARS. The clinical and symptom scores could be used in nonendemic areas to screen for the probability of

SARS in febrile patients with recent contact with SARS or travel history to endemic areas.

Validation of a Novel Severe Acute Respiratory Syndrome Scoring System
Su C-P, Chiang W-C, Ma MH-M, et al (Natl Taiwan Univ, Taipei)
Ann Emerg Med 43:34-42, 2004   7–8

Background.—There have been efforts to develop rapid laboratory tests for severe acute respiratory syndrome (SARS), but it is not yet practical or economical to use these laboratory tests for screening large numbers of people. The criteria promulgated by the World Health Organization have remained the sole screening tool for many hospitals. As SARS has developed into a significant global public health concern, screening tools that have acceptable sensitivity and make use of easily available symptomatic and laboratory items are highly desired, particularly for use in mass screening. A previous pilot study developed 2 SARS screening scores for the prediction of SARS among febrile patients seen at the ED. These scoring systems were validated with a different set of patients.

Methods.—All adult patients seen at the ED of a university-based hospital in Taiwan were prospectively enrolled. Two previously developed SARS screening scores, a 4-item score and a 6-item score, were applied to all the patients. The final diagnosis of SARS was made on the basis of criteria developed by the Centers for Disease Control and Prevention.

Results.—A total of 239 adult patients (117 men and 122 women) were enrolled in the study, 82 of whom were finally diagnosed with SARS. Compared with the SARS patients in the derivation cohort, patients in the validation cohort were older, more likely to acquire the disease locally, and were more likely to have cough before or during fever. For non-SARS patients, cases in the validation cohort had less cough and coryza but more diarrhea. The sensitivity for the 4-item score was 96.3% and the specificity was 51.6%. Sensitivity and specificity for the 6-item score were 92.6% and 71.2%, respectively. When the clinical score was applied to all patients with a positive symptom score, the combined sensitivity was 90.2% and the combined specificity was 80.1%.

Conclusions.—A scoring system for the detection of SARS was validated. The scoring systems used in this study could be applied to mass screening for SARS in future outbreaks.

Establishing a Clinical Decision Rule of Severe Acute Respiratory Syndrome at the Emergency Department

Wang T-L, Jang T-N, Huang C-H, et al (Shin-Kong Wu Ho-Su Memorial Hosp, Taipei, Taiwan; Taipei Municipal Chung-Shin Hosp, Taiwan; Taipei Municipal Wan-Fang Hosp, Taiwan; et al)
Ann Emerg Med 43:17-22, 2004 7–9

Background.—It has been established that the causative agent in severe acute respiratory syndrome (SARS) is a coronavirus. Recent epidemiologic studies in Hong Kong and Canada have demonstrated the clinical characteristics and important laboratory findings of SARS. Whether a scoring system established for SARS could improve the sensitivity and specificity of the World Health Organization (WHO) criteria was determined.

Methods.—A scoring system for SARS was designed by multivariate analysis and stepwise logistic regression. The system was based on the clinical characteristics and initial laboratory findings of 175 suspected cases of SARS defined by the WHO criteria. The scoring system was applied to a series of 232 consecutive patients (the validation group) who met the WHO criteria of suspected cases from April 21 to May 22, 2003. The final diagnosis of SARS was determined by the results of real-time polymerase chain reaction and paired serum.

Results.—The scoring system for SARS was defined as radiographic findings of multilobar or bilateral infiltrates (3 points), sputum monocyte predominance (3 points), lymphocytopenia (2 points), history of exposure (1 point), lactate dehydrogenase more than 450 U/L (1 point), C-reactive protein more than 5.0 mg/dL (1 point), and activated partial thromboplastin time more than 40 seconds (1 point). Among patients in the validation group, 60 of 232 were confirmed as having SARS. The other 172 patients tested negative for SARS. The total points on the scoring system for SARS at initial presentation were significantly higher in the SARS group than in the non-SARS group. At the cutoff value of 6 points, the sensitivity and specificity of the scoring system for SARS in diagnosis of the disease were 100% and 93%, respectively. The positive and negative predictive values of the SARS scoring system were 83% and 100%, respectively.

Conclusion.—The scoring system that has been developed for SARS was shown to be valuable in making a rapid, reliable clinical decision to help ED physicians detect cases of SARS more accurately in an endemic area.

An Emergency Department Response to Severe Acute Respiratory Syndrome: A Prototype Response to Bioterrorism

Tham K-Y (Tan Tock Seng Hosp, Singapore)
Ann Emerg Med 43:6-14, 2004 7–10

Background.—In March 2003, the small nation-state of Singapore was confronted with an outbreak of atypical pneumonia that was eventually named severe acute respiratory syndrome (SARS). The application of an ED response plan at 1 hospital to manage the SARS outbreak was described.

Methods.—The ED of the study hospital implemented protection procedures for the staff, patients, and the facility as a whole. Infection control measures were also implemented, as were disaster-response workflow changes. SARS cases in the hospital were centralized by the Singapore Ministry of Health, and the ED became the national screening center. A screening questionnaire and a set of admission criteria were applied after assessment of clinical features and chest radiograph findings.

Results.—For the duration of the SARS outbreak that commenced on March 13 and ended on May 31, 2003, the ED screened a total of 11,461 persons for SARS, 1386 (12.9%) of whom were admitted to exclude SARS and 235 (17%) were confirmed as having SARS. Among the 10,075 patients discharged from the ED were 28 reattending patients who were admitted and diagnosed with SARS for an undertriage rate of 0.3%. The sensitivity of ED admission for SARS was 89.4%, and the specificity was 89.7%. The positive predictive value was 17%, and the negative predictive value was 99.7%. There were no patients who contracted SARS as a result of an ED visit. One ED nurse with undiagnosed diabetes mellitus was treated for suspected SARS after full implementation of protective measures.

Conclusions.—The SARS outbreak was not a bioterrorism event, but the disaster response of the ED was applicable to the outbreak's management. The screening questionnaire and admission criteria used in this study facilitated the screening, treatment, and safe discharge of the majority of ED patients.

▶ These first 3 articles (Abstracts 7–7 to 7–9) describe efforts during the SARS epidemic to characterize the disease process and establish criteria for screening for SARS. The last article (Abstract 7–10) describes how 1 system response to SARS could be a model for chemical and biological terrorism.

Clearly, while management was largely supportive for these patients, it was essential to be able to identify patients at risk and isolate those patients from others who also might use prehospital and ED care. The screening method developed as reported in the first paper (and validated in the second paper) is particularly useful to early care. They found that among those patients with fever more than 38°C and likely SARS exposure, the presence of 4 symptoms was 100% sensitive and 76% specific for diagnosing SARS. This symptom screening tool is very useful for medics and ER triage staff to quickly identify cases and isolate them to protect staff and other patients. These symptoms are infrequent cough before or during the fever, diarrhea, muscle aches, and either sore throat or rhinorrhea.

Tham's report (Abstract 7–10) describes how a hospital could be mobilized to manage a chemical or biologic disaster. Note that the key elements of this mobilization were rapid communication and a flexibility of resources. Isolation/decontamination space was important and a decision to close the ED to general patients was made so that this ED became the main SARS "hospital" for the region. Once patients were identified by screening tools as being at risk for SARS, they would be transported to this ED for further evaluation and care.

The lessons: Successful screening tools depend on our identifying patterns and easily sharing patient contact experiences in some regional way. Providing the facilities to manage such epidemics/disasters requires agreements between hospitals, transport services, and public media. Each hospital needs to have focused disaster leadership, and each site needs to inventory physical and staff resources. Every hospital needs to practice its disaster response plans (the Singapore hospital had a drill just days before the SARS epidemic hit).

N. B. Handly MD, MSc, MS

▶ Tham's report is useful reading for those who think they may ever have to deal with a widespread communicable disease, bioterrorism or otherwise. In this era of emergent diseases with the potential for rapid globalization as the persistent threat of bioterrorism as a weapon of mass destruction, this audience includes everyone engaged in the practice of emergency medicine. The problem with disaster medicine, particularly bioterrorism, is the difficulty in conducting research. Contributions such as this evaluation of the response to outbreaks such as SARS are likely one of our best tools in improving our planning for the outbreaks we hope to never see.

S. L. Werner, MD

Ultrasonography of the Internal Jugular Vein in Patients With Dyspnea Without Jugular Venous Distention on Physical Examination
Jang T, Aubin C, Naunheim R, et al (Washington Univ, St Louis)
Ann Emerg Med 44:160-168, 2004   7–11

Background.—Jugular venous distention can be difficult to recognize in patients with dyspnea. Whether US of the internal jugular vein or inferior vena cava can help assess jugular venous distention in patients with dyspnea was examined.

Methods.—The participants in this pilot study were 8 patients aged 32 to 85 years who were seen in the ED with dyspnea but whose physical examination results were negative for jugular venous distention. An ED sonographer blinded to the other clinical findings used US to assess each patient's internal jugular vein and inferior vena cava. Imaging findings were compared with other clinical data, including the initial B-type natriuretic peptide (BNP) level and the diagnosis at hospital discharge.

Results.—At hospital discharge, 5 patients had probable or confirmed congestive heart failure (CHF). Four of these 5 patients had initial BNP levels greater than 500 pg/mL; the initial BNP level in the patient with probable CHF was 439 pg/mL. US of the internal jugular vein showed central venous pressure was elevated ($\geq$12 cm H_2O) in all 5 of these patients, and was <12 cm H_2O in the 3 patients without CHF. US findings in the internal jugular vein correlated significantly with BNP levels ($r = 0.67$). In contrast, US of the inferior vena cava showed a moderately increased central venous pressure in only 3 of these 5 patients.

Conclusion.—US of the internal jugular vein in the ED can identify patients with dyspnea caused by cardiogenic pulmonary edema but whose physical examination fails to reveal jugular venous distention.

▶ An innovative use for bedside US, worthy of a larger study to include the feasibility of its use by emergency physicians with limited US training and experience. Another recent *American Journal of Cardiology* study using US to make the diagnosis of CHF/pulmonary edema found that the presence of a "comet-tail" sign during lung US correlated well with the finding of pulmonary edema on chest x-ray.[1]

S. L. Werner, MD

Reference

1. Jambrik Z, Monti S, Coppola V, et al: Usefulness of lung comets as a nonradiologic sign of extravascular lung water. *Am J Cardiol* 93:1265-1270, 2004.

Diagnostic Value of B-Type Natriuretic Peptide and Chest Radiographic Findings in Patients With Acute Dyspnea
Knudsen CW, Omland T, Clopton P, et al (Ulleval Univ, Oslo, Norway; Hôpital Bichat, Paris; Univ of Cincinnati, Ohio; et al)
Am J Med 116:363-368, 2004   7–12

Introduction.—Early diagnosis of heart failure may be challenging in patients seen in the ED with acute dyspnea. B-type natriuretic peptide (BNP) is primarily a ventricular-derived cardiac neurohormone secreted in response to ventricular volume and pressure overload. Increased circulating BNP levels are seen in patients with heart failure. Radiographic findings and circulating BNP levels as an adjunct to clinical findings were compared in patients seen in the ED for acute dyspnea.

Methods.—The diagnostic performance of radiographic evidence of cardiomegaly/redistribution and BNP levels of 100 pg/mL or more as indicators of heart failure were examined in 880 patients with acute dyspnea seen in 5 US and 2 European teaching hospitals. The BNP levels were ascertained by means of a rapid, point-of-care device. Two cardiologists who were blinded to the results reviewed all clinical data and categorized patients as having or not having acute heart failure (447 and 443 patients, respectively).

Results.—Three-factor analyses revealed that BNP levels of 100 pg/mL or more contributed significantly to the prediction of heart failure over each of the radiographic indicators. Multivariate logistic regression analyses revealed that both BNP levels of 100 pg/mL or more (odds ratio [OR], 12.3; 95% confidence interval [CI], 7.4-20.4) and radiographic findings of cardiomegaly (OR, 2.3; 95% CI, 1.4-3.7), cephalization (OR, 6.4; 95% CI, 3.3-12.5), and interstitial edema (OR, 7.0; 95% CI, 2.9-17.0) added significant, predictive information concerning historical and clinical predictors of heart failure.

Conclusion.—Among patients seen in the ED for acute dyspnea, BNP levels and chest radiographs provide complementary diagnostic information that could be beneficial in the early evaluation of heart failure.

▶ This is a report of a multicenter study of the diagnostic utility of BNP.

Regression analysis was used to determine BNP's performance in diagnosing acute chronic heart failure (CHF) independently of findings of chest radiographs and of elements of history and physical examination.

It should be noted that this study was not an assessment of how well the BNP level would work in the ED. While BNP levels were assayed with a point-of-care system, the assay was not done at the bedside nor was it done in real time with the initial management of the patient. Additionally, some samples were frozen and later centrifuged—a step that could not likely be done in all EDs.

Another part of the study that does not reflect typical care in the ED was that the official reading from a radiologist was used. In many settings, it is neither possible nor practical to wait for the official reading before initiating treatment. Does the BNP level give us a unique description of the disease process? This also is worth investigating. In one study cited by the authors, a 5-point clinical score had equivalent diagnostic accuracy to the BNP level.

The sample exclusion criteria also remove some of our most complicated dyspneic patients: those with acute coronary syndrome, and/or renal failure. It is in these patients that we often need the most help in differentiating acute CHF from other processes.

To test the ED utility of BNP, one should consider all steps performed by ED staff in real time—and see if BNP levels actually change management. This study protocol would require collecting the emergency physician's initial pretest probability of acute CHF, then again after gathering history and physical elements and radiographic findings, then after the BNP level. If it can be shown that management is changed significantly, then it would be reasonable to add BNP levels to the ED workup.

Serial BNP levels are perhaps more meaningful in following the course of treatment (to assess the success of in-patient management) and to establish the final diagnosis. However, there is no proof that BNP levels will change what we do in the ED.

N. B. Handly, MD, MSc, MS

Reference

1. Yamamoto K, Burnett JC Jr, Bermudez EA, et al: Clinical criteria and biochemical markers for the detection of systolic dysfunction. *J Card Fail* 6:194-200, 2000.

8 Emergency Center Activities

Clinical Skills

Resuscitating the Physician-Patient Relationship: Emergency Department Communication in an Academic Medical Center
Rhodes KV, Vieth T, He T, et al (Univ of Chicago; Indiana Univ, Indianapolis; Univ of Toronto)
Ann Emerg Med 44:262-267, 2004   8–1

Background.—The ED presents unique challenges to effective communications between patients and health care providers. In an effort to improve communications and provide more effective health care, provider-patient communications in an urban academic medical center ED were analyzed.

Methods.—A total of 93 ED encounters (62 to obtain medical history and perform physical examination, 31 to discuss discharge instructions) at an inner-city academic medical center ED were audiotaped during a 2-month period. Participants included 93 nonemergency adult patients, 24 emergency medicine residents, and 8 nurses. Encounters were coded to study the timing and nature of the encounter.

Results.—The 93 nonemergency patients (mean age, 45 years) were mostly women (68%) and mostly black (84%), whereas the residents (most often postgraduate year 2 or above) were mostly men (70%) and mostly white (80%). Among the 62 encounters for obtaining the medical history and physical examination, residents introduced themselves by name in only 65% of encounters, and in only 8% of encounters did residents indicate their training status. The mean length of the history and examination was 7.5 minutes (range, 1-20 minutes). Most residents (63%) started the interview with an open-ended question, but only 15% of patients were allowed to complete their response; the mean time to interruption (typically by a closed question) was 12 seconds. Among the 31 encounters for discussing discharge instructions, the mean duration of the instruction was 76 seconds (range, 7-205 seconds). Only 55% of patients were given a diagnosis at discharge, but 90% were prescribed medications. Verbal instructions about the frequency, dose, duration of therapy, and possible adverse events of therapy (if prescribed) were provided in less than 50% of encounters. The expected course of illness was discussed in 16% of encounters, instructions for self-care were discussed in 48% of encounters, and symptoms that should prompt a return to the ED were discussed in 65% of encounters. Furthermore, in only 16% of encounters were patients asked whether they had any questions, and in none of the encounters were patients asked whether they understood the diagnosis or the discharge plan.

Conclusion.—The provider-patient encounters examined were brief, with frequent interruptions, and often lacked important health care information. Improvements in these areas are key to improving provider-patient relationships and, ultimately, patient-oriented care.

▶ Communication with patients in the ED is an area ripe for research and improvement. Although physician sampling was based on convenience, the findings ring true. This type of discourse analysis is very time-consuming and requires careful training and monitoring to ensure that the data are meaningful. A number of tools, such as ATLAS.ti,[1] are available to organize coding projects, but automated analysis of verbal data is still far off. Eighty percent intercoder correlation is quite good and probably reflects the relatively clear and simple domains that were coded.

This research will influence the way we practice when communication behaviors can be linked to patient outcomes and satisfaction, as well as the amount of testing (and retesting) performed, and the amount of time (including revisits) it takes to successfully resolve a patient's problem. My bias is that better communication skills up front save a great deal of "rework" later on, and I hope more researchers join this line of work to test that hypothesis.

W. P. Burdick, MD, MSEd

Reference

1. ATLAS.ti The Knowledge Workbench. Demo Version: WIN 4.2 available through www.atlasti.de Scientific Software Development, Berlin.

Communicating Life-Threatening Diagnoses to Patients in the Emergency Department

Takayesu JK, Hutson HR (Massachusetts Gen Hosp, Boston; Harvard Med School, Boston)
Ann Emerg Med 43:749-755, 2004

8–2

Background.—The disclosure of a new, life-threatening diagnosis is a difficult task for the physician and a traumatic experience for the patient and the family. The emergency physician must be prepared to respond to the wide range of reactions from both the patient and family that such a disclosure will provoke. Complicating this situation is the limited time that the emergency physician has to spend with the patient, the strained resources of a busy ED, and, often, the inability to make a definitive diagnosis on the basis of the ED workup and evaluation. A case in which a new, life-threatening illness required disclosure to the patient and family was presented. Guidelines were given, and 10 specific recommendations were presented for the emergency physician, emphasizing patient- and family-centered disclosure of the life-threatening diagnostic findings.

> *Case Report.*—Woman, 47, came to the ED with complaints of persistent right–upper-quadrant abdominal pain of 1-month duration. She reported a family history of colon cancer, with her father dying of the disease at 44 years of age. The physical examination was notable for periumbilical and left–lower- quadrant tenderness, and the laboratory studies were notable for a white blood cell count of 16,000/mm^3. An abdominal CT scan in the ED showed multiple hypodense circular lesions in the liver, a finding that was consistent with metastatic adenocarcinoma of the colon. The primary care physician was unavailable for consultation, and the emergency physician was unsure of how to approach the patient with these troubling findings.

Conclusions.—Disclosure of new life-threatening illnesses to patients in the ED should involve a team of physicians, nurses, social workers and other health-care professionals to ensure that the patients' concerns are addressed adequately, and specific plans can be discussed for continued inpatient or outpatient care.

▶ The communication challenges facing emergency physicians are not unique but are made more difficult by the setting in which we practice. Without a prior relationship, establishing rapport and trust quickly is a critical skill for all of our patient interactions. Once established, subsequent communication of a treatment plan or of bad news will be much easier. In this matter, I am reminded of Peabody's essay[1] on the care of the patient. He wrote "the secret of the care of the patient is caring for the patient." That care can be manifested by some simple behaviors—greeting the patient by his or her full name, shaking hands, greeting other family members in the room, making eye contact, and most importantly, sitting down. It always amazes me how bright, resourceful medical professionals are stumped by the lack of an immediately available chair. I have simple advice for these frustrated individuals: find one.

W. P. Burdick, MD, MSEd

Reference

1. Peabody FW: The care of the patient. *JAMA* 88:877-882, 1927.

General Competencies Are Intrinsic to Emergency Medicine Training: A Multicenter Study

Reisdorff EJ, Hayes OW, Reynolds B, et al (Michigan State Univ, Lansing; William Beaumont Hosp, Royal Oak, Mich; Wayne State Univ, Detroit; et al)
Acad Emerg Med 10:1049-1053, 2003   8–3

Background.—The Accreditation Council for Graduate Medical Education (ACGME) has endorsed 6 areas, known as general competencies, that must be embraced by residency programs. These domains are patient care, medical knowledge, practice-based learning and improvement, interpersonal communication skills, professionalism, and systems-based practice. These general competencies (GCs) will be used to determine whether a program is adequately preparing physicians for a contemporary medical and public environment. Whether these 6 domains formed an intrinsic part of emergency medicine (EM) residency training was determined.

Methods.—A global assessment evaluation device was used in this multicenter observational, cross-sectional study that compared GC acquisition between first-, second-, and third-year (EM1, EM2, and EM3) residents. The study participants were 5 postgraduate year (PGY) 1 to PGY 3 allopathic EM programs. Each resident was rated on every item. A rating of 5 was set as the anticipated achievement for the average EM resident for all levels of training. A score of 5 was the midpoint; a level of 6 meant an above-average level of performance for the resident; a score of 7 was suggestive of excellence, and a level of 8 or 9 indicated that the resident's performance was exceptional. Residents were not scored on the basis of their own level of training but were compared with all residents at all levels of training.

Results.—In the 5 EM programs, 150 residents were evaluated. The GC scores were patient care: EM1, 4.92; EM2, 5.79; and EM3, 6.40; medical

TABLE 2.—General Competency Scoring Results†

	EM1*	EM2*	EM3*
Patient Care	4.92	5.79	6.40
	(4.81, 5.03)	(5.70, 5.88)	(6.31, 6.49)
Medical Knowledge	4.90	5.80	6.46
	(4.83, 4.97)	(5.74, 5.86)	(6.40, 6.52)
Practice-based Learning and Improvement	4.60	5.48	6.16
	(4.41, 4.79)	(5.32, 5.64)	(5.99, 6.33)
Interpersonal and Communication Skills	4.99	5.39	6.01
	(4.88, 5.10)	(5.29, 5.49)	(5.89, 6.13)
Professionalism	5.43	5.68	6.27
	(5.31, 5.55)	(5.59, 5.77)	(6.16, 6.38)
Systems-based Practice Improvement	4.80	5.48	6.21
	(4.71, 4.89)	(5.40, 5.56)	(6.14, 6.28)

*Values are reported as mean (95% confidence interval).
†In all comparisons, $P < .001$ (ANOVA).
(Courtesy of Reisdorff EJ, Hayes OW, Reynolds B, et al: General competencies are intrinsic to emergency medicine training: A multicenter study. *Acad Emerg Med* 10:1049-1053, 2003.)

knowledge: EM1, 4.90; EM2, 5.80; and EM3, 6.46; practice-based learning and improvement: EM1, 4.60; EM2, 5.48; and EM3, 6.16; interpersonal and communication skills: EM1, 4.99; EM2, 5.39; and EM3, 6.01; professionalism: EM1, 5.43; EM2, 5.68; and EM3, 6.27; and systems-based practice: EM1, 4.80; EM2, 5.48; and EM3, 6.21 (Table 2). Analysis of variance showed statistically significant differences for all GCs.

Conclusions.—A global assessment device demonstrated that emergency medicine residents from several residency programs showed statistically significant progressive acquisition of the ACGME GCs. GCs may be an intrinsic component in the training of emergency medicine residents.

Integrating the Accreditation Council for Graduate Medical Education Core Competencies Into the Model of the Clinical Practice of Emergency Medicine

Chapman DM, Hayden S, Sanders AB, et al (Washington Univ, St Louis; Univ of California, San Diego; Univ of Arizona, Tucson; et al)
Ann Emerg Med 43:756-769, 2004   8–4

Background.—The approach to medical education and assessment of physician competency is in the midst of an ongoing transformation. This transformation is occurring as a response to public pressure for greater accountability from the medical profession. During the past 5 years, the Accreditation Council for Graduate Medical Education (ACGME) has implemented the Outcomes and General Competencies projects to better ensure that physicians are appropriately trained in the knowledge and skills of their specialties. The core competencies have been crucial to the development of the Model of Clinical Practice of Emergency Medicine (Model). An Emergency Medicine Competency Task Force (Taskforce)was formed by the Residency Review Committee-Emergency Medicine to determine how these general competencies fit in the Model. The approach the Taskforce used to integrate the ACGME core competencies into the Model was described.

Overview.—The Model was developed by a consensus of major organizations in emergency medicine. Among the contents of the Model were a list of 3 acuity frames, 14 physician tasks, and hundreds of conditions and diseases that comprise the clinical practice of the specialty of emergency medicine. In addition to its use as part of its blueprint for developing written and oral certification examinations, the Model is used by residents in emergency medicine as the basis for didactic study. However, although many uses for the Model have been identified, a critical missing link is that competencies are not specifically addressed by the Model. The Model defines the specialty of emergency medicine, so there is a need to determine whether the core competencies can be integrated into the Model.

Conclusions.—The ACGME 6 core competencies—patient care, medical knowledge, practiced-based learning, interpersonal skills, professionalism, and systems-based practice—are an inherent part of the practice of emergency medicine. These 6 core competencies are embedded in the Model.

▶ Although board-certified emergency physicians already in practice may not immediately understand the relevance of these 2 articles (Abstracts 8–3 and 8–4) to themselves, I would recommend that they read both articles and familiarize themselves with the 6 general competencies. The article by Chapman and colleagues (Abstract 8–4), in particular, presents a very thorough explanation with easy-to-understand examples of the 6 general competencies in which all physicians who are certified in an American Board of Medical Specialty will soon be required to demonstrate ongoing activity. It's encouraging to note that Reisdorff et al (Abstract 8–3) demonstrates improvement in each general competency as residents advance through training.

R. K. Cydulka, MD, MS

▶ Practicing physicians should note that the general competencies concept is jointly endorsed by the ACGME and the American Board of Medical Specialties. This means that specialty boards, including the American Board of Emergency Medicine, will be moving to incorporate them into the specialty recertification process. The competencies are much broader than medical knowledge—they include communication, self-directed learning, cultural awareness, ethics, and quality improvement. As continuing professional development (previously known as recertification) evolves, it will be grounded in these concepts.

W. P. Burdick, MD, MSEd

Hand Hygiene Among Physicians: Performance, Beliefs, and Perceptions
Pittet D, Simon A, Hugonnet S, et al (Univ of Geneva Hosps)
Ann Intern Med 141:1-8, 2004   8–5

Introduction.—The issue of hand hygiene promotion is a major challenge worldwide. Physician adherence to hand hygiene continues to be low in most hospitals. Risk factors for nonadherence were examined, along with beliefs and perceptions linked with hand hygiene among physicians.

Study Design.—Individual observation of hand hygiene practices during routine patient care were observed in 163 physicians participating in a cross-sectional survey in a large university hospital.

Methods.—Relevant risk factors were recorded. A self-reported questionnaire was used to measure beliefs and perceptions concerning hand hygiene. Logistic regression was used to identify variables independently correlated with adherence.

Results.—Adherence with hand hygiene recommendations was 57% and varied widely across medical specialties (Table 2). Multivariate analysis revealed that adherence was correlated with the awareness of being observed, the belief of being a role model for other colleagues, a positive attitude toward hand hygiene after patient contact, and easy access to hand-rub solu-

TABLE 2.—Distribution of Opportunities and Adherence With Hand Hygiene Among Physicians at University of Geneva Hospitals

Variable	Physicians	Opportunities for Hand Hygiene	Adherence to Hand Hygiene	P Value
	n (%)		%	
Sex				0.076
Male	103 (63)	617 (70)	53.2	
Female	60 (37)	270 (30)	67.0	
Age				>0.2
21-30 y	49 (33)	175 (21)	62.3	
31-40 y	75 (51)	457 (56)	56.9	
≥41-50 y	24 (16)	185 (23)	51.4	
Professional status				0.024
Professor or attending physician	18 (12)	146 (18)	49.3	
Fellow or resident	115 (76)	630 (76)	57.1	
Medical student	18 (12)	52 (6)	78.9	
Medical specialty				<0.001
Internal medicine	32 (20)	134 (15)	87.3	
Surgery	25 (15)	173 (19)	36.4	
Intensive care unit	22 (14)	91 (10)	62.6	
Pediatrics	21 (13)	109 (12)	82.6	
Geriatrics	10 (6)	59 (7)	71.2	
Anesthesiology	15 (9)	120 (14)	23.3	
Emergency medicine	16 (10)	42 (5)	50.0	
Other	22 (14)	159 (18)	57.2	
Hand-rub solution at bedside				0.12
No		156 (18)	46.8	
Yes		727 (82)	59.4	
Hand-rub solution in pocket				<0.001
No		729 (83)	52.1	
Yes		152 (17)	81.6	
Hand-rub solution available (bedside or pocket)				0.004
No		118 (13)	34.8	
Yes		759 (87)	60.5	
Use of gloves				>0.2
No		749 (84)	59.2	
Yes		138 (16)	47.8	
Activity Index*				0.03
≤5 opportunities/h		425 (48)	63.3	
>5 opportunities/h		462 (52)	52.0	
Level of risk for cross-transmission				<0.001
Low-medium		700 (79)	62.9	
High		187 (21)	36.9	

*Refers to opportunities for hand hygiene per hour of patient care and represents the hand hygiene workload.
(Courtesy of Pittet D, Simon A, Hugonnet S, et al: Hand hygiene among physicians: Performance, beliefs, and perceptions. *Ann Intern Med* 141:1-8, 2004.)

tions. Risk factors for nonadherence were a high workload, activities linked with a high risk for cross-transmission, and certain technical medical specialties, including surgery, anesthesiology, emergency medicine, and intensive care medicine.

Discussion/Conclusion.—The direct observation of physicians may have affected both adherence to hand hygiene and responses to the self-reported questionnaire. Physician adherence to hand hygiene is linked with work and system constraints, along with knowledge and cognitive factors. Physicians who work in technical specialty areas need to be targeted for improvement in hand hygiene. It may be useful to reinforce the idea that each individual can influence the behavior of colleagues.

▶ Attitude is almost everything. The chances of a physician adhering to hospital guidelines for hand washing had the strongest association with attitude, not with knowledge. If physicians had a positive attitude toward hand hygiene after patient contact or before manipulation of IV devices, they were 2 to 3 times more likely to wash their hands.

But clearly, this article indicates that it is more that just attitude. The pace of technical activity was inversely related to hand washing, unfortunately. Important to note is that availability of "hand-rub solution," that is, the waterless washing solutions, made a substantial difference in adherence. I have found this in my own practice—where hand-rub solutions are available around the ED, it is very easy to "wash" one's hands while moving on to the next patient.

W. P. Burdick, MD, MSEd

Predictors of Emergency Department Patient Satisfaction: Stability Over 17 Months

Boudreaux ED, d'Autremont S, Wood K, et al (UMDNJ, Camden, NJ; Louisiana State Univ, Baton Rouge, La)
Acad Emerg Med 11:51-58, 2004   8–6

Background.—The research on patient satisfaction with emergency care has been steadily increasing in the past 10 years. Many studies have used multivariate data analytic strategies to identify factors that are most predictive of global satisfaction. However, inconsistencies in the findings from these studies are quite common, and firm conclusions are difficult to make. The contradictory findings in the literature about ED patient satisfaction may be the result of methodologic differences between studies and actual differences in the predictors. The stability of predictors of ED patient satisfaction across multiple assessments during 17 months was assessed.

Methods.—The study was conducted among all patients who came to emergency care to the study hospital during 4 designated periods for 17 months. The study participants were contacted by telephone to assess several factors, including demographics, visit characteristics, perceived waiting times, subjective quality of care indicators, and overall satisfaction. Logistic regressions were computed to predict overall satisfaction for each of the 4 periods. Results were compared across the assessments, both visually and using an aggregated logistic regression, to determine the consistency of the final equations. Then a comparison was made of interpretations that were based on traditional *P*-value cutoffs and odds ratios (ORs).

Results.—Using a *P*-value cutoff strategy of $P < .05$, the researchers noted common discrepancies in the predictors of overall satisfaction. Six indicators, including age, perceived wait before bed placement, perceived wait before physician evaluation, physician care, discharge instructions, and waiting time satisfaction, were found to be statistically associated with satisfaction for only 1 of the 4 assessments. However, examining the size of the ORs associated with each predictor showed far fewer discrepancies. Physician care was the only factor that appeared to have large differences in the strength of its relation to overall satisfaction, and this finding was confirmed by aggregated logistic regression analysis.

Conclusions.—The use of *P*-value cutoffs as the sole criterion for interpreting the relative importance of most variables used to determine ED patient satisfaction is not advised because it may result in spurious conclusions of discrepant findings. However, some determinants of ED satisfaction likely differ to a significant degree on the basis of the cohort that is being analyzed. It is crucial to avoid overgeneralizing conclusions derived from a single ED patient satisfaction study, particularly when studies are cross-sectional and use a single site.

▶ Boudreaux and colleagues' findings leave me wondering why hospital administrators place so much value in such unreliable instruments. This study and many others lead me to believe that if as much money and attention were devoted to improving ED staff morale and ED staff behavior toward patients as is now committed to paying consultant firms to develop, analyze, and publish these surveys, patient satisfaction would skyrocket. Many of the issues seem to boil down to remembering the golden rule—do unto others as you would want done onto you. So, when the ED is backed up, and you and the rest of the staff are really tired, and all of you have several more shifts in a row to look forward to this week, remember that caring for the ill is a privilege. Always treat your patients with kindness, gentleness, and respect.

R. K. Cydulka, MD, MS

Emergency Medicine and Society

Estimating the Degree of Emergency Department Overcrowding in Academic Medical Centers: Results of the National ED Overcrowding Study (NEDOCS)

Weiss SJ, Derlet R, Arndahl J, et al (Univ of California Davis Med Ctr, Sacramento; Harbor/Univ of California, Los Angeles; Truman Med Ctr, Kansas City, Mo; et al)

Acad Emerg Med 11:38-50, 2004   8–7

Introduction.—The problem of overcrowding in EDs has long been the focus of articles in the lay press and in academic journals, and few of the issues of concern have improved over the past decade. Because there is no standard definition of "overcrowding," the National ED Overcrowding Study sought to develop a simple screening tool to determine the degree of overcrowding at an academic institution.

Methods.—The National ED Overcrowding Study was divided into 2 phases. In the first, a 23-question site-sampling form was completed, with a total of 336 site-samplings conducted at 8 academic medical centers. Samplings were conducted at 42 computer-generated random times over a

3-week period. The outcome variable was the degree of overcrowding as assessed by the charge nurse and ED physicians.

Specific objective data applied in the full model were indexed to site-specific demographics. A multiple linear regression model compared outcome and objective data to determine predictive validity of the full model. Because the full model was accurate but impractical in an ED setting, a 5-question reduced model was calculated with the use of a backward step-down procedure.

Results.—The average academic ED had 50 ED beds and 500 beds in the hospital. Most of the hospitals included in the analysis were tertiary-care centers. Overcrowding occurred from 12% to 73% of the time in the study institutions (mean, 35%); 2 hospitals were overcrowded more than 50% of the time. A comparison of objective and outcome data yielded an R^2 of 0.49, indicating a good degree of predictive validity. The 5-question reduced model predicted the full model with 88% accuracy.

Conclusion.—The precise definition of ED overcrowding is a matter of debate. More than a dozen possible causes were incorporated into a sampling form, and a 5-question model was found to determine overcrowding at academic EDs with a high degree of reliability and discrimination. Conditions of overcrowding included a lack of available ED beds, closing of the ED because of saturation, a full waiting room and long waits to see a physician, and delays in other areas such as laboratory and radiology services.

Emergency Department Crowding: Consensus Development of Potential Measures
Solberg LI, Asplin BR, Weinick RM, et al (HealthPartners Med Group, Minneapolis; Clinics and HealthPartners Research Found, Minneapolis; Regions Hosp, St Paul, Minn; et al)
Ann Emerg Med 42:824-834, 2003   8–8

Introduction.—Overcrowding of EDs has become a major health care problem in the United States. The causes are complex and involve both increased patient demand and decreased hospital capacity. A national group of experts was called upon to develop measures of ED and hospital work flow to be used by policymakers to better understand and address the issue.

Methods.—The 74 experts developed 113 potential measures with the use of a conceptual model of ED crowding that segmented the measures into input, throughput, and output categories. Group consensus methods were then employed by the 10 core investigators to revise and consolidate these measures into a refined set. The resulting 30 measures were rated by all 74 experts. Each measure was compared to a standard to obtain numeric ratings for feasibility, cost efficiency, early warning potential, a summary rating of operational usefulness, and research potential. Eight additional measures were subsequently developed and rated by all reviewers.

Results.—Fifteen input measures based upon the concepts of patient demand, ED capacity, and patient complexity were identified. Examples of measures included are patient volume and episodes of ambulance diversion. The 9 throughput measures addressed ED efficiency and ED workload, with measures such as ED bed placement time and ED occupancy rate. Fourteen output measures addressed hospital efficiency and capacity. Examples are rate of ED transfer to another facility and hospital occupancy rate.

Conclusion.—The measures developed by these experts should be useful in the management or prevention of ED crowding. They require testing and use for operational and research purposes, yet the measures represent the start of a process for addressing the problem of ED crowding.

▶ I suspect that our dealing with ED overcrowding is like a person's taste in art: One may not know how to talk about what it is, but one "knows it when one sees it." Overcrowding is becoming more notable as EDs close and the number of patients who leave without being seen and ED boarding occur. The Joint Commission on Accreditation of Healthcare Organizations has recognized that ED overcrowding is not an ED-created problem but a hospital problem.

The first article (Abstract 8–7) uses a subjective measure of overcrowding (the consensus opinion of a physician and a nurse) at multiple times and at 8 different academic ED sites. This overcrowding estimate was then fitted to a model using objective data at the time of estimation. Parameters of the model included the numbers of patients waiting or in process in the ED, the times required for each process, and the amount of ED/ancillary staffing. The authors do also review diversion status while questioning whether it is a cause or consequence of crowding. Nevertheless, this work is useful to easily describe a crowding index—if this index, based on the gold standard of opinions of doctors and nurses, can be accepted by other parties, such as hospital administrators.

The second article (Abstract 8–8) identifies a number of measures that could be used to identify overcrowding. An expert panel was invited to define overcrowding measures that could be organized into 3 process steps: those that lead to patients coming to the ED; those that influence the times of ED workup, and those that influence disposition/discharge. Each expert was called upon to review the overall list of measures for usefulness, cost effectiveness, and ability to be easily measured. The final number of measures was reduced to a set of 38 and are made available for research and discussion.

Note that the National ED Overcrowding Study report can only explain about 50% of the variability of the overcrowding outcome with their complete model. There might be value in including some other measures of the Solberg et al article, such as patient complexity.

As more EDs move to computerized patient tracking, these studies will be easier to conduct. Then we need to determine the effect that overcrowding has on outcomes, such as patient care, and bring further to the table other forces such as hospital administration and payers into the discussion.

N. B. Handly, MD, MSc, MS

▶ Weiss and colleagues (Abstract 8–7) present an excellent first step in quantifying overcrowding. Although no clear cut definition currently exists for overcrowding, most ED personnel seem to know it when they see it. This study (minus the detailed survey development methodology, which is of interest to researchers only) should be required reading for administrators whose responsibilities include management and oversight of the ED.

R. K. Cydulka, MD, MS

The Overcrowded Emergency Department: A Comparison of Staff Perceptions
Reeder TJ, Burleson DL, Garrison HG (East Carolina Univ, Greenville, NC; Pitt County Mem Hosp, Greenville, NC)
Acad Emerg Med 10:1059-1064, 2003   8–9

Background.—Interest in ED overcrowding and its potential negative impact on the health care safety net has been increasing. A report from the Institute of Medicine cited ED overcrowding as 1 of the reasons that the health care safety net is in jeopardy. Overcrowding in the ED has also become a topic in the popular press. Many causes and contributing factors related to ED overcrowding have been detailed, but no widespread agreement has been reached as to exactly when acute demand for ED services has exceeded capacity. The perceptions of physicians and nursing staff regarding real-time demands and capacity of an ED were determined. The use of ED data to calculate proposed demand ratios called Real-time Emergency Analysis of Demand Indicators (READI) scores was assessed, and the READI scores were compared with ED staff perceptions of demand and capacity.

Methods.—A computerized clinical management system was used to provide data about ED demand and capacity. Physicians and staff charge nurses were surveyed about their perceptions of ED demand and capacity. The results were compared with mathematical READI scores, which were proposed to objectively assess ED demand. Kappa scores were used to measure interrater reliability between the physicians' and charge nurses' assessment of demand and between the staff assessments and the READI scores.

Results.—In a comparison of respondents who indicated that demand had or had not exceeded capacity, 1 of the READI ratios, the bed ratio, showed a significant difference in mean, 0.245, between groups (Fig 1).

Conclusions.—Real-time data may be useful in predicting ED demand and resource needs. Subjective assessment of excess ED demand did not correlate between physician groups or between physicians and charge nurses. A trend was noted toward prediction of excess demand with 1 of the READI scores, but these scores did not correlate with staff perceptions.

$$BR = (\text{number of patients in ED} + \text{predicted arrivals}$$
$$- \text{predicted departures})/\text{ED spaces}$$
$$AR = \Sigma(\text{triage category})(\text{number at each category})/$$
$$\text{number of patients}$$
$$PR = \text{arrivals per hour}/\Sigma PPH \text{ for each physician}$$
$$DV = (BR + PR) \times AR$$

FIGURE 1.—Formulas for READI scores. *Abbreviations: BR*, Bed ratio; *AR*, acuity ratio; *PR*, provider ratio; *DV*, demand value; *PPH*, patient seen per hour; *READI*, Real-time Emergency Analysis of Demand Indicators. (Courtesy of Reeder TH, Burleson DL, Garrison HG: The overcrowded emergency department: A comparison of staff perceptions. *Acad Emerg Med* 10:1059-1064, 2003.)

▶ The idea was great, but the execution was flawed. Reeder and colleagues were on the right track when they sought to develop a mathematical model to predict overcrowding, but their model is overly simplistic and doesn't include a number of key variables. Furthermore, the low response rates during busy times make it tough to determine if agreement between nursing and physician perceptions of overcrowding are better when it really matters. Finally, discounting nursing and physician perceptions of overcrowding seems naive. If the charge nurse or attending physician or resident physician filling out the survey states that he or she feels that demand exceeds capacity during the shift, it's true because it's their reality. In other words, even if the rest of the department is fairly quiet, but the attending physician is overwhelmed with 3 critically ill or injured patients, then that attendant's demand has exceeded his or her capacity, and help is needed because he or she can't care for any other patients. Issues such as this need to be addressed in the model.

R. K. Cydulka, MD, MS

Performance, Training, Quality Assurance, and Reimbursement of Emergency Physician–Performed Ultrasonography at Academic Medical Centers
Moore CL, Gregg S, Lambert M (Yale Univ, New Haven, Conn; Resurrection Med Ctr, Chicago)
J Ultrasound Med 23:459-466, 2004   8–10

Background.—US has become a widely used diagnostic tool in many specialties. However, the amount and character of the training required to attain competence in performing and interpreting US remain a controversial issue. In recent years, hospital privileging and credentialing issues have gained prominence. Emergency physician–performed US (EPPUS) is increasingly being incorporated into the curriculum of emergency medicine residency programs in the United States. Bedside EPPUS when used by emergency physicians has been shown to be helpful in diagnosing and excluding a variety of emergent conditions. The current state of bedside EPPUS in terms of prevalence, training, quality assurance, and reimbursement at emergency medicine residency programs was determined.

Methods.—A 10-question Web-based survey was e-mailed to US/residency directors at 122 emergency medicine programs in the United States.

Results.—The response rate was 84%. Of the programs responding, 92% reported that 24-hour EPPUS was available. A slight majority of programs (51%) reported that a credentialing/privileging plan was in place at their hospital, and 71% of programs had a quality assurance/image review procedure in place. Guidelines specific to emergency medicine for 150 US examinations and 40 hours of instruction were met by 39% and 22% of residencies, respectively, although only 13.7% of programs were completing the 300 examinations recommended by the American Institute of Ultrasound in Medicine. Only 16% of programs reported that they were currently billing for EPPUS. Of those programs not billing, 12% planned to bill within 1 year, and 37% planned to bill at some future date.

Conclusions.—At academic medical centers, performance and training in EPPUS continue to increase. The number of residency programs that meet specialty-specific guidelines has more than doubled in the past 4 years; however, only a small number currently meet guidelines from the American Institute of Ultrasound in Medicine. At present, only 16% of programs are billing for EPPUS, but most programs plan to do so in the future.

▶ Clearly, this study shows that there is considerable variability in the training of our staff and residents. There appear to be inadequate quality assurance (QA) processes in place (only 70% of respondents have a QA process). Even if there was complete QA compliance, there do not seem to be clear standards for training. About 40% are using the American College of Emergency Physicians standard of 150 scans with 16 hours of didactic time.

An interesting question to be answered is, what are the obstacles that academic ED programs must overcome to reach minimal standards of performance? The hospital credentialing system, specialty turf wars, or the cost are 3 possible hurdles.

Billing for US occurs in about 16% of respondents. The income from these procedures could finance some portion of US training programs. However, billing still might be affected by credentialing problems, whether by hospitals or insurance companies. (At our residency program, we were notified that a number of our bills were rejected from one insurance company because we were not identified as approved providers of US procedures. After a thorough inspection, we were added to the list for that company.) Another obstacle to billing is that the insurance system will only accept one bill for the procedure; that is, they will not pay both an ED and a competing bill from radiology. Agreements with the radiologists at your hospital about using limited or reduced services identifiers for *Current Procedural Terminology (CPT)* codes for ED US can help, since bills for a limited or reduced services study and a full study will both be paid in most cases for the same day.

N. B. Handly, MD, MSc, MS

▶ Emergency medicine residencies continue to make progress toward the residency review committee requirements for US education. As more residents complete their programs with solid US skills, we will need to begin to answer the questions of whether these skills are being utilized and expanded upon in the community, and of the impact of emergency physicians performing limited US on patient care and outcomes beyond the academic setting.

S. L. Werner, MD

"You Are Commanded to Appear": The Subpoena and the Emergency Medicine Resident
Reiley DG, Guldner GT, Leinen AL (Univ of California, San Francisco)
Ann Emerg Med 42:843-846, 2003   8–11

Background.—Receiving a subpoena can be stressful. Frequently asked questions were addressed to help resident physicians respond to a subpoena.

Discussion.—A subpoena does not mean a physician is being sued. A subpoena is the mechanism by which attorneys require witnesses to testify in criminal or civil court cases. Without such a mechanism, many witnesses would refuse to testify because of time constraints, financial concerns, or other reasons, and justice would not be served. The right to a fair trial takes precedence over the rights of witnesses to not be bothered. Subpoenas provide information to the witness about what he or she needs to do to comply, including the time and place that the witness must appear, the name of the court issuing the subpoena, the title of action, and the name of the court in which the case is pending. In addition, the subpoena specifies whether the witness is to provide testimony, records, or both. If documents are required, a time frame is given. The 3 main types of subpoena are "testimony only," "business records," and "records and testimony." The rights and duties of the witness and the penalties for noncompliance are explained.

Emergency physicians may receive a subpoena for criminal or civil cases. Treating a victim of violence may lead to a subpoena to testify later. Occasionally, an emergency physician may be asked to help establish some element of a civil case, in which 1 or more persons are usually suing another for damages. The prosecutor or the defense attorney may issue a subpoena to a physician.

"Witness of fact" differs from "expert witness." The former is anyone who has first-hand information about a case. By contrast, an expert witness generally has no first-hand information but reviews records and provides opinions to the court. An expert witness is asked for his or her opinion and generally charge several hundreds of dollars an hour. A witness of fact will be asked questions about what happened in a particular case and is not paid as an expert witness. Sometimes, a witness of fact receives a small fee but may have to specifically ask about it.

Occasionally, a physician will receive a subpoena that does not seem reasonable, such as a demand to appear in the court the next day with no prior notice or to testify in a court hundreds of miles away. When this happens, a physician can make an objection to the court. Consulting with the hospital attorney about the requirements of a particular state may be helpful in such situations.

It is generally unnecessary for a physician to have his or her own attorney when responding to a subpoena, but certain situations arise in which a physician's testimony may be used against him or her. Physicians who have any concerns that they may become defendants in particular cases should consider having their own attorneys present.

Conclusions.—Most emergency physicians have received or will receive a subpoena. Physicians need to be aware of their rights and obligations to avoid unnecessary hardships associated with a subpoena.

▶ Although this article was written for residents, it provides a nice overview of the subpoena process that is informative and worth reading.

R. K. Cydulka, MD, MS

The Demands of 24/7 Coverage: Using Faculty Perceptions to Measure Fairness of the Schedule
Zwemer FL Jr, Schneider S (Univ of Rochester, NY)
Acad Emerg Med 11:111-114, 2004   8–12

Background.—Equitable scheduling of faculty providing clinical coverage in EDs 24 hours, 7 days a week, is a challenge. Most ED care occurs during personally valuable times, such as weekends and evenings. Objective criteria were developed to evaluate schedule fairness.

Methods.—The 7 daily shifts were categorized as weekday, weekend, holiday, or teaching-conference coverage. Twenty-six faculty members use visual analog scales to assign perceived stress levels to the different shifts (ShiftStress). In 1998 and 1999, faculty schedules were measured (ShiftScores). The ShiftScore distribution of faculty was determined quarterly. In 1999, schedules were modified to reduce the interindividual ShiftScore standard deviation.

Findings.—Perceived stress increased in progression from day to evening to night and from weekday to weekend to holiday. Through the intervention, the interindividual ShiftScore standard deviation was decreased by 21%. Survey results obtained after the intervention demonstrated no change in perceived equality or satisfaction.

Conclusions.—Despite scheduling modifications that increased equitability in the schedule using objective measures, faculty did not perceive any improvement in scheduling. Further research is needed to identify other predictors of stress, fairness, and satisfaction with the demanding clinical schedule of emergency medicine faculty.

▶ Although it's difficult to predict whether Zwemer and Schneider's data are generalizable to any ED but their own, their findings highlight a few opinions (untested) of mine: (1) Some people understand the schedule and are generally satisfied with it. (2) Some people are stressed and unhappy with the schedule no matter how hard you try to appease them. (3) It's difficult to develop a schedule that physicians think is fair, not stressful, and satisfying when trying to cover an ED 24/7. Be nice to your scheduler! It's a tough job.

R. K. Cydulka, MD, MS

Accuracy of Emergency Medical Information on the Web
Zun LS, Blume DN, Lester J, et al (Finch Univ, North Chicago; Mount Sinai Hosp, Chicago)
Am J Emerg Med 22:94-97, 2004   8–13

Background.—The Internet contains an estimated 7000 to 100,000 health- and medicine-related Web sites. About one third of patients in the United States look for health information on the Internet, compared with only 1% to 2% in the United Kingdom. Many US patients turn to the Internet because of their frustration with the lack of personal attention and detail received from health care providers. Unfortunately, the accuracy of Web-site information has not been determined. The gold standards of emergency medicine (EM) information on 4 common emergencies were compared with the information provided for the same emergencies on popular health care Web sites.

Methods.—Gold standard checklists were developed for influenza, febrility in a child, chest pain, and stroke on the basis of information from the American Stroke Association; the American Heart Association; the National Heart, Lung and Blood Institute; and the American College of Emergency Physicians. The 20 most visited health information Web sites were reviewed. Eight of these sites were excluded because they were not intended for laypersons. Information appearing from January 18-30, 2002, was analyzed.

Findings.—The most complete Web site was MEDLINEplus, which contained 74.8% of the checklist items. MayoClinic.com contained 54.5%, and Medscape contained 50.9%. Half of the Web sites contained only 35% to 50% of the checklist items, including WebMD (46.9%), InteliHealth (45.5%), HealthWorld Online (44.8%), Yahoo! Health (41.3%), AllHealth.com (40.6%), and Health.excite.com (36.4%). The least complete 3 sites were Healthcentral.com (35%), Drkoop.com (35%), and AskDrWeil (26.8%). In 11 of the 12 Web sites, information on stroke was most complete. Information provided on 4 Web sites was questionable or gave some concern. Certification was not associated with completeness of content.

Conclusions.—Most Web sites are not good sources of information for laypersons to find out what to do in case of a medical emergency. Few Web sites analyzed contained a significant amount of information on the 4 emergencies investigated. Furthermore, some of the information provided on the Internet is potentially dangerous.

▶ I like Zun and colleagues' message, but I am unsure of their methodology. First, I would have liked to see the checklists, especially for pediatric fever.

Second, the lack of weighting for checklist items and lack of interrater reliability are significant methodologic concerns. Despite these problems, Zun addresses an increasingly important issue: medical and emergency medical information posted on the internet may be incorrect and, in fact, dangerous. This is of much concern as the lay population becomes increasingly computer literate.

R. K. Cydulka, MD, MS

Characteristics of Occasional and Frequent Emergency Department Users: Do Insurance Coverage and Access to Care Matter?
Zuckerman S, Shen Y-C (Urban Inst, Washington, DC)
Med Care 42:176-182, 2004   8–14

Background.—Between 1992 and 2001, ED visits increased by 20% in the United States. However, in any given year, most people do not use an ED. Research has shown that, in 1999, about 1 in 5 adults sought care at an ED, with about 7% seeking ED care 2 or more times during a 12-month study period. How insurance coverage, access to care, and other individual characteristics are related to differences in ED use among the general population was investigated.

Methods.—Data were obtained from the 1997 and 1999 National Survey of America's Families, a nationally representative sample. On the basis of the number of ED visits during the 12 months preceding the survey, people were classified into 3 groups: non-ED users (with no visits), occasional ED users (with 1 or 2 visits), and frequent ED users (with 3 or more visits). A multinomial logit model was used to estimate the effect of insurance status and other factors on ED use levels.

Findings.—Persons with fair or poor health were 3.64 times more likely than others to be frequent users compared with nonusers. Uninsured and privately insured adults had the same risk of being frequent users. However, publicly insured adults were 2.08 times more likely to be frequent users. Adults making 3 or more visits to physicians during the 12-month period were 5.29 times more likely to be frequent ED users than those making no visits to physicians.

Conclusions.—Contrary to popular belief, the uninsured do not appear to use ED care more than insured populations. In addition, frequent ED users do not appear to use ED visits as a substitute for primary care visits. Rather, they are a less healthy population who need and use more care overall.

▶ This nicely done study by Zuckerman and Shen emphasizes several important points: (1) Frequent users of the ED are sicker and probably more chronically ill than non-ED users or occasional ED users; (2) adhering to the simplistic idea that decreasing ED visits for nonurgent problems will fix ED overcrowding ignores the real issue: our health care system is broken; and (3) ED overcrowding needs to be addressed on multiple fronts.

R. K. Cydulka, MD, MS

Pharmaceutical Advertising in Emergency Departments

Marco CA (St Vincent Mercy Med Ctr, Toledo, Ohio)
Acad Emerg Med 11:401-404, 2004   8–15

Background.—The pharmaceutical industry has traditionally spent substantial amounts of money to market prescription drugs. In recent years, the spending on marketing of these drugs has increased dramatically, growing 70% from 1996 to 2000. An estimated 84% of pharmaceutical marketing is directed at physicians. The frequency of items containing pharmaceutical advertising in clinical EDs was identified.

Methods.—This observational study was conducted by emergency physician on-site investigators, who quantified a variety of items containing pharmaceutical advertising present in 65 clinical EDs in the United States at specified representative times and days. The data collection form used in this study was designed to record measurements of specific items containing pharmaceutical advertising, including books, pens, mugs, brochures, literature, samples, food, and other items.

Results.—Measurements were obtained by 65 on-site investigators in 22 states. Most of the EDs in this study were community EDs (87% community and 14% university or university affiliated), and most were in urban settings (50% urban, 38% suburban, 13% rural). Measurements were obtained for 42 items per ED containing pharmaceutical advertising in the clinical area. The most commonly observed items were pens, product brochures, stethoscope labels, drug samples, books, mugs, and published literature.

EDs that had a policy restricting pharmaceutical representatives in the ED had significantly fewer items containing pharmaceutical advertising than EDs without such a policy. No differences were observed in quantities of pharmaceutical advertising in the community compared with university settings, in rural versus urban settings, or annual ED volumes.

Conclusion.—Many items containing pharmaceutical advertising are frequently observed in EDs. Policies that restrict pharmaceutical representatives in the ED are associated with reduced pharmaceutical advertising.

▶ Marco has demonstrated how deeply and subtly the pharmaceutical industry has infiltrated our work environment with their advertisements. They're everywhere. Although Marco's sample may not be representative of all EDs, physicians must be vigilant to remain unbiased in their treatment practices.

R. K. Cydulka, MD, MS

Prevalence of Information Gaps in the Emergency Department and the Effect on Patient Outcomes

Stiell A, Forster AJ, Stiell IG, et al (Ottawa Health Research Inst; Univ of Ottawa, Ont, Canada; Inst for Clinical Evaluative Sciences, Toronto)
Can Med Assoc J 169:1023-1028, 2003   8–16

Background.—Information gaps may occur when patients attend multiple sectors of the health system, resulting in fragmented care when clinical information gathered by one health care provider is not communicated to others involved in a patient's care. The prevalence of physician-reported information gaps for patients who present to an ED at a teaching hospital was investigated.

Methods.—All information gaps identified by the emergency physician immediately after patient assessment were recorded for 1002 visits to the ED by 983 patients. When an information gap was present, the physician was asked to identify the required information and indicate why it was required and how important it was to the patient's care. Patient charts were reviewed to measure the severity of illness and to determine whether the patient was referred to the ED by a community physician. Multiple linear regression was used to determine whether information gaps were associated with length of stay in the ED.

Results.—At least 1 information gap was identified in 323 (32.3%) of the 1002 visits. Information gaps were associated with the severity of illness and were significantly more common in patients who had serious chronic illnesses, who arrived by ambulance, who had visited the ED or had been hospitalized recently, patients in monitored areas in the ED, and older patients. Aspects of care most commonly adversely affected by information gaps were medical history (58%) and laboratory test results (23.3%) and were thought to be essential to patient care in 47.8% of the cases.

The presence of information gaps was not associated with admission to the hospital. After adjustment for important confounders, including patient sex, previous hospital admissions, diagnosis, and severity of illness, it was found that stays in the ED were 1.2 hours longer on average for patients with an information gap than for those who did not have such a gap.

Conclusion.—Information gaps were found in nearly one third of patients seen in the ED. These information gaps were found to occur more commonly in sicker patients and were independently associated with a prolonged stay in the ED.

▶ Stiell and colleagues' report on information gaps in the ED is certainly not news for anyone who works in an ED. We work daily with incomplete information, especially when caring for patients sent in from places where this information could have and should have been sent with the patient. Personally speaking (but not studied), I find much less of a problem with information gaps now that our hospital system's records are electronic and instantly available and hope that all systems follow suit. The availability of these records allows for more informed medical decision making and safer patient care practices.

R. K. Cydulka, MD, MS

How Patients and Visitors to an Urban Emergency Department View Clinical Research
Wilets I, O'Rourke M, Nassisi D (Mount Sinai School of Medicine, New York)
Acad Emerg Med 10:1081-1085, 2003   8–17

Background.—Many challenges are involved in the recruitment of patients into medical studies, and studies involving emergency medicine (EM) present even greater challenges to patient recruitment. The acuity of patient illnesses, the limited time frame in which to receive consent from patients, and the lack of prior relationship between the patient and physician-investigator are the most significant of these challenges. Further complicating the recruitment of patients for EM research is a level of mistrust among patients of minority groups, who may equate participation in medical research with experimentation and exploitation. A successful research agenda is dependent on the understanding that EM investigators have of how their patients perceive research and what their concerns may be regarding involvement in research. Views regarding clinical research were assessed by obtaining current opinions from an urban, largely minority population within 1 ED.

Methods.—Two focus groups of ED patients and visitors were conducted. Data from these focus groups were used to develop a 27-item interview that investigated views about clinical research and knowledge of human subjects' protections.

Results.—The study included 172 patients and visitors who were interviewed within an adult ED. The diversity of the patient population was reflected in the composition of the study group, which was 38% African American, 32% Hispanic, 25% white, and 6% other. When asked why a person might choose to participate in medical research, 46% of respondents said to benefit mankind, 26% said to improve one's own health, 18% cited access to medical care, 17% said financial incentive, and 11% said curiosity. When asked how one might define research participation, 38% cited fear, 24% cited lack of interest in research, 10% cited medical mistrust, 9% indicated not wanting to feel like a "guinea pig," 6% indicated lack of time, and 5% suggested privacy concerns. When asked about the meaning of informed consent, 32% responded that they did not know. One quarter of the respondents did not know that they could withdraw from a study. Most (96%) of the respondents endorsed a statement about the potential benefit of research for themselves or their loved ones, but a substantial proportion (49%) of respondents equated research subjects with "guinea pigs."

Conclusions.—Many persons hold a favorable view regarding clinical research, but apparently, a level of medical mistrust exists. The sources of the mistrust—concerns about human experimentation and the limited understanding of human subject protections—indicate a need to improve informed consent.

▶ This study by Wilets and colleagues serves as a reminder to those of us who conduct clinical research that we need to be more vigilant in ensuring that our study participants understand the consent process, subject rights, and patient protection processes.

R. K. Cydulka, MD, MS

Violence Prevention in the ED: Linkage of the ED to a Social Service Agency
Zun LS, Downey LA, Rosen J (Finch Univ, Chicago; Mount Sinai Hosp, Chicago; Boys & Girls Clubs of Chicago)
Am J Emerg Med 21:454-457, 2003   8–18

Background.—There have been many calls for psychosocial assessment and referral of victims of violence in the acute care setting, but there has been little attention to this topic. Interpersonal violence is an ongoing problem in the United States, particularly among young persons in inner-city minority communities, but the psychosocial needs of this population are not being adequately addressed. A review of the emergency medicine literature has found few prior studies providing psychosocial services with or without a linkage of an ED to a social service agency. A program was described to link young persons who are victims of violence to a health care system and a social service agency in an effort to meet their psychosocial needs.

Methods.—An unvalidated screening tool was developed by a multidisciplinary team that was composed of an emergency physician, a social worker, and a public health scientist. A total of 188 patients aged 10 to 24 years who were victims of interpersonal violence (with the exception of child abuse, domestic violence, or sexual assault) were randomly assigned to either a treatment or a control group. Those in the treatment group were given an assessment, case management, and referral to appropriate resources.

Results.—The majority of the patients were male (82.5%); 65.4% were African American and 31.4% were Hispanic. After 6 months, 78 (81.3%) of 96 young persons in the treatment group made 1 or more contacts with their case manager and made use of social service, health care, and other referrals. The most frequently used services were education (21.6%), job readiness (19.1%), and mental health services (11.9%). Services were used by 9 (9.8%) of 92 patients in the control group, and most of these referrals were for social services (7 of 9 patients); the remaining were health care–related referrals. This difference in service utilization between the 2 groups was found to be significant, and there was a strong positive correlation between using services and case management.

Conclusions.—The results of this study showed that the linkage of an ED and a social service agency increased the number of resources used by young victims of interpersonal violence. Additional studies of the effects of such an intervention in the ED are recommended.

▶ Screening systems without treatment programs are futile. ED physicians have questioned taking the time to screen victims of intentional violence if nothing can be done after the ED visit to specifically interrupt the repeat violence/revenge pattern. However, Zun et al reported a study of the effect of assigning a case manager to victims of violence (life or limb threatening) on the outcome of use of postdischarge social support services. It should be noted that this outcome is not the same as showing there was a decrease in the re-incidence of violence.

The control group was given a list of support services at discharge. In the treatment group, each patient was assigned to a case manager for 6 months. The case manager performed an assessment of service needs and then made referrals to health and social services at the hospital, the Boys and Girls Clubs of Chicago, or other community resources according to the results of an unvalidated assessment tool.

After 6 months, patients were interviewed to determine the amount and types of services used. Of those patients not lost to follow-up, 92 of the nonmanaged patients and 96 of the case-managed patients responded. Approximately 10% of all patients meeting inclusion standards and consenting were lost to follow-up. Case management was strongly correlated with self-reported use of social services (83% of case-managed patients reported use of referral service compared with about 10% of self-reported use of referral services by non-case-managed patients). One of the problems with self-reporting is that we cannot tell if there was a bias of "normative behavior," in that the patients felt they were expected to say they had used services as part of their relationship with the case manager. It is unknown how many patients actually went to services, whether services were delivered, and most importantly whether the use of services prevented further injury.

I look forward to studies linking these referral interventions with a decrease in repeat injury or participation in revenge injuries or death. It will be hard to connect one with the other, but it will be worth it.

N. B. Handly, MD, MSc, MS

The Influence of Gender and Race on Physicians' Pain Management Decisions
Weisse CS, Sorum PC, Dominguez RE (Union College, Schenectady, NY; Albany Med Ctr, NY)
J Pain 4:505-510, 2003   8–19

Background.—There is increasing evidence in the literature that both women and minorities in pain are treated less aggressively than men and nonminorities with comparable medical conditions. Studies of gender differences in pain management have examined treatment regimens prescribed to patients in a wide variety of medical situations, including postsurgical care for appendectomies and coronary bypass and for more chronic conditions such as metastatic cancer pain and AIDS. There have also been reports of gender differences in the dosage of analgesic administered. Disparities in pain treatment by race have also been reported.

A previous study of whether patient race and gender would influence physicians' pain treatment decisions in an experimental setting found evidence of gender and racial differences in pain management when physician gender was considered. Whether gender or race influence physicians' pain management decisions was examined in a national sample.

Methods.—A national sample of 712 practicing physicians (414 men and 272 women) was used in this study. Medical vignettes were used to vary patient gender and race experimentally while maintaining symptom presentation constant. Treatment decisions were assessed by calculating the maximum permitted doses of narcotic analgesic (hydrocodone) prescribed for initial pain treatment and follow-up care.

Results.—There were no overall differences by patient gender or race in decisions to treat or in maximum permitted doses. However, for persistent back pain, female physicians prescribed lower doses of hydrocodone, particularly to male patients. For renal colic, lower doses were prescribed for black versus white patients when the patient was female; however, the reverse was true when patients were male.

Conclusion.—The findings in this study challenge an extensive body of literature suggesting that physicians treat women and minorities less aggressively for pain. The results have provided further evidence that pain treatment decisions are influenced by physician gender.

▶ Weisse and colleagues' findings have been described by others looking at pain management.[1] It's not surprising that men and women have different prescribing habits, as there is a growing body of literature to suggest that physician gender and patient gender interact in unique ways. Look for more work in this area.

R. K. Cydulka, MD, MS

Reference

1. Tamayo-Sarver JH, Dawson NV, Hinze SW, et al: The effect of race/ethnicity and desirable social characteristics on physicians' decisions to prescribe opioid analgesics. *Acad Emerg Med* 10:1239-1248, 2003.

SUBSPECIALTY EMERGENCY MEDICINE

9 Pediatric Emergency Medicine

Successful Treatment of Long QT Syndrome-Induced Ventricular Tachycardia With Esmolol
Balcells J, Rodriguez M, Pujol M, et al (Hosp Vall d'Hebron, Barcelona)
Pediatr Cardiol 25:160-162, 2004   9-1

Background.—IV beta blockade is a seldom-used strategy in pediatric patients because situations that would warrant rapid beta blockade are restricted. In addition, IV propanolol is difficult to titrate, and its long half-life is a contraindication to use in unstable patients. Symptomatic long QT syndrome is a clear indication for beta blockers, yet the IV route is not normally used because beta blockade is usually indicated for prevention of recurrences of ventricular arrhythmia. The unusual presentation of recurrent bursts of nonsustained ventricular tachycardia after cardiac arrest in a pediatric patient with secondary long QT syndrome is a clinical situation in which rapid and precise titration of an IV beta blocker may be desired. Esmolol is a cardioselective beta-blocker with very rapid onset of action and short half-life because of its metabolism by blood-borne esterases. A case in which a young boy with secondary long QT syndrome and ventricular tachycardia was successfully treated with esmolol is presented.

Case Report.—Boy, 4 years, was referred to a pediatric ICU (PICU) after resuscitation from cardiac arrest. The boy's medical history included spastic diplegia, mild mental retardation, and previous admission to the hospital for an episode of mental torpor and rhabdomyolysis. At that time, he was treated with lidocaine for long QTc interval. He was discharged from the PICU after 6 days and discharged from the hospital 2 days later on oral propanolol for 6 weeks as well as oral thyroxine. The patient experienced cardiac arrest caused by pulseless ventricular tachycardia at home 5 weeks after cessation of oral propranolol. He was successfully resuscitated in the ED, stabilized with lidocaine infusion, and admitted to the PICU. Control of tachyarrhythmias was unsatisfactory, and the decision was made to quickly titrate beta blockade with an IV infusion of esmolol (Table 1). After control of arrhythmia was obtained with

TABLE 1.—Continuous Infusion of Esmolol

	Dose of Esmolol (Concentration 10 mg/mL)		
Weight (kg)	50 µg/kg/min	200 µg/kg/min	300 µg/kg/min
3	0.9*/21.6†/7‡	3.6/86.4/29	5.4/130/43
5	1.5/36/7	6/144/29	9/216/43
10	3/72/7	12.5/300/30	18.8/451/45
20	6.2/149/10	25/600/40	37.5/900/60§
30	10/240/14	40/960/56§	60/1400/82§
50	16.6/398/21	66.6/1800/84§	100/2400/126§
70	20.8/500/24	83.3/2000/95§	125/3000/142§

*Infusion rate (mL/h).
†Volume of fluid infused in 24 hours (mL).
‡Volume of infusion administered compared with volume of maintenance fluids (percentage).
§Volume infused in 24 hours exceeds 45% of maintenance fluids.
(Courtesy of Balcells J, Rodriguez M, Pujol M, et al: Successful treatment of long QT syndrome-induced ventricular tachycardia with esmolol. *Pediatr Cardiol* 25:160-162, 2004.)

esmolol, the drug was tapered and stopped. Lidocaine infusion was also reduced and stopped 13 days after PICU admission, and the patient was discharged from the PICU on oral propranolol and thyroxine. The boy remained well and euthyroid on oral propranolol and thyroxine at 15 months after esmolol treatment, with no episodes of tachyarrhythmia and no neurologic sequelae from his arrest.

Conclusions.—Esmolol is safe and useful in the treatment of critically ill children with nonsustained ventricular tachycardia and secondary long QT syndrome, as these patients may benefit from rapid institution and precise titration of beta blockade. Specific considerations for the safe use of esmolol in children can be drawn from published experience and should be taken into consideration when dealing with pediatric patients.

▶ IV beta blockers are used often in adults; however, that is not the case in children. This case report presented a 4-year-old boy who had a cardiac arrest caused by pulseless ventricular tachycardia. After a successful resuscitation, his ECG had a long QTc of 530 ms (normal value is less than 450 ms) and bursts of nonsustained ventricular tachycardia. Esmolol was used to control this arrhythmia.

Esmolol is a great option in this case because of its very short half-life and its selectivity. In children, its use has proven to be safe and with similar pharmokinetic properties with the exception that the half-life is even shorter (less than 5 minutes). The authors' recommendations for esmolol infusion (Table 1) take into account the differences between adults and children. This case report demonstrates that esmolol should be considered in the right scenario in children, thus adding another medication to our pediatric pharmacologic armamentarium.

E. C. Quintana, MD, MPH

A Comparison of High-Dose and Standard-Dose Epinephrine in Children With Cardiac Arrest
Perondi MBM, Reis AG, Paiva EF, et al (Univ of São Paulo, Brazil; Univ of Pennsylvania, Philadelphia; Univ of Arizona, Tucson)
N Engl J Med 350:1722-1730, 2004   9–2

Background.—It is known that the administration of epinephrine during CPR consistently improves coronary and cerebral perfusion. The American Heart Association (AHA) guidelines for pediatric advanced life support have recommended the use of the standard dose of epinephrine administered IV. However, when resuscitation efforts in a pediatric patient with cardiac arrest are unsuccessful despite the administration of an initial dose of epinephrine, it is unclear whether the next dose of epinephrine should be the same (standard) dose or a higher dose. The hypothesis that for children with in-hospital cardiac arrest, rescue therapy with high-dose epinephrine would improve the survival rate at 24 hours when compared with that of the continued use of the standard dose was tested.

Methods.—A prospective, randomized, double-blind trial was conducted to compare high-dose epinephrine (0.1 mg/kg of body weight) with standard-dose epinephrine (0.01 mg/kg body weight) as rescue therapy for in-hospital cardiac arrest. The study included 68 children. The primary outcome measure was survival at 24 hours after the cardiac arrest.

Results.—The survival rate at 24 hours was less for the patients receiving a high dose of epinephrine as rescue therapy compared with that for the patients receiving the standard dose (2.9% in the high-dose group vs 20.6% patients in the standard therapy group. After adjustment for differences in the groups at the time of arrest, the high-dose group tended to have a lower 24-hour survival rate. The 2 treatment groups were not significantly different in their rate of return of spontaneous circulation. None of the patients in the high-dose group and only 4 of the patients in the standard-dose group survived to hospital discharge. Cardiac arrest was precipitated by asphyxia in 30 patients. None of the 12 who were assigned to high-dose epinephrine were alive at 24 hours, compared with 7 (38.9%) of the 18 standard-dose patients who were still alive at that time.

Conclusions.—These findings are not supportive of any benefits of high-dose epinephrine rescue therapy for in-hospital cardiac arrest in children after failure of an initial standard dose of epinephrine. It is suggested that high-dose therapy may be worse than standard-dose therapy for these children.

▶ CPR with the adjunctive medications, such as epinephrine and atropine, has improved coronary and cerebral perfusion in cardiopulmonary arrest in children. Standard-dose epinephrine is 0.01mg/kg/dose; in contrast, high-dose is 0.1 mg/kg/dose. Multiple studies in adults, children, and animals showed that high-dose epinephrine did not improve outcomes in comparison to those from standard-dose epinephrine. However, rescue therapy using high-dose epinephrine has not been studied previously. This double-blinded randomized study looked at the efficacy of using high-dose epinephrine after the initial standard-dose as a rescue medication. The rate of survival at 24 hours was lower in the high-dose rescue epinephrine group than in the standard-dose group, even after adjustment for other variables (such as sex, race, location of arrest, and initial cardiac rhythm). At 6-month follow-up, 4 children survived to hospital discharge with 2 of 4 neurologically normal. Despite these findings, the authors still speculate that some patients (eg, prolonged, untreated cardiac arrests, cardiac surgery, and ventricular fibrillation) would benefit from high-dose epinephrine.

E. C. Quintana, MD, MPH

▶ Perondi and colleagues report disappointing outcomes for the use of high-dose epinephrine after in-hospital cardiac arrest in children. I'm particularly interested in the physiology of this, but circumstances obviously precluded them from studying such parameters. Most disappointing, but not surprising, is the low overall survival rate in these very sick kids.

R. K. Cydulka, MD, MS

Inequalities in Cycle Helmet Use: Cross Sectional Survey in Schools in Deprived Areas of Nottingham
Kendrick D, for the "Lids for Kids" Project Team (Nottingham, England)
Arch Dis Child 88:876-880, 2003   9–3

Background.—Recent studies in the United Kingdom have shown that although 86% of 11-year-old children ride a bicycle and 69% own a helmet, only 30% of these children regularly wear it. Of the more than 7000 patients with bicycle-related head injuries admitted to National Health Service hospitals in the United Kingdom from 1991 to 1995, mortality rates were 4 times greater for children in the lowest socioeconomic class. Cycle helmet ownership and the use among children in a deprived area were described, and the association between helmet ownership and use and socioeconomic deprivation was evaluated.

Methods.—A cross-sectional survey was conducted in 28 primary schools in deprived areas of the city of Nottingham. A total of 1061 school children in year 5 were studied.

Results.—The children residing in a deprived area were less likely to own a bike and more likely to ride a bike they owned 4 days a week or more. Half (52%) of the children owned a helmet, but only 29% of these children always wore their helmet. Children in deprived areas were less likely to own a helmet, but those that owned a helmet were not less likely to always wear one. Family encouragement and parental warning of the dangers of not wearing a helmet were found to be associated with increased helmet ownership rates, and family encouragement and best friends wearing helmets were associated with higher rates of helmet use.

Conclusions.—Programs intended to prevent head injury among children riding bicycles will have to address the inequality in helmet ownership that exists between children who reside in deprived and nondeprived areas. Strategies to increase family encouragement to wear a helmet may be useful, as may strategies that recognize the importance of the attitudes and behaviors of peers, such as peer education programs. There is a need for additional work to assess the character of the variation in exposure to risk of cycling injury with deprivation.

Parental Knowledge and Children's Use of Bicycle Helmets

Bernstein JD, Harper MA, Pardi LA, et al (Children's Hosp Med Ctr, Akron, Ohio)
Clin Pediatr (Phila) 42:673-677, 2003   9–4

Background.—Of the 4.4 million sports and recreation related injuries in the 5- to 14-year-old population, 24% to 40% are caused by bicycle-related injury. The protective effect of helmet use has been documented in numerous studies, with decreases of 65% to 86% in the incidence of head injury in some studies. Whether parental knowledge of helmet safety is associated with helmet use in children and whether there is a relation between helmet ownership and other safety behaviors were evaluated.

Methods.—A total of 341 surveys were distributed to parents of third through fifth graders at 2 elementary schools in Akron, Ohio. The surveys consisted of 22 questions regarding demographic information, child safety behaviors, bicycle helmet ownership and use, and potential barriers to helmet ownership. Parents were also asked whether a bicycle helmet law exists in Akron and whether they believe the helmet provides protection from head injury.

Results.—Of the 215 surveys (63%) returned, 97% of parents believed that a helmet provides protection from injury, and 49% of parents reported that their child owns a helmet. Among helmet owners, 27% reported that the child wears it more than 75% of the time. Use of seat belts was associated with helmet ownership and frequency of wearing a helmet.

Conclusion.—A barrier exists between bicycle helmet ownership and use of the helmet, even though parents appear to be aware of the benefits of helmet use.

Contracting With Children and Helmet Distribution in the Emergency Department to Improve Bicycle Helmet Use

Bishai D, Qureshi A, Cantu N, et al (Johns Hopkins Univ, Baltimore, Md; Union Mem Hosp, Baltimore, Md)
Acad Emerg Med 10:1371-1377, 2003   9–5

Introduction.—The correct use of bicycle helmets can prevent or reduce the severity of brain injury in the event of a crash. Bicycle-related injuries peak in children between 10 and 14 years old, yet children in this age group often fail to wear a helmet. A trial of counseling for children seen at an ED sought to determine whether such an intervention might increase self-reported bicycle helmet use.

Methods.—The prospective trial was conducted between August 2000 and October 2001. Participants were patients, 5 to 15 years old, who came to the ED of an urban community hospital without a life-threatening condition and who had ridden a bicycle in the past 6 months. The patients were assigned by odd- or even-numbered date of admission to an intervention consisting of discussion of a handout on injury prevention for children and signing of a behavioral contract promising to always use a helmet when bicycling (even-numbered day). Half of the children in the intervention group were fitted with a free helmet if they did not already own one. A control group (odd-numbered day) received only a photograph of the hospital.

Results.—A follow-up, conducted by telephone 1 month later, was available for 148 (67%) of the 222 enrolled children. Only 69 of respondents reported riding a bike in the month after the ED visit: 31 from the control group and 38 from the intervention group (including 20 fitted with a helmet). The rate of self-reported helmet use was greater in the intervention group (66%) than in the control group (42%), and effectiveness of the intervention was independent of helmet ownership status at baseline.

Conclusion.—Brief interventions given to children who happened to be seen at the ED for a variety of reasons helped increase the rate of bicycle helmet use. The counseling session was brief and able to be delivered by staff members without specialized training.

▶ It is intuitive for us EM physicians to recommend that the protective effects of the bicycle helmet be used. However, the implementation of helmet use has been and continues to be a challenge. Bernstein et al (Abstract 9–3) showed that parental awareness of protection from head injuries by bike helmets does not positively predict its usage. Additionally, there is concern regarding socioeconomic reasons for lack of bike helmet use in underserved areas (Abstract 9–4). It has been suggested that the ED would be the ideal location for a prevention injury initiative.

There is skepticism about the ED-implemented prevention injury programs. This study (Abstract 9–5) done in children from 5 to 15 years old determined that "ordinary" staff—physicians, nurses, or physician assistants—rather than specially trained behavioral change counselors can be used to deliver effective preventive intervention for self-reported helmet use. Contracting and counseling increased the report of helmet use by 4.5 times when compared to those without contract or counseling. The ramifications of this result are significant. It could potentially prevent bicyclist's deaths and bicycle-injury ED-related visits. This study reinforces the belief that injury prevention could be incorporated into the clinical practice of a busy ED, provided adequate resources.

E. C. Quintana, MD, MPH

A Randomized, Double-blinded, Placebo-controlled Trial of Phenytoin for the Prevention of Early Posttraumatic Seizures in Children With Moderate to Severe Blunt Head Injury

Young KD, Okada PJ, Sokolove PE, et al (Univ of California, Los Angeles; Univ of Texas, Dallas; Univ of California, Sacramento; et al)
Ann Emerg Med 43:435-446, 2004   9–6

Background.—Posttraumatic seizures after head injury contribute to morbidity in children with head injury. Prophylactic phenytoin is effective in reducing early posttraumatic seizures in adults and has been recommended for children. The effect of prophylactic phenytoin in preventing early posttraumatic seizures in children with moderate to severe blunt head injury was investigated in a multicenter, randomized, placebo-controlled, double-blind clinical trial.

Study Design.—The study group consisted of 102 children younger than 16 years with acute blunt head injury who had a Glasgow Coma Score of 10 or less for patients aged 4 years or older, or a Children's Coma Scale score of 9 or less for those younger than 4 years, and a pulse rate greater than 60 beats/min. The median age of the patients was 6.1 years, and 68% were boys. The patients were randomly assigned to receive either phenytoin or placebo within 60 minutes of arrival at the ED. The primary end point was the occurrence of a posttraumatic seizure within 48 hours. Secondary end points included survival to discharge and neurologic outcome at 30 days.

Findings.—During the 48-hour observation period, 7% of the patients who received phenytoin and 5% of those who received placebo had posttraumatic seizures. No significant differences in survival or neurologic outcome at 30 days were noted between these 2 groups.

Conclusions.—The rate of early posttraumatic seizures after moderate to severe blunt head injury was low in this pediatric patient group. There was no evidence that phenytoin reduced the rate of posttraumatic seizures. Therefore, routine prophylaxis with phenytoin cannot be recommended for pediatric patients with blunt head trauma.

▶ A major cause of morbidity and mortality in children is head trauma, which could lead to significant long-term neurologic sequelae. Children's brains may have a higher rate of edema and intracranial deposition of heme (iron), thus reacting differently than adults' acutely injured brains. Posttraumatic seizures are commonly seen in moderate to severe blunt head injuries; however, the use of phenytoin to reduce this complication has not been evaluated.

The primary end point of this study was to determine whether any seizures occurred within 48 hours postinjury in a group using phenytoin or placebo stratified by age and Glasgow/Children's Coma Scale points. A low rate of early posttraumatic seizures in children was observed, which was lower than previously reported rates. There was no significant difference in the rate of posttraumatic seizures in either the phenytoin or placebo group (3/47 and 3/56, respectively). At the 30-day end point, only 3% of children had a posttraumatic seizure. In summary, prophylactic phenytoin does not appear to decrease posttraumatic seizures in children who sustain moderate to severe blunt head trauma.

E. C. Quintana, MD, MPH

Procedural Sedation for Children With Special Health Care Needs
Sacchetti A, Turco T, Carraccio C, et al (Our Lady of Lourdes Med Ctr, Camden, NJ; Univ of Maryland, Baltimore, Md; Morristown Mem Hosp, NJ)
Pediatr Emerg Care 19:231-238, 2003   9–7

Introduction.—Children with special health care needs (CSHCN) because of persistent underlying medical conditions are seen with increased frequency at the ED. The medical treatment of these patients is the subject of considerable research, yet little information has been published on the management of their procedural sedation or analgesia (PSA). The issue of PSA for CSHCN is discussed under 7 headings as follows: (1) patient assessment; (2) monitoring; (3) neurologic developmental and behavioral conditions; (4) cardiovascular lesions; (5) respiratory problems; (6) endocrine or metabolic problems; and (7) hematologic or oncologic problems.

Observations.—The initial assessment of CSHCN is similar to that of any other child, encompassing the chief complaint, relevant history, physical examination, and assignment of an American Society of Anesthesiologists classification. The ED physician may be able to obtain information from the child's parents, physician, and/or from standard reference texts and Internet sites. Entering the specific condition in MEDLINE, with the word "and" followed by the specific PSA drug to be considered, may determine the safety of a given agent in an urgent situation. The IV route offers optimal flexibility for titration in cases of CSHCN. Some agents (Table 3) are recommended for specific health care needs, but these may not always be the first agent of choice for every child.

The extent to which a patient is monitored is generally more conservative in CSHCN, but some form of continuous cardiorespiratory monitoring is needed. Because many of these children undergo many painful procedures, the child or caretaker may have preferences for PSA on the basis of past successes. Ketamine, which can produce vivid dreams, should probably be avoided in children with psychiatric histories. No single approach is possible for children with cardiac lesions because of the wide spectrum of possible conditions. With most of the pure sedatives, procedural sedation has a higher risk of cardiovascular depressions. Propofol should be used with caution or avoided entirely in children with known asthma. Children with endocrine problems are unlikely to have problems with commonly used sedation and analgesia medications, but it is difficult to select drugs for those with metabolic disorders. In children with hematologic or oncologic problems, involvement of other organ systems must be considered.

Conclusion.—The safe and effective management of children with special health care needs requires the ED physician to have an effective understand-

TABLE 3.—PSA Options

Special Health Care Need	Simple Analgesia	Anxiolysis/ Agitation	Painless Procedural Sedation	Painful Procedural Sedation	Extended ED Sedation
Neuropsych	Morphine, fentanyl, hydromorphone	Lorazepam, pentobarb, droperidol	Pentobarb, propofol, methohex	Ketamine/midaz, fentanyl/ Midaz, etomidate	Propofol, lorazepam, droperidol
Cardiovascular	Fentanyl, morphine, PCA	Morphine, lorazepam, diazepam	Fentanyl, ketamine, midazolam	Ketamine, fentanyl/midaz, etomidate	Lorazepam, propofol, ketamine
Respiratory	Morphine, hydromorphone, PCA	Morphine, lorazepam, diazepam	Ketamine, etomidate, propofol*	Ketamine, fentanyl/midaz, etomidate	Propofol,* lorazepam, diazepam
Endocrine/Metabolic	Morphine, hydromorphone, PCA	Pentobarb,† lorazepam, diazepam	Propofol, pentobarb,† midazolam	Ketamine, fentanyl/midaz, remifentil	Propofol, lorazepam,† ketamine
Heme/Oncologic	Morphine, hydromorphone, PCA	Lorazepam, diazepam, pentobarb†	Propofol, pentobarb,† midazolam	Ketamine, fentanyl/midaz, etomidate	Propofol, lorazepam, ketamine

*Avoid in sulfite sensitive asthmatics.
†Avoid in porphyria.
Abbreviations: PSA, Procedural sedation or analgesia; *PCA*, patient controlled analgesia pump; *Pentobarb*, pentobarbital; *Methohex*, methohexital; *Midaz*, midazolam.
(Courtesy of Sacchetti A, Turco T, Carracio C, et al: Procedural sedation for children with special health care needs. *Pediatr Emerg Care* 19:231-238, 2003.)

ing of PSA options. This specialized knowledge will be an ongoing emergency medicine expectation.

► Children with special health care needs are increasing over the last few years due to advances in medical care. These children with moderate to severe chronic medical conditions can create a challenge if procedural sedation is needed. One of the challenges is recognizing the behavioral and physiologic differences in many of these children. The use of Internet Web sites and text may provide information regarding rare and complex congenital diseases or syndromes that will aid in the selection of sedation agents. The selected route of administration could make the selection difficult. IV route is ideal because it offers the titratable option; however, IV access could be challenging in these special health care children, who have undergone multiple admissions, procedures and IV access in the past. This article reviews general categories of special care for these children. The table with the procedural sedation options is a good summary of general agents to use.

E. C. Quintana, MD, MPH

Cardiac Troponin I as a Predictor of Respiratory Failure in Children Hospitalized With Respiratory Syncytial Virus (RSV) Infections: A Pilot Study

Moynihan JA, Brown L, Sehra R, et al (Loma Linda Univ, Calif; St Louis Children's Hosp)
Am J Emerg Med 21:479-482, 2003   9–8

Introduction.—The value of cardiac troponin I is used infrequently for pediatric patients in the ED, but this serum marker may be of assistance in predicting respiratory failure in children admitted with respiratory syncytial virus (RSV) infection. The use of the value of cardiac troponin I for stratifying the risk of children with RSV infection was assessed.

Methods.—A pilot study, conducted at a tertiary care children's hospital, prospectively enrolled a convenience sample of patients between December 1, 2000, and February 1, 2002. The children were all admitted through the ED with a diagnosis of RSV infection. A cardiac troponin I value was obtained in addition to standard therapy and diagnostic testing. Any value greater than normal (>0.3 ng/mL according to the manufacturer) was defined as a "positive cardiac troponin I." Patients with respiratory failure were those who underwent endotracheal intubation and mechanical ventilation.

Results.—Of 25 children, 10 (40%) had a positive cardiac troponin I, and 3 (12%) of these 25 children met the study criteria for respiratory failure. All 3 neonates (≤28 days old) had a positive cardiac troponin I; 2 were intubated. But among patients younger than 12 months versus those 12 months or older, similar proportions were cardiac troponin-positive (41% and 38%, respectively). The third patient with a positive value and respiratory failure was 15 months old. A positive troponin I value demonstrated a sensitivity of 100%, a specificity of 68%, a positive predictive value of 30%, a negative predictive value of 100%, and an accuracy of 72% in the prediction of respiratory failure.

Conclusion.—Cardiac troponin I is a readily available test that can be easily added to the routine laboratory tests ordered for children ill enough to be hospitalized. This serum marker has a high degree of discriminatory power in selecting those children with respiratory failure, but better data on its normal values in infants and a study with a greater number of patients are needed before the clinical use of cardiac troponin I becomes routine in children with RSV infections.

▶ This study used troponin I as a marker for respiratory failure in children with RSV. It is well known that RSV can cause respiratory failure, and cardiac dysfunction. Could this serum marker widely used for acute coronary syndrome workup also be used in the pediatric ED? This pilot study found that 0.3 ng/mL or less (normal) will yield a sensitivity of 100% with a specificity of 68%. Sensitivity and specificity increases to 100% if the cutoff of 0.7 ng/mL is used. Pretty impressive results.

The innovative use of troponin I warrants caution. This study had a convenience small sample. Additionally, clinicians were not blinded to their data. Selection bias could not be eliminated. There are currently no normal ranges defined for troponin I in children, a fact that affects the interpretation of these findings. Still, this could be the beginning of exploring this test as a marker for other uses in the ED.

E. C. Quintana, MD, MPH

Antiemetic Use for Acute Gastroenteritis in Children
Li S-TT, DiGiuseppe DL, Christakis DA (Univ of Washington, Seattle)
Arch Pediatr Adolesc Med 157:475-479, 2003   9–9

Introduction.—In the United States, acute gastroenteritis (AGE) accounts for about 20% of all outpatient visits for children younger than 5 years. A 1996 practice guideline from the American Academy of Pediatrics did not routinely recommend antiemetics for this age group because of a lack of evidence of benefit and a concern for potential adverse effects. Nevertheless, some physicians continue to prescribe antiemetics for young children with AGE. The patterns of use and the factors associated with the prescribing of antiemetics were analyzed in a retrospective cohort study of pediatric patients.

Methods.—The study included 20,222 children, 1 month to 18 years old, who were enrolled in Washington State's Medicaid program and who had an initial first diagnosis of gastroenteritis, diarrhea, or vomiting during 1998. An antiemetic was considered to be prescribed if dispensed within 3 days of the initial diagnosis of AGE. Data analyzed included patient demographic variables, urban or rural residency, and adverse events.

Results.—Within 3 days of diagnosis, 1802 (8.9%) children seeking ED care for AGE had 1813 prescriptions filled for an antiemetic. Most prescriptions (92%) were for promethazine therapy. Children for whom an antiemetic prescription were filled were older, less likely to be cared for by a pediatrician, spoke Spanish as the primary language, and lived in a rural area. The incidence of adverse events and the risk of subsequent health care use did not differ between children who had an antiemetic prescription filled and those who did not.

Conclusion.—Approximately 9% of children seen at the ED with gastroenteritis, diarrhea, or vomiting filled a prescription for an antiemetic. Variables associated with antiemetic prescription filling were older age, provider other than a pediatrician, Spanish as the primary language, and rural residency. Providers other than pediatricians may be unaware of guidelines that do not support antiemetic use. However, among these patients, adverse events related to antiemetic use appeared to be rare.

▶ Acute gastroenteritis (AGE) is a common pediatric chief complaint. Most children are treated with supportive care only. In contrast to adults, antiemetic medications are not routinely recommended in children because of the lack of evidence of any benefit and potential adverse effects. This study found that 8.9% of more than 20,000 children had an antiemetic prescription filled within

3 days of their gastroenteritis diagnosis. The most commonly used medication was promethazine. Older children who were treated by an emergency medicine physician, and had Spanish as a primary language were more likely to have their prescriptions filled. Only 7 children reported adverse effects, which included extrapyramidal or dystonic reactions, and unspecified "allergic reaction."

Even though the American Academy of Pediatrics' guidelines discourages the use of antiemetics, there may be several reasons for their use. The lack of awareness of such guidelines may be a significant reason. Because of the lack of studies of antiemetic use and safety in children, physicians may use their own anecdotal evidence to justify their use. It is possible that the subgroup of children visiting the ED had more severe symptoms in contrast to those in the primary care physician's offices. Nonetheless, the low number of adverse reactions to antiemetic medications should be interpreted with caution. Children with significant dehydration and failure of oral hydration therapy may be those who would benefit from hospitalization for IV hydration, rather than from antiemetics.

E. C. Quintana, MD, MPH

Risk Factors for Tobacco Use by Utilizers of the Pediatric Emergency Department
Mahabee-Gittens EM, Berz K, Pickup T (Cincinnati Children's Hosp Med Ctr)
Clin Pediatr (Phila) 42:653-656, 2003   9–10

Introduction.—The prevalence of adolescent smoking in the United States has increased markedly in recent years. Families who come to the ED are at high risk for tobacco use, and their ED contact can offer an important opportunity for tobacco education and prevention. A cross-sectional study conducted at the Cincinnati Children's Hospital Medical Center ED investigated the prevalence of current tobacco use and risk factors for smoking among older children and adolescents.

Methods.—Eligible participants ranged from 9 to 17 years old and had come to the pediatric ED with nonurgent complaints. A self-administered survey designed specifically for the study was given to a convenience sample from September to December 2001. Respondents were divided into 3 groups according to survey responses: regular smokers, who had smoked at least 1 cigarette within the past week; experimenters, who had smoked at least 1 puff of a cigarette; and nonsmokers.

Results.—The mean age of study participants was 13.4 years; 50% were male, 46% white, and 48% African American. Responses identified 21 (7%) regular smokers, 57 (18%) experimenters, and 236 (75%) nonsmokers. Smoking rates did not differ by sex, but experimenters and regular smokers were significantly older than nonsmokers (14.8 vs 13 years). Most regular smokers were white (95.2%). Compared with nonsmokers, experimenters and smokers were more likely to have a parent or friends or both who smoked and were less likely to report participation in organized sports or interest in a hobby. None of the regular smokers of cigarettes used other forms of tobacco. Reasons cited for smoking included stress (24%), peer pressure (24%), and addiction (29%). Most smokers (62%) said they wanted to quit smoking.

Conclusion.—The use of tobacco among these older children and adolescents was related to parental and peer group smoking. Rates of smoking among parents of children seen at the ED were as high as 54.1%. The pediatric ED may provide an opportunity for health care providers to offer tobacco education and prevention to high-risk children.

▶ This cross-sectional study evaluated the prevalence of tobacco use in pediatric ED patients. White, older patients (≥14 years) with at least 1 smoker parent and at least 1 smoker friend or peer are the at-risk population for tobacco use. Stress, peer pressure, and addiction were reasons stated for smoking. Recent work has explored the ED's importance in providing public health services. This study provided baseline information that could be used for developing prevention and educational programs in our ED.

E. C. Quintana, MD, MPH

Piroxicam Gel, Compared to EMLA Cream Is Associated With Less Pain After Venous Cannulation in Volunteers
Dutta A, Puri GD, Wig J (Postgraduate Inst of Med Education and Research, Chandigarh, India)
Can J Anesth 50:775-778, 2003   9–11

Background.—Pain during venous cannulation is a continuing problem in surgical patients and continues to be a frequent complaint after discharge. One of the mechanisms of pain is local inflammation at the cannulation site. The incidence of peripheral venous thrombophlebitis is 10% to 57% in patients with peripheral IV lines. Local anesthetics in a variety of forms are commonly used to overcome pain on cannulation. The analgesic efficacy and anti-inflammatory effects of topical piroxicam gel versus eutectic mixture of local anesthetic (EMLA) cream to the peripheral venous cannulation site were evaluated and compared in adult volunteers.

Methods.—Piroxicam gel and EMLA cream were randomly applied to the dorsum of the right and left hand of 10 volunteers, with 1 hand of each patient serving as a control. A venous cannula was inserted (with no IV infusion) and then removed after 1 hour. Pain scores and signs of inflammation were noted at the cannulation site up to 48 hours.

Results.—Pain scores were higher for the hands with piroxicam gel on cannulation and on advancement of the cannula. After cannulation, pain scores were significantly higher with EMLA. Blanching was present at all the peripheral venous sites treated with EMLA cream. Signs of inflammation were no more frequent with EMLA than with piroxicam. However, induration was more frequent with EMLA at 6 hours after cannulation.

Conclusions.—In this study of volunteers, the use of EMLA cream was associated with less pain on cannulation and cannula advancement compared with piroxicam gel. It would appear from these findings that topical application of piroxicam gel before peripheral venous cannulation alleviates pain and possibly inflammation in the period after the cannulation.

▶ Amid the ongoing challenge of patient care and satisfaction, Dutta et al compare topical piroxicam and EMLA for pain control in volunteers receiving IV cannulation.

Random application of each of the agents to the dorsum of left and right hands was made 1 hour prior to IV placement. (This regimen of applying medication 1 hour prior to IV placement would not be practical in an ED.) Patients were excluded from the study if the IV catheter could not be successfully positioned on the first attempt. IV catheters were removed after 1 hour. Outcomes were patient-rated pain and signs of inflammation up to 48 hours after cannulation.

At the time of skin puncture and during catheter advancement, EMLA provided better pain control; after catheter removal, piroxicam gel provided better relief and showed less evidence of inflammation (erythema and edema).

There appears to be 2 different pain processes: one that responds to the immediate trauma and another related to inflammatory changes after injury. In short-procedure/same-day surgery, it might be possible to coordinate patient flow well enough to administer a mixture of EMLA and a nonsteroidal anti-inflammatory drug topically. However, in the ED, there is no way to delay IV placement 1 hour. We might consider giving a nonsteroidal anti-inflammatory to all patients receiving at IV to control the inflammatory changes that occur after the injury.

As a methodologic critique, it might have been more useful to look at the outcomes based on intention to treat and not exclude patients in whom catheters could not be placed in 1 attempt. This would tell us much more about real-world situations.

N. B. Handly, MD, MSc, MS

Diagnosis and Management of Acute Otitis Media
Lieberthal AS, for the Subcommittee on Management of Acute Otitis Media
Pediatrics 113:1451-1465, 2004   9–12

Background.—Acute otitis media is the most common infection for which antibacterial agents are prescribed for children in the United States. Thus, the diagnosis and management of acute otitis media is of great significance in regard to the health of children, the cost of care, and the overall use of antibacterial agents. The purpose of this clinical practice guideline is to provide a specific definition of acute otitis media and to address pain management, initial observation versus antibacterial treatment, appropriate choices of antibacterials, and preventive measures. This guideline is intended to provide recommendations to primary care clinicians for the management of children from 2 months through 12 years of age with un uncomplicated acute otitis media.

Methods.—This clinical practice guideline was developed by the Subcommittee on Management of Acute Otitis Media of the American Academy of Pediatrics and the American Academy of Family Physicians. The subcommittee used an extensive systematic literature review. Conclusions were based on the consensus of the subcommittee after the review of newer literature and reevaluation of the evidence.

Results.—Six recommendations were developed. First, the diagnosis of acute otitis media should be made after confirmation of a history of acute onset, identification of signs of middle ear effusion, and evaluation for the presence of signs and symptoms of middle ear inflammation. Second, management should include an assessment of pain; if pain is present, the clinician should recommend treatment to reduce pain. Third, observation without the use of antibacterial agents is an option for selected children with uncomplicated acute otitis media on the basis of diagnostic certainty, age, illness severity, and assurance of follow-up. Amoxicillin should be prescribed for most children when a decision is made to treat with an antibacterial agent. Fourth, the patient who does not respond to treatment within 48 to 72 hours should be reassessed to confirm acute otitis media. If confirmed, patients who were initially managed with observation should receive antibacterial therapy, and those who were managed with an antibacterial agent should begin treatment with a different agent. Fifth, prevention of acute otitis media should be encouraged through reduction of risk factors. Sixth, no recommendations for complementary and alternative medicine are made for the treatment of acute otitis media because only limited and controversial data have been presented.

Conclusion.—Evidence-based recommendations are provided for the definition and management of acute otitis media in children from 2 months through 12 years of age without signs or symptoms of systemic illness unrelated to the middle ear.

▶ These guidelines are worth reading since we see so many patients with otitis media. As far as I'm concerned, the key messages to take home are: (1) not all patients with otitis media need antibiotics immediately—many cases will resolve without them; (2) address the child's pain—the child will appreciate it, and parents can get some rest.

I suppose the real question is this: do the pros of immediate antibiotic use (shorter duration of pain, crying, and fever) outweigh the risk of diarrhea?

R. K. Cydulka, MD, MS

Management and Outcomes of Care of Fever in Early Infancy

Pantell RH, Newman TB, Bernzweig J, et al (Univ of California, San Francisco; Stanford Univ, Calif; American Academy of Pediatrics, Elk Grove Village, Ill; et al)
JAMA 291:1203-1212, 2004   9–13

Introduction.—Febrile infants frequently lack suggestive clinical symptoms or findings, making it a challenge to distinguish between a minor febrile illness and one that is life-threatening. The practice patterns of office-based pediatricians in the treatment of febrile infants and the clinical outcomes resulting from their care have yet to be systematically examined. To characterize the management and clinical outcomes of fever in infants, develop a clinical prediction model for the identification of bacteremia or bacterial meningitis, and compare the accuracy of various strategies, a prospective cohort study was performed.

Methods.—The study included analysis of data collected from the offices of 573 practitioners from the Pediatric Research in Office Settings (PROS) network of the American Academy of Pediatrics in 44 states, the District of Columbia, and Puerto Rico. A consecutive group of 3066 infants, 3 months or younger, with temperatures of at least 38°C seen by PROS practitioners between February 28, 1995, and April 26, 1998, was evaluated. The primary outcome measures were management strategies, illness frequency, and rates and accuracy of treating bacteremia or bacterial meningitis.

Results.—The PROS physicians hospitalized 36% of infants, performed laboratory testing in 75%, and initially treated 57% of infants with antibiotics. Most infants (64%) were treated exclusively outside of the hospital. Bacteremia was identified in 1.8% of infants (2.4% of those tested) and bacterial meningitis in 0.5%. Well-appearing infants 25 days or older with fever of less than 38.6°C had an incidence of 0.4% for bacteremia or bacterial meningitis. The incidence of other illnesses included urinary tract infection, 5.4%; otitis media, 12.2%; upper respiratory tract infection, 25.6%; bronchiolitis, 7.8%; and gastroenteritis, 7.2%. Practitioners followed current guidelines in 42% of febrile events. In the initial visit, physicians treated 61 of 63 cases of bacteremia or bacterial meningitis with antibiotics. Neither current guidelines nor the model developed in this study performed with greater accuracy than observed practitioner management.

Conclusion.—Pediatric physicians in the United States use individualized clinical judgment in the treatment of fever in early infancy. Relying on current clinical guidelines would not have improved care in this cohort. Instead, it would have resulted in more hospitalizations and laboratory testing.

▶ It's nice to see a study that supports physician judgment during patient care. It's a different world since the practice guideline for the management of infants and children 0 to 36 months of age with fever without source was published.[1] The *Hemophilus influenzae* type B vaccine and the pneumococcal conjugate vaccine are routinely administered. As such, meningitis is now more commonly a disease of adults than of infants.

Please keep in mind the following: Just as the guidelines created using ED data turned out to be not so generalizable to an outpatient office setting, the results of this study may not be so generalizable to an ED setting. For starters, I suspect that more children visiting the ED may be bacteremic than described in this study of outpatient office visits. More important, close reliable follow-up is the essential component of proper care for febrile young infants and, unless this can be guaranteed, it is wise to err on the side of caution.

R. K. Cydulka, MD, MS

Reference

1. Baraff LJ, Bass JW, Fleisher GR, et al: Practice guideline for the management of infants and children 0 to 36 months of age with fever without source. Agency for Health Care Policy and Research. *Ann Emerg Med* 22:1198-1210, 1993.

Topical Ciprofloxacin/Dexamethasone Otic Suspension Is Superior to Ofloxacin Otic Solution in the Treatment of Children With Acute Otitis Media With Otorrhea Through Tympanostomy Tubes
Roland PS, Kreisler LS, Reese B, et al (Univ of Texas, Dallas; Virginia ENT Associates, Richmond; Florida Otolaryngology Group, Orlando, Fla; et al)
Pediatrics 113:e40-e46, 2004   9–14

Introduction.—Otorrhea is a common complication seen in children who have undergone insertion of a tympanostomy tube into the eardrum for treatment of recurrent otitis media with effusion. The safety and efficacy of topical ciprofloxacin/dexamethasone otic suspension were compared with those of ofloxacin otic solution as therapy for acute otitis media (AOM) with otorrhea through tympanostomy tubes (AOMT) in pediatric patients.

Methods.—The study included 599 children (mean age, 2.45 years) at 39 centers in the United States and Canada. Eligible children were 6 months to 12 years old who had an AOMT episode lasting 3 weeks or less. Both treatment groups had more boys than girls, but the groups were similar in age, ethnicity, affected ear(s), and discharge volume. The children were assigned randomly to ciprofloxacin 0.3%/dexamethasone 0.1% otic suspension 4 drops daily for 7 days or ofloxacin 0.3% otic solution 5 drops twice daily for 10 days. Patients were evaluated at baseline and at days 3, 11, and 18 by observers blinded to the treatment assignments. Oral acetaminophen for pain relief was the only other drug allowed during the study period. Audiologic evaluations were conducted at baseline and the final test of cure (TOC) visit. Primary efficacy variables were clinical response to therapy, microbiologic response, and treatment failure rate.

Results.—Clinical cure at the TOC visit was achieved in 90% of patients in the ciprofloxacin/dexamethasone group versus 78% in the ofloxacin group. Ciprofloxacin/dexamethasone was also superior in fewer treatment failures (4% vs 14% with ofloxacin), more rapid resolution of symptoms (median, 4 days vs 6 days) and microbiologic success at the TOC visit (92%

versus 81.8%). Both regimens were safe and well tolerated, and neither was associated with hearing loss.

Conclusion.—Topical ciprofloxacin/dexamethasone was safe and superior in all measures of outcome to topical ofloxacin in the treatment of AOMT in children. The combination regimen is expected to yield important medical and economic benefits.

▶ It is common for the cases of AOM to have otorrhea through their tympanostomy tubes. The expected bacterial pathogens are *Streptococcus pneumoniae, Staphylococcus aureus, Pseudomonas aeruginosa, Haemophilus influenzae* and *Moraxella catarrhalis*. This randomized, prospective, observer-masked, multicenter study demonstrated that ciprofloxacin/dexamethasone had fewer treatment failures, and decreased time to cessation of otorrhea. The adverse reactions were mild and unrelated to the treatment (abdominal pain, pneumonia, and cellulitis). The strength of the study is in its methodology and sample size, thus, leading to an advantage in clinical, therapeutic, and economic benefits.

E. C. Quintana, MD, MPH

Adenoviral Infections in Children: The Impact of Rapid Diagnosis
Rocholl C, Gerber K, Daly J, et al (Brown Univ, Providence, RI; Primary Children's Med Ctr, Salt Lake, Utah; Univ of Utah, Salt Lake City)
Pediatrics 113:e51-e56, 2004   9–15

Introduction.—Adenovirus (ADV), a well-known cause of respiratory illness in children, may be underdiagnosed in clinical practice. Rapid testing for ADV became available at the Primary Children's Medical Center (PCMC) in Salt Lake City in December 2000. To review the characteristics of ADV infection in children, the microbiology records of PCMC patients who tested positive by direct fluorescent assay (DFA) or culture for ADV between December 12, 2000, and May 23, 2002, were reviewed.

Methods.—Testing for respiratory viruses during the study period was performed at the discretion of the attending physician. In most cases, DFA was requested for infants younger than 90 days with fever and for infants and children brought to the PCMC ED with acute respiratory illness. Data obtained from records included demographic and clinical information and the impact of rapid viral testing on patient care.

Results.—Viral testing performed on 4568 nasal wash specimens during the 17-month period yielded 1901 (42%) findings positive for respiratory viruses. Of the 1901 children with positive specimens, 143 (7.5%) had ADV infection; 89 cases (62%) were identified by DFA and 54 (38%) by culture. Results were obtained within a mean of 4 hours by DFA; viral culture results required a mean of 9 days. The mean age of ADV-positive patients was 23 months. Most (80%) were previously healthy, and 56% required admission; the mean length of hospitalization for children with ADV was 3.4 days. Fever (31%), bronchiolitis (24%), and pneumonia (14%) were the most common diagnoses. Forty-six percent of ADV-positive children were given anti-biotics initially, yet only 2 (1.4%) had documented bacterial infection. Management was changed in 36% as a result of positive ADV DFA results, and the change may have been life-saving in a child with fulminant hepatitis.

Conclusion.—Because ADV infection can appear in previously healthy children and be serious in nature, early diagnosis is important. DFA is a reasonably sensitive and rapid way to detect ADV infection, which can mimic bacterial infection and Kawasaki disease.

▶ ADVs can cause a significant number of respiratory illnesses, such as bronchiolitis or pneumonia. However, its diagnosis is impractical when cultures are sent. The results are not available for days. However, the use of a rapid test could possibly impact the management of fever in children. This study looked at the impact in patient care using DFA rapid ADV test.

Their findings were interesting. All patients were evaluated for infection, as well as for ADVs, with blood, urine and CSF cultures. Only 1.4% of children had a culture-confirmed bacterial infection. A positive ADV DFA test changed the patient's care in 31% of cases. These changes consisted in stopping antibiotics or hospital discharge. For example, 4 of 5 children who were admitted with suspected Kawasaki disease and were found to have a positive DFA ADV test had their immunoglobulin therapy withheld. Positive results could aid in excluding Kawasaki disease from ADV infection in immunocompetent children. ADV DFA rapid testing could be an additional marker in our armamentarium in the fever workup.

E. C. Quintana, MD, MPH

Evaluation of the Efficacy of Treatment of Kawasaki Disease Before Day 5 of Illness
Fong NC, Hui YW, Li CK, et al (Princess Margaret Hosp, Hong Kong)
Pediatr Cardiol 25:31-34, 2004   9–16

Background.—The first report of Kawasaki disease was published in 1967. Many cases have been diagnosed since then, particularly in Asia. The clinical diagnosis is based on the presence of 5 of 6 classical features—fever for 5 days or longer with 4 other features, including polymorphic rash, conjunctival congestion, cervical lymphadenopathy of 1.5 cm or greater, changes in extremities, and oral mucosal changes. The cause of Kawasaki disease is unknown, but the underlying pathogenesis is related to vasculitis of small and medium-size arteries. The accepted treatment is a single dose of immunoglobulin and an anti-inflammatory dose of aspirin during the acute stage within 10 days of illness, followed by an 8-week course of an antiplatelet dose of aspirin that is continued for as long as a coronary aneurysm is present. As this disease becomes more familiar to pediatricians and to the general public, there is a tendency to diagnose and treat it early. However, it is not known whether early treatment results in early recovery and fewer coronary artery complications. The efficacy of treating Kawasaki disease earlier than day 5 of illness with a standard dose of immunoglobulin and aspirin was evaluated.

Methods.—A case-control study was conducted of patients with Kawasaki disease admitted to Princess Margaret Hospital from 1994 to 1999. Patients were excluded if they had pretreatment coronary aneurysm or were treated after day 10 of illness. All the patients received immunoglobulin (2 g/kg) and aspirin (80 to 100 mg/kg/d) until fever subsided for 48 hours. Immunoglobulin retreatment was administered for persistent fever 48 hours after the first dose of immunoglobulin or recrudescent fever. The case group was comprised of 15 patients who received treatment earlier than day 5 of illness, and the control group was comprised of 66 patients who were treated on or after day 5. The age, sex, duration of posttreatment fever, need for additional immunoglobulin, and coronary artery status were noted. Treatment efficacy was assessed by the duration of posttreatment fever and the prevalence of coronary artery aneurysms.

Results.—Eighty-one patients were included in the study: 15 patients in the case group and 66 in the control group. No significant difference was noted in age and sex between the case and control groups. Persistent or recrudescent fever 48 hours after the first dose that required immunoglobulin retreatment was observed in 33% of the case group and 8% of the control group. Coronary aneurysms were present in 13% of the case group and 5% of the control groups.

Conclusions.—Treatment of Kawasaki disease before day 5 of illness was associated with persistent/recrudescent fever that required retreatment. However, no significant increase in the prevalence of coronary aneurysm was observed when retreatment was given.

▶ Kawasaki disease is a clinical syndrome in which the blood vessel damage (vasculitis) is believed to be caused by circulating antibodies or immune complexes. The diagnostic criteria include fever for 5 days or more, which is the most consistent manifestation, and 4 of 5 of the following criteria: (1) bilateral conjuntival injection, (2) oropharyngeal mucosal changes (erythematous and/or fissured lips, strawberry tongue or injected pharynx), (3) extremity changes (erythema, edema, or desquamation of hands or feet), (4) nonvesicular polymorphous rash, or (5) cervical lymphadenopathy larger than 1.5 cm. Although the cause of Kawasaki disease is unknown, it is suggested that bacterial/viral toxin may be involved. Nonetheless, Kawasaki disease has a common pathophysiology of immune-mediated vasculitis after a wide range of infections. Laboratory studies will show leukocytosis with a left shift with thrombocytosis, and elevation of acute phase reactants (ESR, C-reactive protein). General management includes IV immunoglobulins within 10 days of disease onset, aspirin, and an extensive cardiac evaluation. Cardiac complications are common; therefore evaluation is tailored toward elucidation of these abnormalities. Respectively, ECGs and echocardiograms could show prolonged P-R intervals and nonspecific ST changes, and left ventricular function reduction. This study demonstrated that early treatment shortened hospitalization, mul-

tiple courses of immunoglobulin, and steroid use; however, there was no significant difference in the rate of coronary aneurysm at the 1-year follow-up.

E. C. Quintana, MD, MPH

Azithromycin Compared With β-Lactam Antibiotic Treatment Failures in Pneumococcal Infections of Children

Gonzalez BE, Martinez-Aguilar G, Mason EO Jr, et al (Baylor College of Medicine, Houston; Instituto Mexicano del Seguro Social, Durango, Mexico)
Pediatr Infect Dis J 23:399-405, 2004   9–17

Background.—*Streptococcus pneumoniae* is the most common cause of
meningitis and bacteremia without a source in children under 24 months of
age. *S pneumoniae* is also the major bacterial cause of acute sinusitis, acute
otitis media, and pneumonia in the pediatric population. In the United
States, approximately 35% of pneumococcal clinical isolate are resistant to
penicillin and 26% are resistant to erythromycin. A decrease in the in vitro
activity of many antimicrobial agents against *S pneumoniae* has been documented in the last decade, but some investigators have questioned the clinical significance of this resistance. Whether treatment failures occurred more
commonly with azithromycin than with β-lactam antibiotics in children
who had invasive pneumococcal disease develop within 30 days of receiving
prior antimicrobial therapy was determined.

Methods.—A retrospective review was conducted of the medical records
of children evaluated at 1 institution from 1996 to 2002 who received anti-
microbials (azithromycin or a β-lactam antibiotic) and had invasive pneumococcal disease develop within 30 days. Treatment failure was defined as
development of invasive pneumococcal infection in a patient taking antimi-
crobials or within 3 days of stopping azithromycin treatment or within 1 day
of stopping β-lactam treatment.

Results.—There were 21 children with similar demographic features who
had invasive pneumococcal disease develop within 1 month of receiving
azithromycin and 33 children who had invasive pneumococcal disease develop within 1 month of receiving a β-lactam antibiotic. The rate of treatment failure was 52% in the azithromycin group and 33% in the β-lactam
group. Among the treatment failures in the azithromycin group, 8 of 11 were
caused by pneumococci with the macrolide-resistant phenotype, 2 with the
macrolide-, lincosamide-, and streptogramin B-resistant (MLS$_\beta$) phenotype,
and 1 by a macrolide-susceptible organism. Among the treatment failures in
the β-lactam group, 7 resulted from a penicillin-resistant isolate, 3 had an
intermediately susceptible isolate, and 1 had a susceptible isolate.

Conclusions.—Treatment failures in patients who had invasive disease
develop within 1 month of antimicrobial treatment occur with similar frequency in patients who receive β-lactam antibiotics and in those who receive
azithromycin. Macrolide-resistant organisms are not more likely to be re-

covered after a macrolide treatment failure than a penicillin-nonsusceptible isolate being recovered after a β-lactam treatment failure.

▶ *Streptococcus pneumoniae* is a common cause for meningitis, bacteremia, acute sinusitis, pneumonia, and acute otitis media. Unfortunately, its resistance to both penicillin and erythromycin is increasing. Azithromycin has become more popular because of its once-a-day dosing. This article suggested that the treatment failures between azithromycin and β-lactam antibiotics were similar. Caution is warranted with these results because of the small sample sizes and low power. Still, this is an option that should be considered next time one treats *S pneumoniae* infection.

E. C. Quintana, MD, MPH

Headache and Backache After Lumbar Puncture in Children and Adolescents: A Prospective Study
Ebinger F, Kosel C, Pietz J, et al (Univ of Pediatric Hosp, Heidelberg, Germany)
Pediatrics 113:1588-1592, 2004   9–18

Background.—Lumbar puncture is one of the most frequently performed invasive diagnostic procedures in children and adolescents, yet there have been few studies devoted to the indications for and method of lumbar puncture in pediatric patients and to postpuncture complaints, which have been recognized since the end of the nineteenth century. Postpuncture complaints are generally believed to be rare in children and adolescents, but their exact incidence is unknown. The frequency of postlumbar puncture headaches or backaches among general pediatric and neuropediatric patients and factors that might influence their occurrence was investigated.

Methods.—The study group for this 12-month investigation was comprised of 112 patients ages 2 to 16 years. The patients were evaluated for factors that might influence the rate of postpuncture complaints, including age, gender, use of local anesthesia, cannula gauge, bevel orientation, number of puncture attempts, volume of CSF aspirated, and cell count in CSF.

Results.—Headaches were experienced by 27% (including positional headache in 9%), and 40% had backache develop. Frequency of complaints increased with increasing age of the patients. In older children, girls reported complaints more frequently than did boys. Patients with higher cell counts in CSF had more frequent headaches than did patients without pleocytosis. Outcome was not influenced by cannula gauge or bevel orientation.

Conclusions.—The frequency of positional and nonpositional headaches after lumbar puncture is lower in children than in adults. Backaches are a significant component of postpuncture morbidity. The incidence of postpuncture complaints increased in this study with puberty, and at puberty, girls were more prone to development of postpuncture headaches. Recommendations regarding cannula gauge or bevel orientation in lumbar puncture that have developed from studies in adults have not been confirmed in children.

▶ This is one of the most commonly performed invasive procedures in the ED. Many adults have headaches and backaches develop. It is believed that it is a rare occurrence in children. The exact incidence is unknown. This study investigated the frequency of postlumbar puncture headache or backache and any modifying factors that influence their occurrence. Fifty-three percent of patients' complaints were of at least 1 pain-related symptom (either headache or backache), which were present by the second day after puncture. This finding was statistically significant in patients older than 10 years and in those with CSF pleocytosis. There was a trend that noted that older girls reported more symptoms than did boys; however, this was not statistically significant. The gauge of the lumbar needle, orientation of bevel (cranial vs lateral), the need for multiple puncture attempts, or the amount of CSF aspirated at the lumbar puncture did not produce significant differences in symptoms. Anesthetic cream was not associated with backaches, but with positional headaches. The authors of this study theorize that the result was due to the patients' characteristics rather than the cream itself.

E. C. Quintana, MD, MPH

Azithromycin Is as Effective as and Better Tolerated Than Erythromycin Estolate for the Treatment of Pertussis
Langley JM, and the Pediatric Investigators Collaborative on Infections in Canada (Dalhousie Univ, Halifax, Canada)
Pediatrics 114:e96-e101, 2004   9–19

Background.—Universal immunization against *Bordetella pertussis* (whooping cough) infection has resulted in dramatic reductions in the incidence of pertussis. However, outbreaks continue to occur in countries with excellent vaccine coverage. Treatment of the infection ameliorates the severity of symptoms during the catarrhal phase of pertussis, but it has no effect on established paroxysmal or convalescent phases. Erythromcyin, which is recommended for treatment of pertussis to prevent transmission of infection, is poorly tolerated because there are gastrointestinal side effects. The safety and efficacy of erythromycin were compared with azithromycin for the treatment of pertussis.

Methods.—The large, randomized controlled trial enrolled children from primary care practices in 1 American and 11 Canadian urban centers. All the children were age 6 months to 16 years and had had cough illness that was suspected to be or was confirmed to be pertussis. The children were randomly assigned to receive either azithromycin (10 mg/kg on day 1 and 5 mg/kg on days 2 to 5 as a single dose) or erythromycin estolate (40 mg/kg/day in 3 divided doses for 10 days), with stratification by center. The primary outcome measure was bacteriologic cure of infection as determined by cultures of nasopharyngeal aspirates. Adverse events, such as nausea, vomiting, diarrhea, or any gastrointestinal complaint, were determined by a parent-completed diary that was reviewed with study personnel during study visits.

Results.—A total of 477 children was enrolled. Of these, 114 (24%) grew *B pertussis* from nasopharyngeal specimens, including 58 of 239 patients in the azithromycin group (24%) and 56 of 238 patients in the erythromycin group (23%). Gastrointestinal adverse events were reported less frequently in the azithromycin group (18.8%) than in the erythromycin group (41.2%). Children who were randomly assigned to azithromycin were much more likely to have complied with antimicrobial therapy over the treatment period: 90% of children in the azithromycin group took 100% of prescribed doses, whereas only 55% of children in the erythromycin group took 100% of prescribed doses.

Conclusions.—Azithromycin was found to be as effective as erythromycin for the treatment of pertussis in children, with a lower incidence of gastrointestinal adverse effects compared with erythromycin. Compliance with azithromycin was also better than that for erythromycin in this study.

▶ Despite immunization, pertussis outbreaks still occur. Pertussis (whooping cough) is a respiratory infection caused by *B pertussis*. It can be divided into 3 stages. First stage (catarrhal stage), which presents as mild cough, conjunctivitis, and coryza, can last 1 to 2 weeks. The second stage (paroxysmal stage), which presents as increasing severe cough, can last 2 to 4 weeks. This stage with its prolonged spasms of coughing with a sudden inflow of air produces the characteristic "whoop" sound of the whooping cough. The examination is entirely normal in between these coughing spasms. The third stage (convalescent stage), which presents with a waning of cough intensity, could last several more weeks. The most common life-threatening complication is airway obstruction, thus leading to respiratory arrest. Young infants and any child who presents with cyanosis or any other complications (bacterial pneumonia, seizures, encephalitis) need admission for observation and treatment. Treating with erythromycin is to prevent transmission of the infection by eradicating the bacteria from the nasopharynx. However, the use of erythromycin is poorly tolerated because of significant gastrointestinal side effects, thus leading to poor compliance.

This study evaluated the safety and efficacy of azithromycin with erythromycin in a large, randomized trial across Canada. At the end of therapy, there was 100% bacterial eradication in both groups with no recurrence. There were less gastrointestinal effects, such as nausea, and diarrhea, with azithromycin when compared with erythromycin estolate. Compliance to medication was greater with azithromycin versus erythromycin. In conclusion, azithromycin was found to be as effective as erythromycin in the treatment of pertussis.

E. C. Quintana, MD, MPH

Effect of Dextromethorphan, Diphenhydramine, and Placebo on Nocturnal Cough and Sleep Quality for Coughing Children and Their Parents

Paul IM, Yoder KE, Crowell KR, et al (Pennsylvania State College of Medicine, Hershey)

Pediatrics 114:e85-e90, 2004   9–20

Background.—Cough is one of the most troubling symptoms in children with upper respiratory tract infections (URIs) and prompts more ambulatory health care visits than any other symptom in the United States. Cough is particularly bothersome at night because it often has an adverse effect on sleep for both the ill children and the parents. Thus, many parents will administer the over-the-counter (OTC) medications diphenhydramine or dextromethorphan before bedtime to children with cough to improve their own sleep and functioning during the following day. Whether the commonly used OTCs diphenhydramine and dextromethorphan are superior to placebo for the treatment of nocturnal cough and sleep difficulty associated with URIs and whether parents have improved sleep quality when their children received the medications when compared with placebo were determined.

Methods.—Parents of 100 children with URIs were questioned to determine the frequency, severity, and bothersome nature of nocturnal cough in their children. Their responses were recorded on 2 consecutive days, initially on the day of presentation, when no medication had been given the previous evening, and then again on the subsequent day, when either medication or placebo was given before bedtime. Sleep quality was assessed on both nights for both the child and the parent.

Results.—All outcomes were significantly improved for the entire cohort on the second night of the study, when either medication or placebo was administered. However, neither diphenhydramine nor dextromethorphan produced a superior benefit when compared with placebo for any of the outcomes studied. Insomnia was reported more frequently in children who were given dextromethorphan, and drowsiness was reported more commonly in patients who were given diphenhydramine.

Conclusions.—Diphenhydramine and dextromethorphan are not superior to placebo in providing nocturnal symptom relief for children with cough and sleep difficulty as a result of an URI. The administration of these medications to children with cough do not provide improved quality of sleep for their parents when compared with placebo. These findings, the potential for adverse effects, and the individual and cumulative cost of these medications should be considered by each clinician before these drugs are recommended to families.

▶ Children's cough is a complaint that can present at night in the ED because it affects both children's and parents' sleep and awake patterns. This study evaluated the most commonly used medications for nocturnal cough for URIs in improving sleep quality when compared with placebo. The treatment of cough is not supported by the American Academy of Pediatrics mainly because there is a lack of proven benefit and the possibility for toxicity and overdose. Survey questions assessed nocturnal cough and sleep quality for both child and parent. All groups showed dramatic improvement cough frequency, impact on child and parent sleep, and "bothersome" nature of cough and severity of cough. When separated by treatment group (diphenhydramine, dextromethorphan, and placebo), there was no statistical difference among the groups. The most common adverse effects were hyperactivity, insomnia (dextromethorphan), and drowsiness (diphenhydramine); however, there was no significant difference between the treatment groups.

Several limitations should be noted. First, these responses are a subjective report by parents, and they could be inaccurate. The answers were paired and compared with their own responses from the previous night, thus eliminating this limitation. In addition, there was no reassurance that parents were compliant to medication administration. Telephone follow-up was the only reassurance of this compliance. Still, the overall results in this study were remarkable. They are reassuring to clinicians that regardless of treatment, the improvement of symptoms occurs with time alone, as expected with the natural history of URIs.

E. C. Quintana, MD, MPH

Difficulty in Obtaining Peak Expiratory Flow Measurements in Children With Acute Asthma
Gorelick MH, Stevens MW, Schultz T, et al (Med College of Wisconsin, Milwaukee; Univ of Washington, Seattle; Children's Hosp of Philadelphia; et al)
Pediatr Emerg Care 20:22-26, 2004   9–21

Background.—National guidelines for the treatment of acute asthma have specified measurement of peak expiratory flow rate (PEFR) as a more valid and reproducible measure of airway obstruction than clinical examination. However, compliance with this recommendation has been found to be low. One study among pediatric emergency physicians had reported that respondents obtained PEFR in only 60% of eligible patients. One reason for low compliance with PEFR recommendations in children may be uncertainty regarding their ability to perform the maneuver, which is effort-dependent and requires a significant degree of coordination. In particular, the ability of children to perform PEFR during ED treatment of acute asthma has not been well studied. The frequency with which children 6 years and older with acute asthma can perform PEFR in an ED was determined.

Methods.—This prospective cohort study of children with acute asthma included all children ages 2 to 18 years treated at an urban pediatric ED for an acute exacerbation of asthma during randomly selected days over 12 months. PEFR was to be measured in all children age 6 years and older before therapy and after each treatment with inhaled bronchodilators. PEFR measurements were obtained by registered respiratory therapists, who determined whether patients were able to adequately perform the maneuver.

Results.—A total of 456 children with a median age of 10 years was enrolled in the study. Of these children, 291 (64%) had PEFR measured at

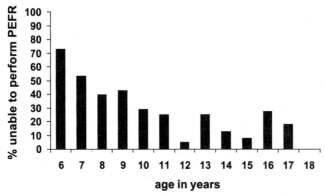

FIGURE 1.—Proportion of patients unable to perform PEFR maneuver properly, by age. (Courtesy of Gorelick MH, Stevens MW, Schultz T, et al: Difficulty in obtaining peak expiratory flow measurements in children with acute asthma. *Pediatr Emerg Care* 20:22-26, 2004.)

least once. Of the patients in whom PEFR was attempted at least once, only 190 patients (65%) were able to perform adequately. At the beginning of therapy, 54% of eligible patients were able to perform PEFR. Of the 120 patients who were unable to perform initially, 76 had another attempt at the end of ED treatment, of whom 55 (72%) were still unable to perform. A total of 149 patients had attempts at PEFR at both the start and end of treatment; of these, only 71 patients (48%) provided valid information on both attempts. The patients who were unable to perform PEFR were younger than patients who are able to perform successfully and younger than those with no attempts (mean 8.7 ± 2.8 years vs 11.2 ± 3.2 years and 10.0 ± 3.4 years, respectively) (Fig 1). Children admitted to the hospital were more likely to be unable to perform PEFR (46%) than those discharged from the ED (13%).

Conclusions.—It is difficult to obtain adequate peak expiratory flow measurements in children with acute asthma. Treatment and research protocols should not rely exclusively on PEFR for the evaluation of asthma severity in these patients.

▶ PEFR is recommended and accepted as an objective and reproducible measurement of asthma airway obstruction when compared with clinical findings; however, compliance to its use is low. One of the major objections to the use in children is its difficulty to use and teach in the ED. This study enrolled children older than 6 years to determine whether PEFR could be reliably performed while receiving asthma treatment in the ED. There was no consistent pattern regarding which patients had PEFR attempted. Those children who did not have PEFR performed were less likely to be admitted to the hospital (18%, $P =$ .001). Although a significant proportion of patients were unable to perform PEFR properly, as per respiratory therapists, children younger than 10 years had greater difficulty in obtaining a reliable measurement (Fig 1). An additional PEFR attempt did not improve the performance. This study concluded that

PEFR during the treatment of asthma exacerbation in the ED visit is difficult and should not be exclusively used as a marker for severity.

E. C. Quintana, MD, MPH

A Randomized Trial of Nebulized Epinephrine vs Albuterol in the Emergency Department Treatment of Bronchiolitis
Mull CC, Scarfone RJ, Ferri LR, et al (Alfred I du-Pont Hosp for Children, Wilmington, Del; Children's Hosp of Philadelphia; Children's Hosp, Boston; et al)
Arch Pediatr Adolesc Med 158:113-118, 2004   9–22

Background.—The efficacy of inhaled β_2-agonists in infants with bronchiolitis has not been proved, despite their widespread use for bronchodilation in these patients for more than 4 decades. Whether nebulized epinephrine is more efficacious than nebulized albuterol in the ED treatment of moderately ill infants with bronchiolitis was determined.

Methods.—The study included 66 patients age 0 to 12 months with new-onset wheezing, an antecedent upper respiratory tract infection, and a clinical score of 8 to 15 on the Respiratory Distress Assessment Instrument. The patients were randomly assigned to receive either 0.9 mg/kg of nebulized 2.25% racemic epinephrine (34 patients) or 0.15 mg/kg of nebulized 0.5% albuterol sulfate (32 patients) at 0, 30, and 60 minutes. The main outcome measures were clinical score and respiratory rate. The secondary outcome measures were room air oxygen saturation, elapsed time to meeting clinical criteria for ED discharge, hospitalization rate, and proportion of patients relapsed within 72 hours of ED (relapse rate).

Results.—Both treatments showed a similar pattern of change in mean clinical score, respiratory rate, and room air saturation over time, with no significant differences between the groups by these same measures at any time. The median time at which infants were well enough for discharge from the ED was 90 minutes in the epinephrine-treated group versus 120 minutes in the albuterol-treated group. The rate of hospitalization was 47.1% in the epinephrine-treated group versus 37.5% in the albuterol-treated group. The relapse rate was 18.8% in the epinephrine-treated group and 42.1% in the albuterol-treated group. There were few adverse events in either group.

Conclusions.—In a group of infants with bronchiolitis, those patients treated with epinephrine were well enough for ED discharge significantly earlier than the patients treated with albuterol. However, epinephrine was not found to be more efficacious than albuterol in the treatment of moderately ill infants with bronchiolitis.

▶ This prospective, randomized, double-blinded study investigated the efficacy of epinephrine versus albuterol for treatment of moderately ill infants with bronchiolitis. There were no statistically significant differences in hospitalization rate, adverse reactions, or relapse rate between both treatment groups. Interestingly enough, the median time for discharge in the epinephrine group (90 minutes) was less than albuterol. However, the use of epinephrine did not produce any significant clinical benefits over albuterol. Since the publication and preparation of this article, further prospective studies have shown similar findings of early discharge for those infants with bronchiolitis treated with epinephrine. Therefore, one should consider epinephrine as a viable treatment alternative of infants moderately ill with bronchiolitis.

E. C. Quintana, MD, MPH

Meta-analysis of Cephalosporin Versus Penicillin Treatment of Group A Streptococcal Tonsillopharyngitis in Children
Casey JR, Pichichero ME (Univ of Rochester, NY)
Pediatrics 113:866-882, 2004   9–23

Background.—Penicillin has long been the most commonly used antibiotic for group A β-hemolytic streptococcal (GABHS) tonsillopharyngitis. Since the 1980s, however, there have been increasing reports of GABHS resistance to penicillin. Cephalosporins have been successfully used to treat GABHS tonsillopharyngitis since the 1970s. The relative efficacy of these 2 drugs against GABHS tonsillopharyngitis in children was examined in a meta-analysis.

Methods.—Databases (MEDLINE, Embase), relevant reference lists, and meeting abstracts were searched to identify relevant randomized controlled trials. Only trials comparing the efficacy of 10 days of oral cephalosporin versus penicillin in patients younger than 18 years with culture-proven GABHS tonsillopharyngitis were included. Study quality was evaluated according to the Jadad scale. Clinical cure rates and bacteriologic cure rates (as assessed by throat culture) were compared between the 2 drug groups. In addition, the influences of careful clinical illness descriptions, compliance, GABHS serotype, GABHS carriers, and timing of the test-of-cure visit were examined in sensitivity analyses.

Results.—A total of 35 published trials involving 7125 children were included in analyses. The mean quality score was 2.3, and about one third of studies had a Jadad score of greater than 2. The summary odds ratio (OR) for clinical cure (30 studies, 6448 patients) was 2.34 in favor of cephalosporin therapy. The summary OR for bacteriologic cure (all 35 studies) was 3.02 in favor of cephalosporin therapy. When the cephalosporins were analyzed individually, both clinical and bacteriologic cure rates were superior with the first-generation (ORs, 2.36 and 2.41, respectively), the second-generation (ORs, 2.36 and 2.68), and the third-generation (ORs, 3.28 and 3.93) cephalosporins compared with penicillin. Bacteriologic cure rates among these 3 generations of drugs did not differ significantly. Comparing the trials published in the 1970s, 1980s, and 1990s, the bacteriologic cure rate for penicillin tended to decrease over time. In sensitivity analysis, bacteriologic cure rates were significantly better with cephalosporin than with penicillin among the double-blind studies (OR, 2.31), the high-quality trials (Jadad score >2; OR, 2.50), trials with well-defined clinical status (OR, 2.12), trials with detailed compliance monitoring (OR, 2.85), trials with GABHS serotyping (OR, 3.10), trials that excluded GABHS carriers (OR, 2.51), and trials with a test-of-cure 3 to 14 days after treatment (OR, 3.53). Sensitivity analyses of clinical cure rates also consistently showed an advantage for cephalosporins over penicillin.

Conclusion.—The likelihood of clinical and bacteriologic cure is 2 to 3 times greater when an oral cephalosporin is used to treat children with GABHS tonsillopharyngitis.

▶ There has been a diminishing trend of bacterial cure of group A streptococcal pharyngitis using penicillin. This trend has been steady since the mid 1970s. This meta-analysis showed that there is a significant bacteriologic and clinical cure rate using cephalosphorins, regardless of the individual type. However, the studies available for this meta-analysis were poor. Practically speaking, one should consider cephalosporins in treating strep pharyngitis. Cephalosporins may increase compliance (taste, dosing), thus decreasing overall resistance and the carrier state, and improving clinical cure.

E. C. Quintana, MD, MPH

Streptococcal Intertrigo: An Underrecognized Condition in Children
Honig PJ, Frieden IJ, Kim HJ, et al (Univ of Pennsylvania, Philadelphia; Univ of California, San Francisco; Univ of Virginia, Richmond)
Pediatrics 112:1427-1429, 2003   9–24

Background.—Group A β-hemolytic streptococci (GABHS) cause several widely known skin infections. Less well known is the streptococcal skin infection GABHS intertrigo, an underrecognized cause of intertriginous eruptions. The typical presentation and clinical course of GABHS intertrigo in 3 patients were described.

Patients and Findings.—The 3 patients were 2 girls and 1 boy, aged 3 months, 5 months, and 5 months, respectively. The condition manifested as intense, fiery-red erythema and maceration in the intertriginous folds of the neck, axillae, or inguinal spaces. Also characteristic were a distinctive foul

---

TABLE 2.—Distinguishing Features of Candidal and GABHS Intertrigo

	Intertriginous Location	Presence of Satellites	Foul Odor	Typical Treatment
Candidal Intertrigo	Yes	Common	Rare	Topical nystatin or triazole (clotrimazole, econazole)
GABHS Intertrigo	Yes	Rare	Common	Topical mupirocin oral penicillin or cephalexin; topical hydrocortisone 1%

Abbreviation: GABHS, Group A β-hemolytic streptococci.
(Courtesy of Honig PJ, Frieden IJ, Kim HJ, et al: Streptococcal intertrigo: An underrecognized condition in children. *Pediatrics* 112:1427-1429, 2003. Reproduced by permission of *Pediatrics*. Copyright 2003 by the American Academy of Pediatrics.)

odor and an absence of satellite lesions. Specific clinical features were identified that help differentiate GABHS intertrigo from other conditions that mimic it (Table 2). In all patients, topical and oral antibiotic treatment with or without concomitant low-potency topical steroid application was successful.

Conclusions.—A variety of common childhood cutaneous infections result from GABHS. Infants and young children may be especially susceptible to GABHS intertrigo, an underrecognized condition in this patient population.

▶ Intertrigo is created when opposing skin folds are irritated by trapped moisture and friction. Young infants with their short and chubby necks are particularly susceptible. It may present as intensely red erythema and macerated skin, without any satellite lesions, in the folds of the neck, axillae, and inguinal area. There are several bacterial superinfections that should be considered when faced with this presentation: group A streptococci, *Staphylococcus aureus*, *Pseudomonas*, *Proteus* spp, and *Candida albicans*. A distinct and foul odor on examination suggests group A streptococcal intertrigo. Streptococcal intertrigo has been underdiagnosed in contrast to candidal intertrigo. Successful treatment with topical mupirocin and oral penicillin with confirmatory cultures of the affected areas can most clearly distinguish between these 2 common pathogens.

E. C. Quintana, MD, MPH

Pseudotumor Cerebri in Children With Sickle Cell Disease: A Case Series
Henry M, Driscoll MC, Miller M, et al (Children's Natl Med Ctr, Washington, DC)
Pediatrics 113:e265-e269, 2004   9–25

Background.—Sickle cell disease (SCD) is a hereditary hemoglobin disorder that affects 1 in 400 African American births. Pseudotumor cerebri (PC), or benign intracranial hypertension, is characterized by increased intracranial pressure in the absence of a space-occupying lesion or obstruction to the CSF pathway. PC has been reported to be associated with various forms of anemia. Three cases of PC in association with SCD were reported.

Case Report.—Girl, 9½ years, who had SCD-SC and was obese, presented with a worsening headache, blurred vision, and photophobia of 3 days' duration. She had no fever or signs of head trauma, and there was no family history of headache or migraine. Neuroimaging studies were negative. Her headaches were treated with nonsteroidal and narcotic medications, but she was seen again after 6 months with worsening symptoms. Ophthalmologic examination found bilateral papilledema, sluggish pupils, and bilateral blind-spot enlargement. Lumbar puncture revealed an opening pressure of 44.5 cm H_2O. PC was diagnosed and acetazolamide was prescribed. She has been using acetazolamide for 10 months, but her opening pressure remains high.

Discussion.—All 3 patients with SCD and PC had an elevated opening pressure during lumbar puncture. Results of neuroimaging studies were negative in all cases. Bilateral papilledema was detected in all 3 patients. Symptoms in 2 patients disappeared completely with administration of acetazolamide, whereas 1 patient had symptom improvement. None of the patients had permanent visual field deficits.

Conclusions.—Complaints of severe headache among patients with SCD may be related to PC. These patients should have neuroimaging to rule out other causes of headache and should be evaluated by both a neurologist and an ophthalmologist. PC responds well to carbonic anhydrase inhibitors, but these drugs must be used with caution in patients with SCD.

▶ Patients with SCD can present with many complaints, but headache is a concerning one. It could be attributable to anemia or cerebrovascular disease; however, this article reported 3 cases in which PC was diagnosed. All cases presented with headache and changes in vision, most commonly blurry vision. Lumbar puncture opening pressures were between 29 and 44.5 cm H_2O (normal, ≤ 20 cm H_2O). CT, MR angiography, and MRI showed no evidence of thrombosis or vessel abnormalities. Improvement of symptoms was achieved with acetazolamide orally.

PC is a condition that presents with headache, papilledema, diplopia (caused by cranial nerve VI palsy), and altered visual and light perception. Even though symptoms may spontaneously resolve, treatment with acetazolamide or furosemide is successful in most cases. Acetazolamide should be used with caution in children with SCD because it may potentiate the effects of dehydration in sickled red blood cells. Lumbar puncture is therapeutic in the short term. There is an association with obesity, but the real relationship is not clear. PC has been reported in several medical conditions, including anemia, and now, SCD. These cases remind us that other etiologies, such as PC, should be considered when facing a child with SCD who presents with severe headache.

E. C. Quintana, MD, MPH

A Randomized, Placebo-controlled Trial of the Effect of Antihistamine or Corticosteroid Treatment in Acute Otitis Media
Chonmaitree T, Saeed K, Uchida T, et al (Univ of Texas, Galveston)
J Pediatr 143:377-385, 2003   9–26

Introduction.—The most frequent reason for antibiotic prescription in the United States is childhood acute otitis media (AOM). Treatment failures and recurrent infections, along with persistent effusions, remain common. Treatment with adjunctive drugs antihistamine and corticosteroid was evaluated to determine whether these agents can improve immediate and long-term outcomes in patients with AOM.

Methods.—The study included 179 children with AOM, 3 months to 6 years old, who were at risk for recurrent AOM episodes. All children received 1 dose of IM ceftriaxone and then were selected randomly in a double-blind placebo-controlled trial to treatment for 5 days with either chlorpheniramine maleate (0.35 mg/kg per day) or prednisolone (2 mg/kg per day) or both or placebo. The primary outcome measures were rate of treatment failure during the first 2 weeks, duration of middle ear effusion, and incidence of recurrences of AOM to 6 months.

Results.—Clinical outcomes and recurrence rates did not vary significantly with the type of treatment. Children who received antihistamine alone experienced a longer duration of middle ear effusion (median, 73 days), compared to that experienced by participants in other treatment groups (median, 23-36 days; $P = .04$). Temporary normalization of tympanometric findings on day 5 occurred more often in the corticosteroid-treated group ($P = .04$).

Conclusion.—Five-day treatment with antihistamine or corticosteroid, in addition to antibiotic, did not benefit AOM outcomes. Antihistamine treatment during an acute episode of AOM is not recommended because it may prolong the duration of middle ear effusion. The efficacy of 7- to 10-day treatment of AOM with corticosteroid, in addition to antibiotic, should undergo further investigation.

▶ One of the most common reasons for use of oral antibiotics is AOM. Recurrence, failure, and chronic effusions are also common. Concurrent bacterial and viral infections can induce the production of histamine and leukotrienes—powerful inflammatory mediators. This study evaluated the improvement of AOM by reducing the initial degree of inflammation using antihistamines and oral corticosteroids. AOM was diagnosed by signs, symptoms, and pneumatic otoscopy to identify middle ear effusion. This study showed no benefit to a 5-day course of antihistamine and/or corticosteroids in the immediate- or long-term treatment of AOM. It was found that antihistamines actually lengthened the duration of the middle ear effusion. The use of corticosteroids had a "rebound effect" by reaccumulating the middle ear effusion, after an initial reduction of fluid. For now, this practice is not supported by clinical studies. Further studies may be warranted before we use antihistamine and corticosteroids with antibiotics for the treatment of AOM.

E. C. Quintana, MD, MPH

Parental Presence During Invasive Procedures in Children: What Is the Physician's Perspective?
Waseem M, Ryan M (Lincoln Med and Mental Health Ctr, Bronx, NY)
South Med J 96:884-887, 2003   9–27

Background.—Parental presence during care of children in the ED can reduce both parental and children's anxiety, but remains controversial among

ED staff. Physicians' views on parental presence during procedures in the ED were investigated in an ED-based observational study.

Study Design.—A questionnaire was sent to the directors of 80 EDs with pediatric or emergency medicine residencies or pediatric emergency medicine fellowship training programs to determine whether parents were present during procedures, as well as their opinions regarding the presence of parents and the effect it had on performance and training of physicians.

Findings.—The response rate to the survey was 77%. More than 87% of physicians allowed parents to be present during simple procedures, but were less likely during more invasive procedures. Less than half of all physicians encouraged parental presence, and 25% discouraged it for all procedures. Almost one third left it to the parents to decide. About 22% found parental presence a distraction, and 12% reported that it made them nervous. Less than half found parental presence helpful. General pediatricians were less likely to encourage parental presence than emergency medicine physicians.

Conclusions.—Most physicians in the ED appear to be comfortable with parental presence during simple procedures, but they are less comfortable during invasive procedures. Physician training also appears to play a role in physician comfort level with parental presence during procedures in the ED.

▶ Despite the increased attention to parental presence during ED invasive procedures, it remains a controversial topic among ED medical staff. This observational survey study asked each department their opinion regarding the presence of parents during a variety of procedures. Physicians were also asked if parental presence had any effect on them.

The results were interesting. Less than half of physicians (41%) encourage, and 25% discourage parental presence during any invasive procedure. Emergency medicine and pediatric emergency medicine physicians were found to encourage parental presence in 56% of cases, in contrast to 20% of pediatricians. Forty-six percent of physicians thought that parents were helpful during the procedure. The other 54% found that parents were distracting, made them nervous, or were not helpful at all.

A more interesting question would have been if physicians' perspectives change based on the invasive procedure being performed and their level of proficiency. For example, if a simple laceration was done, would the physician be more comfortable with the parents being around to help calm the child? In contrast, more intense procedures such as resuscitation would increase both parental and physicians' anxiety. Moreover, no matter how many times parents have seen blood and gory scenes on TV, sometimes it is difficult to predict how they will react to such circumstances.

This study suggests that parental presence during pediatric invasive procedures aids in decreasing the anxiety level in both parents and children alike. In addition, prior physicians' training appears to influence their level of comfort regarding parental presence.

E. C. Quintana, MD, MPH

Do Children Require Hospitalization After Immediate Posttraumatic Seizures?

Holmes JF, Palchak MJ, Conklin MJ, et al (Univ of California-Davis, Sacramento)

Ann Emerg Med 43:706-710, 2004   9–28

Background.—Blunt head trauma is not uncommon in children and is associated with posttraumatic seizures. Most children with minor head trauma have a normal cranial CT but are frequently hospitalized for observation. Whether children with immediate posttraumatic seizure require hospitalization for neurologic observation was investigated in a prospective, observational cohort study.

Study Design.—This study was conducted at an urban Level I trauma center from September 1998 to September 2001. Pediatric patients were eligible for inclusion if they had immediate posttraumatic seizure after blunt head trauma and before ED observation. Data recorded included history, physical examination findings, level of consciousness, and interpretation of CT scans. Patients were followed up in hospital and for at least 1 week after discharge for seizures, neurologic deterioration, and need for neurosurgical intervention.

Results.—During the study period, 2043 children with blunt head trauma were admitted to the ED. Of these children, only 63 (3%) had immediate posttraumatic seizures. These 63 children were 3 to 14 years old and had a median Glasgow Coma Score (GCS) at admittance of 15. Traumatic injuries were detected on cranial CT scans of 10 patients. These 10 patients had a median GCS of 8 and all were hospitalized for a median of 6.5 days. Three had neurosurgical procedures and 2 had repeated seizures. The remaining patients had normal CT scans. Of these patients, 20 were hospitalized for a median of 1.5 days, and the rest were sent home. None of the patients with normal CT scans had further seizures, neurologic deterioration, or neurosurgery.

Conclusions.—Children with immediate posttraumatic seizures and abnormalities of cranial CT scans require hospitalization and neurosurgical consultation. Children who have normal cranial CT scans and neurologic examinations are at low risk for neurologic complications and may be considered for discharge.

▶ This prospective observational cohort study of children younger than 18 years evaluated those who had an immediate posttraumatic seizure after blunt head trauma. Only 63 of 2043 children with blunt head trauma had an immediate seizure. Ninety-eight percent underwent head CT with 16% showing a traumatic brain injury. The most common traumatic injury found was subdural hematoma, followed by depressed skull fracture. All 10 patients with traumatic brain injury on head CT had abnormal GCS score (median score, 8). Eighty-four percent of patients had normal head CT of whom 38% were hospitalized for observation. Only 3 of 20 hospitalized patients had persistent abnormalities in mental status. None of the 20 patients had repeated seizures. Most of the patients discharged home from ED were followed up and reported no further seizures or neurologic/neurosurgical deterioration. This study suggests that children with immediate posttraumatic seizures, a normal head CT, and normal neurologic examination appear to be at low risk for further complications and may not require hospitalization.

E. C. Quintana, MD, MPH

How Much Tachycardia in Infants Can Be Attributed to Fever?
Hanna CM, Greenes DS (Harvard Med School, Boston)
Ann Emerg Med 43:699-705, 2004   9–29

Background.—It is widely believed that pulse rate increases with temperature in young children, yet this topic has not been well studied. Because increased temperature is only 1 of many conditions that can cause tachycardia, the relationship between fever and pulse rate should be better understood. The relationship between naturally occurring fever and pulse rate in children less than 1 year old who came to the ED of Children's Hospital in Boston was analyzed.

Study Design.—From July to December 2001, children less than 1 year old who were brought to the ED had simultaneous rectal temperature and pulse rate assessment. Those children with evident reasons for tachycardia in addition to fever or those who were not calm were excluded from the analysis, leaving a remainder of 490 children for inclusion in the study. The participants were divided into six 2-month-age categories. Linear regression analyses of pulse rate and temperature were performed for each age group.

Results.—For all children older than 2 months, pulse rate increased linearly with increasing temperature, an average of 9.6 beats/min per temperature increase of 1°C. For any temperature, the prediction interval for pulse rate had a 64 beats/min range.

Conclusions.—For children, 2 months to 1 year old, the pulse rate increases linearly with body temperature, although individual pulse rates vary widely. For children less than 2 months old, a linear relationship can not be established.

▶ There are many medical conditions, which could cause tachycardia: hypovolemia, bacterial infection/sepsis, cardiomyopathy, medications, anemia, hypoxia, endocrine, dysrhythmia, and behavioral state. We are taught that fever will increase your child's heart rate; however, there has been sparse clinical data to support such teachings. This study showed that one should expect an increase of almost 10 beats/min for each 1°C in body temperature in children older than 2 months. In infants younger than 2 months, the authors were unable to determine a good linear relationship. It is possible that the immaturity of their autonomic system precludes this association.

E. C. Quintana, MD, MPH

The Use of Restraint for Pediatric Psychiatric Patients in Emergency Departments

Dorfman DH, Kastner B (Boston Univ; Yeshiva Univ, Bronx, NY)

Pediatr Emerg Care 20:151-156, 2004   9–30

Background.—Restraint, either physical or chemical, is a common intervention used to prevent patients from harming themselves or others. The use of restraint for pediatric patients in EDs has not been well characterized. The current pediatric restraint policy in facilities with emergency medicine residencies (EMRs) and in those with pediatric emergency medicine fellowships (PEMFs) was investigated.

Study Design.—A survey was sent to directors of EMRs and PEMFs. Frequency of restraint, staff training, favored positions for physical restraint, and chemical agents used for restraint were assessed.

Findings.—The survey was completed by 41% of EMRs and 66% of PEMFs. The majority of EMRs and PEMFs reported using restraint on pediatric patients infrequently (<5% of patients). The majority had formal policies on physical restraint, but less than half had formal policies on chemical restraint. The majority did not teach their trainees about restraint, although EMRs were more likely than PEMFs to perform restraint training. The supine position was favored for physical restraint, although therapeutic holding was occasionally used for younger children. The majority of EMRs and PEMFs used chemical restraint. The most common agents used were benzodiazepines and butyrophenones, although butyrophenones were often misclassified as phenothiazines.

Conclusions.—Physical and chemical restraints are widely, but infrequently, used in EDs for pediatric patients. Most EDs have a restraint policy, but residents and fellows do not receive training in appropriate restraint use. Chemical restraint agents used for children are similar to those used for adults.

▶ Chemical or physical restraints are options that could be used to prevent patients from harming themselves or others. Even though their use may be idiosyncratic to each institution, the use and safety of restraints have not been studied extensively in children and adolescents. This survey included directors of emergency medicine residencies and pediatric emergency medicine fellowships. The use of physical restraints was more prevalent than the use of chemical restraints. Policies pertaining to physical restraints were more common than those for chemical. Emergency medicine programs were more likely to teach their residents about the appropriate use of restraints in comparison to pediatric emergency medicine fellowships. Most nurses, as a whole, received training in restraints compared to the training of other groups of hospital personnel, including physicians and security.

The current practices of restraints for children and adolescents were as follows. The supine position was favored for physical restraint in all age groups; however, the use of the prone position increased with increasing age. The most common chemical restraint medications used were benzodiazepines and butyrophenones, which are the same type of medications most commonly used in adults. In contrast, the responses in this survey noted that many felt that the use of chemical restraints presented more risks and was more intrusive than physical restraints. As a result, many of the respondents did not chemically restrain children.

This article brings to our attention several facts. First, it is encouraging that these restraints are infrequently used and that there are policies for their use. Second, training in the use of restraints is very limited. This is an area that should be remedied. Third, the medications used for chemical restraints for children and adolescents are similar to those used for adults.

E. C. Quintana, MD, MPH

Visual, Tactile, and Phobic Hallucinations: Recognition and Management in the Emergency Department
Pao M, Lohman C, Gracey D, et al (Children's Natl Med Ctr, Washington, DC; George Washington Univ, Washington, DC)
Pediatr Emerg Care 20:30-34, 2004   9–31

Background.—Physicians in the ED may have to make a differential diagnosis of hallucinations in young children. Amongst the possibilities are visual, tactile, and phobic hallucinations (VTPH) caused by anxiety. A chart review of 10 children who had VTPH during a 24-month period at a single institution was performed, and the case of 1 child representing a prototype of all the cases reviewed is presented.

> *Case Report.*—Girl, 5 years, awoke at 2:45 AM complaining of seeing, feeling, and hearing bugs and bees on her pillow. All medications in the house were out of reach and childproof. A review of symptoms was noncontributory. A physical examination, including neurologic examination, was normal. She was not reassured by attempts to show her nothing was there. A psychiatry consultation found her to be agitated but oriented. No other obsessions, compulsions or pho-

---

TABLE 2.—Classic Profile of Children With VTPH

Young age
Alert, without sensorium changes
Afebrile
Symptoms most prominent at night
Able to convey complaints clearly
Frantic attempts to remove insects, snakes
Child's fear not alleviated by reassurance
Child's fear not amenable to reason
Supportive and appropriately concerned families
No history of abuse, medication reaction, or ingestion
Normal physical examination

(Courtesy of Pao M, Lohman C, Gracey D, et al: Visual, tactile, and phobic hallucinations: Recognition and management in the emergency department. *Pediatr Emerg Care* 20:30-34, 2004.)

bias were noted. Her appetite was fine, and she had been doing well at school. The patient was discharged in 2 days after symptomatic improvement and no recurrences have since occurred.

Conclusions.—Children with VTPH are preschool to early school age; present at night with tactile, visual, and phobic hallucinations, and have no evidence of CNS involvement, fever, ingestion or drug reactions (Table 2). VTPH is a diagnosis of exclusion. Once other causes are eliminated, a child psychiatric consultation can provide the support and reassurance to avoid unnecessary testing and hospitalization.

▶ Hallucinations are well described in the pediatric medical literature. They are often related to a variety of reasons: medication/toxin reactions, high fever, stress/traumatic event or CNS infection. There is a subset of pediatric patients that fit the VTPH. VTPH is a diagnosis of exclusion.

These children need to be screened carefully, for other diagnoses could present as VTPH. For example, visual and tactile hallucinations have been also found in children taking over-the-counter medications, such as decongestants. Children with night terrors present after waking up in the middle of the night with inconsolable crying or screaming, and do not remember the entire event. In contrast, children with VTPH recall the event with detail. Another consideration should be Munchausen's by proxy, in which children have an extensive history of frequent doctor visits, hospitalizations, and procedures/tests. Once all possible underlying causes for these hallucinations have been ruled out, child psychiatry should be involved to provide appropriate support for these children and their families.

E. C. Quintana, MD, MPH

Use of Dosage as a Triage Guideline for Unintentional Cyclic Antidepressant (UCA) Ingestions in Children
Spiller HA, Baker SD, Krenzelok EP, et al (Kentucky Regional Poison Ctr, Louisville; Texas Poison Ctr System, Temple; Univ of Pittsburgh, Pa; et al)
Am J Emerg Med 21:422-424, 2003   9–32

Background.—Pediatric unintentional cyclic antidepressant (UCA) ingestion is a common problem. No commonly accepted triage guidelines for these cases have been reported. A retrospective multicenter case series evaluation was performed for all UCA ingestions among children 6 years old and younger from 1998 through 2000 to develop triage guidelines.

Study Design.—The study group included 246 patients, 7 months to 6 years old, who had ingested a known dose of a single drug, and whose outcome was known. Definitions for outcome were from the Toxic Exposure Surveillance System (TESS). Ingested dose, treatment and outcome were compared for this study group.

Findings.—Of the 246 patients, 136 (55%) were managed in the hospital and 110 (45%) were managed at home. The symptoms included drowsiness, tachycardia, agitation, coma, respiratory depression, and ataxia. The majority of ingestions produced little or no symptoms. The medical outcome was reported as no effect in 75%, minor effect in 23%, moderate effect in 1% and major effect in 1%. The average dosage without an effect was 2.9 mg/kg and with an effect was 6.3 mg/kg. Of those patients with minor symptoms, 75% reported a dose of less than 5 mg/kg. All patients with moderate to major effects reported a dose of more than 5 mg/kg.

Conclusions.—Unintentional cyclic antidepressant ingestions are common among young children, but the majority produce little or no symptoms. Only minor effects were seen in those children who ingested less than 5 mg/ kg. Home monitoring might be appropriate for these children.

▶ Ingestions are a common occurrence in children, especially unintentional ones. Triage guidelines for accidental cyclic antidepressants are not in existence. These ingestions are not without risk—thus, the initial recommendation of an ED evaluation for 6 hours of observation. However, there was a small study in which asymptomatic children with ingestions of less than 5mg/kg could be observed safely at home.[1] This multicenter study used data that included a larger number of children. The ingested amount was known. Of the patients (45%) that were observed at home with a known ingestion of less than 5 mg/kg, only 78% were asymptomatic. Those children who had a major outcome had an ingestion of more than 5 mg/kg. However, it would be wise to recommend ED evaluation when the amount ingested is unknown or when polydrug ingestion is suspected.

E. C. Quintana, MD, MPH

Reference

1. McFee RB, Caraccio TR, Mofenson HC: Selected trycyclic antidepressant ingestions involving children 6 years old or less. *Acad Emerg Med* 8:139-144, 2001.

Development of a Clinical Severity Score for Preseptal Cellulitis in Children
Vu BLL, Dick PT, Levin AV, et al (Univ of Toronto)
Pediatr Emerg Care 19:302-307, 2003   9–33

Background.—Preseptal cellulitis is an infection anterior to the orbital septum, which usually responds to antibiotics. Whether IV antibiotic therapy is necessary is not always clear. The development of an objective clinical scale, the Severity Index (SI), as an outcome measure for the evaluation of treatment options for preseptal cellulitis is discussed.

Study Design.—A panel of 4 physicians from different specialties generated a list of clinical features that could contribute to the assessment of severity of preseptal cellulitis. The clinical relevance of these different clinical features was analyzed by reviewing the published literature and establishing several domains most often used to describe the disease. The clinical features

TABLE 1.—Severity Index for Preseptal Cellulitis in Children

Systemic Features	Category Score		
	0	2	4
Interaction	Alert, smiles	Sleepy but rousable, cries but consolable	Persistently irritable, distressed, or lethargic
Fever	Normal	<39.0°C	>39.0°C

Local Features	Category Score		
	0	1	2
Location	One lid	Two lids	Beyond brow
Erythema	Minimal	Red	Ecchymotic
Extent	Lids open	Opens lids with effort	Unable to open lids
Pain and tenderness	None	Tender to touch	Constant

Note: Total score is simple summation of all categories (maximum 16).
(Courtesy of Vu BLL, Dick PT, Levin AV, et al: Development of a clinical severity score for preseptal cellulitis in children *Pediatr Emerg Care* 19: 302-307, 2003.)

were divided into systemic and local features. As there were more local items, those in the systemic domain were double-weighted. This became the Severity Index (SI) (Table 1). The validity and reliability of the SI was investigated by prospective evaluation of 17 children with preseptal cellulitis. The accuracy of the SI was compared with that of a Global Score that was based on clinical impression.

Results.—The average SI was 2.0 for patients treated exclusively with oral antibiotics and 6.0 for patients treated with IV antibiotics. The SI correlated well with the Global Score. After 24 hours of treatment, the SI was significantly less than before treatment initiation. The agreement between paired SI scores was higher than the agreement between paired Global Scores.

Conclusions.—The development of a pediatric Severity Index for preseptal cellulitis to objectively evaluate clinical status and disease severity over time is discussed. The SI is reliable and valid, with good discriminatory ability and responsiveness to status changes. The SI should be useful for clinical decision making and for assessing the outcome of clinical trials.

▶ The development of an accurate scoring system would allow the development of algorithms, thus providing evidence to determine those children who can safely be discharged for outpatient antibiotic treatment versus those who could not. In this article, a scale was constructed using items seen retrospectively in patients for 1 year. Then, the scale validity and reliability was tested in a prospective cohort group of children between 1 and 16 years old. Those patients who had a severity score of 6.0 were treated with IV antibiotics, whereas those with a score of 2.0 had oral antibiotics. There was a strong correlation. The items used (Table 1) in this severity score scale are a useful tool for evaluating children with preseptal cellulitis.

E. C. Quintana, MD, MPH

The Value of Capnography During Sedation or Sedation/Analgesia in Pediatric Minor Procedures

Yildizdaş D, Yapicioğlu H, Yilmaz HL (Cukurova Univ, Adana, Turkey)
Pediatr Emerg Care 20:162-165, 2004   9–34

Background.—Capnography is used to monitor ventilatory status of intubated patients during anesthesia. The use of capnography during sedation or analgesia for minor pediatric surgical procedures is described. Changes in end-tidal CO_2 levels ($ETCO_2$) associated with the use of different sedation/analgesia strategies are also discussed.

Study Design.—A prospective, randomized clinical trial of 126 pediatric patients who required sedation/analgesia for minor procedures between September 2000 and February 2002 was done. Patients were assigned randomly to ketamine (group K), midazolam (group M), ketamine plus midazolam (group KM), midazolam plus fentanyl (group MF), or propofol (group P). Nasal cannula $ETCO_2$ tracings were recorded on a capnograph before medication and continuing until the patient was awake. The primary outcome was the difference between peak $ETCO_2$ before and during sedation/analgesia.

Results.—Only in the MF and P groups was the average $ETCO_2$ during sedation/analgesia significantly higher than the presedation and postsedation average $ETCO_2$. Of the patients in this series, 21 had respiratory depression or hypoxia, 21 had hypercarbia, and 4 had both.

Conclusions.—Propofol and midazolam plus fentanyl produced a greater incidence of respiratory depression than other forms of sedation/analgesia used for minor pediatric surgery. Capnography effectively provided an early indication of respiratory depression in clinically stable children.

▶ This article supports further use of adjuvant equipment, such as a capnometer, during procedural sedation. It was able to detect hypercapnia in 16.6% of patients. Still, none of these patients were clinically cyanotic, apneic, or unstable. Most of them responded positively to stimuli or oxygen supplementation via cannula for a few minutes. Unfortunately, there was no follow-up or comment to describe whether there were any long-term complications or poor outcomes due to these short episodes of hypercapnia or hypoxia in these children. This is the really interesting question in any procedural sedation. Despite capnometry being useful, the authors of this study noted some technical difficulties with the malposition of the nasal cannula capnometry probe. This is not an uncommon complaint with capnometry. This article reiterates that fact that adjuvant-monitoring tools are always useful, as long as we are aware of the potential technical difficulties that each tool has.

E. C. Quintana, MD, MPH

Apparent Life-Threatening Events in Infants: High Risk in the Out-of-Hospital Environment

Stratton SJ, Taves A, Lewis RJ, et al (Univ of California, Los Angeles; Univ of Southern California, Los Angeles)
Ann Emerg Med 43:711-717, 2004   9–35

Background.—An apparent life-threatening event (ALTE) is defined as an episode that frightens an observer and is characterized by apnea, skin color change, changes in muscle tone, or unexplained choking or gagging in young children. These symptoms have usually dissipated by the time EMS personnel arrive. The demographic characteristics, clinical characteristics, and outcomes were retrospectively determined for a population of infants with ALTEs and for whom an ambulance in an urban EMS system was requested.

Study Design.—The study population consisted of 60 patients younger than 1 year with ALTEs for whom Los Angeles EMS personnel were contacted during January and February 2000. All EMS personnel had been trained in recognition and response to ALTEs. EMS providers prospectively recorded their assessment of physical distress and level of concern about the patient. The EMS prospective assessment was compared with etiologies, diagnoses, and outcomes determined at discharge.

Findings.—Infants who met inclusion criteria had an average age of 3.1 months, and 55% were boys. When EMS providers arrived, 83.3% of the infants appeared to be in no distress, 13.3% were in mild distress, and 3.3% were in moderate distress. Overall, physical appearance, breathing, circulatory signs, respiratory rate, and pulse rate were not abnormal. Almost half of these patients had significant or even life-threatening illnesses, including pneumonia or bronchiolitis, seizures, sepsis, intracranial hemorrhage, bacterial meningitis, dehydration, and severe anemia.

Conclusions.—Even when evaluations by EMS providers appear normal, out-of-hospital ALTEs can be associated with serious illness or injury. Each of these pediatric patients should receive a thorough medical evaluation as rapidly as possible.

▶ This retrospective, outcome-focused, cohort study evaluated the incidence of ALTEs encountered by EMS providers over a 2-month period. The EMS system responded to 804 calls about infants, of which 7.5% met study criteria for ALTEs. Eighty-three percent of infants appeared to be in no distress when evaluated by EMS personnel. The final diagnostic outcomes most commonly found were respiratory (pneumonia, bronchiolitis) or gastrointestinal reflux. Other diagnoses included intracranial bleed caused by shaken baby syndrome, anemia, meningitis, and seizure. Only half of those infants diagnosed with final significant conditions had an abnormal EMS evaluation. Therefore, once there is an EMS call, the signs and symptoms should be considered credible, even when they do not match the observation or clinical impression of EMS personnel. All infants should receive an ED evaluation. Education and monitoring of EMS personnel regarding this deceptively "benign" disease—ALTEs—should be implemented.

E. C. Quintana, MD, MPH

▶ Perhaps this is another demonstration that mother knows best. The high incidence of infants with serious medical problems who, after a caregiver-witnessed apparent ALTE, appeared to be in no distress at the time they were assessed by EMS personnel is concerning. Although this study was small and retrospective, it serves as a reminder to both prehospital providers and emergency physicians of the need for transport and thorough evaluation of infants with a caregiver-witnessed out-of-hospital ALTE.

S. L. Werner, MD

ED Evaluation of Infants After an Apparent Life-Threatening Event
de Piero AD, Teach SJ, Chamberlain JM (George Washington Univ, Washington, DC)
Am J Emerg Med 22:83-86, 2004   9–36

Background.—After an apparently life-threatening event (ALTE), infants often are brought to the ED. The usefulness of the ED in the diagnosis and treatment of these infants was assessed.

Methods.—A retrospective chart review was performed at an urban, tertiary care children's hospital from 1994 through 1998. Inclusion criteria included a history of either apnea monitor alarm or an episode associated with at least 2 of the following conditions: apnea, color change, muscle tone change, choking/gagging, or cardiopulmonary resuscitation. Medical records were abstracted for each patient. A diagnostic intervention was considered part of the ED evaluation if it was ordered in the ED or within the first 6 hours of hospital admission. A positive ED evaluation was the result of an ED diagnostic intervention that resulted in a specific treatment for a defined condition.

Results.—The 5-year study period included 253,408 pediatric patient visits to the ED. The study definition for an ALTE was met by 150 patients. The average age of these patients was 61.7 days, and more than three fourths were admitted to the hospital. Of these patients, 122 had ED diagnostic tests, and 3 positive ED evaluations were done. None of these patients were discharged. Significant medical interventions occurred for 7% of patients. Risk factors for significant interventions included prematurity, positive medical history, and age greater than 60 days.

Conclusions.—The overall rate of positive ED diagnostic evaluations or significant medical interventions is low after an ALTE of infancy. Many of these pediatric patients can be managed with a limited ED diagnostic evaluation followed by observation.

▶ The evaluation of an infant with an ALTE in the ED is common. ALTE is defined as any episode that is frightening to the observer, which has some combination of central or obstructive apnea, color change (commonly, cyanosis), marked muscle tone changes, choking or gagging. It is not uncommon to have as the parental chief complaint fears that the child almost/had died. This study provided further evidence that admission is warranted for children with ALTE; however, the ED diagnostic evaluation in itself is limited. ED tests should be focused, based on the patient's history and physical examination. Cases in this study suggested that prematurity was a risk factor for a significant ED and in-patient evaluation. As another example, this study had several cases where the history and physical examination (H&P) dictated an initiation of treatment in the ED: pertussis (treated with antibiotics), hypoglycemia secondary to di-arrhea (treated with IV glucose), and anemia (treated with several blood trans-fusions). In conclusion, ALTE diagnostic evaluation should be guided by H&P to determine which ED tests need to be ordered, but for the most part, ED evaluation is limited, and in-patient observation and workup is warranted.

E. C. Quintana, MD, MPH

Risk Factors for Emesis After Therapeutic Use of Activated Charcoal in Acutely Poisoned Children
Osterhoudt KC, Durbin D, Alpern ER, et al (Children's Hosp, Philadelphia; Poison Control Ctr, Philadelphia; Univ of Pennsylvania, Philadelphia)
Pediatrics 113:806-810, 2004   9–37

Introduction.—Activated charcoal is often administered to acutely poisoned patients, but vomiting can complicate the effectiveness of this treatment. Some clinicians use antiemetic strategies to reduce the incidence of vomiting. A knowledge of the risk factors associated with vomiting after the administration of activated charcoal might help to identify pediatric patients who would benefit from antiemetic agents. The incidence of vomiting after administration of antiemetics was investigated.

Methods.—The prospective cohort included 275 consecutive patients, 18 years old or younger, who were seen in the ED of a large, tertiary-care children's hospital between January 13, 1998, and July 11, 2000. All received activated charcoal (1 g/kg to a maximum of 50 g) as part of the therapeutic regimen for an acute poisoning exposure. The activated charcoal alternated on an every 2-week basis between preparations with and without sorbitol. Potential risk factors investigated were classified as patient-, poison-, or procedure-specific.

Results.—Fifty-six patients (20.4%) vomited after treatment with activated charcoal, and 55.4% of those who vomited did so before the entire dose of charcoal was administered. The median time between charcoal administration and vomiting was 10 minutes. Significant, independent risk factors for vomiting were previous vomiting (relative risk [RR], 3.41) and nasogastric tube administration (RR, 2.40). Children older than 12 years were more likely to vomit than were younger children, a trend that approached significance. The risk of vomiting was not significantly affected by

TABLE 3.—Unadjusted, Dichotomous, Univariate Estimation of RR of Vomiting Given the Presence of Specific Risk Factors (χ^2 Analysis)

Risk Factor	Prevalence in Study Sample	RR for Vomiting	95% CI
Nausea	9.8%	3.1	1.9-4.8
Previous vomiting	13.5%	3.1	1.9-4.7
Symptomatic poisoning	24.4%	1.7	1.1-2.6
Age >12 y	28.7%	1.6	1.0-2.6
Naso- or orogastric tube administration	42.6%	1.5	0.9-2.3
Emetogenic poison	11.3%	1.5	0.8-2.8
Agitation/crying	27.6%	1.5	0.9-2.4
Intestinal motility-slowing poisons	27.3%	1.4	0.8-2.2
Sorbitol	50.2%	1.3	0.8-2.1
Female gender	47.6%	1.3	0.8-2.0
Reclined position	39.3%	1.3	0.8-2.0
Flavoring agents	42.2%	1.2	0.7-1.9
Physical restraint	34.2%	1.2	0.7-1.9
Depressed consciousness	10.6%	1.0	0.5-2.2
Large charcoal volume	*	0.9	0.5-1.8
Short charcoal administration time	*	0.7	0.4-1.4

Note: Risk factors with less than 5% incidence within study population for which RR data are not provided: infectious symptoms, sedative and/or paralytic administration, antiemetic administration, ipecac use, and chronic gastrointestinal illness.
*Comparison of upper versus lower quartiles.
Abbreviation: RR, Relative risk.
(Courtesy of Osterhoudt KC, Durbin D, Alpern ER, et al: Risk factors for emesis after therapeutic use of activated charcoal in acutely poisoned children. *Pediatrics* 113:806-810, 2004. Copyright 2004. Reproduced with permission.)

sorbitol content of the charcoal, volume of charcoal, or rate of administration (Table 3).

Conclusion.—Administration of activated charcoal has largely replaced gastric emptying as the treatment for poisoning in children. However, vomiting often occurs, reducing the amount of poison adsorbed, increasing the possibility of pulmonary aspiration, and making the therapeutic experience unpleasant. The strongest risk factor for vomiting after charcoal administration is a history of vomiting. This factor and use of a naso- or orogastric tube should be considered in the decision to offer adjuvant antiemetic pharmacotherapy.

▶ The most common medication used for gastrointestinal decontamination for poisoned patients is activated charcoal. However, how many of us have given activated charcoal to a patient with the extremely unpleasant result of vomiting? A large number is the answer, I suspect. Poor taste and the big mess associated with vomiting from the use of charcoal are a common problem in the ED. Commercially, some companies have introduced different flavors to reduce the nasty taste of charcoal. The actual incidence of emesis in the pediatric population for charcoal administration is not known. This study found that about 20% of children would have emesis after charcoal. Those children at the highest risk are those with previous episodes of emesis or use of a nasogastric tube. Personally, I try to avoid using a nasogastric tube as much as possible with trying to make charcoal as enticing as possible: placing the appropriate amount of charcoal in a fast food cup with a lid and straw (kids prefer McDonald's). While the child is watching, add a good squirt of chocolate syrup—yummmmy! Mix and close the lid quickly. Hopefully, this trick will work for you next time in the ED.

E. C. Quintana, MD, MPH

Treatment of Pediatric Migraine Headaches: A Randomized, Double-Blind Trial of Prochlorperazine Versus Ketorolac
Brousseau DC, Duffy SJ, Anderson AC, et al (Med College of Wisconsin, Milwaukee; Brown Univ, Providence, RI)
Ann Emerg Med 43:256-262, 2004   9–38

Introduction.—Migraine headaches are a common cause of visits to the pediatric ED, but few studies have evaluated the treatment of migraine in children. The effectiveness of prochlorperazine was compared with that of ketorolac when used in the ED management of pediatric migraines.

Methods.—The double-blind trial was conducted in the EDs of 2 children's hospitals. It included 62 children (36 girls, 26 boys), 5 to 18 years old, (mean age, 13.7 years) who were seen with headache meeting the Prensky and Sommer criteria for migraine. Once the decision was made to treat with an IV administration of 1 of the study drugs, patients were selected randomly to receive either IV prochlorperazine (0.15 mg/kg) or IV ketorolac (0.5 mg/kg). The Nine Faces Pain Scale was administered to the child at the start of the infusion and at 30 and 60 minutes later. If the initial medication was unsuccessful at relieving pain, the other study drug was given. Treatment success was defined as a reduction of 50% or greater in the Pain Scale score or a complete resolution of symptoms.

Results.—Treatment success 60 minutes after initiation of the first drug was 71% overall, but was higher for the prochlorperazine group (84.8%) than for the ketorolac group (55.2%). The prochlorperazine group also had the greater proportion of children reporting the lowest possible pain score at 60 minutes (33.3% vs 6.9%). Twelve of the 16 children who received the alternative drug met criteria for treatment success 60 minutes later. Thus, by the end of the study, 56 (93%) of 60 children who completed the study were successfully treated. Some headache symptoms recurred in approximately 30% of each group when follow-up calls were made after 48 hours. Two children experienced mild and self-limited side effects.

Conclusion.—IV prochlorperazine was superior to IV ketorolac in the treatment of acute migraine headache in children. Recurrence rates, however, were similar with the 2 drugs.

▶ Migraine headaches are a common presentation in the ED. Prochlorperazine and ketorolac were compared in children presenting with migraine headaches in 2 pediatric EDs. Migraine headaches were defined as recurrent headaches with pain-free intervals with 3 out of the following symptoms: aura, unilateral location, throbbing pulsatile pain, nausea/vomiting/abdominal pain, relief after sleep, and a family history for migraine headaches. Both groups reported a significant decrease of symptoms and pain score. Prochlorperazine showed a higher treatment success at the 60-minute mark. However, there was no difference in the headache recurrence based on a telephone follow-up call.

Unfortunately, this study has several limitations. There was an unusually low report of side effects to either medication. Was it because they had a low sample size, and consequently, lower than 0.8 power? Was it due to their inclusion criteria for migraine headaches? Or was it due to the relatively low use of migraine-specific medication use before the ED visit (32%-35%)? Caution is warranted before one can make this final decision.

E. C. Quintana, MD, MPH

Analgesia for Children With Acute Abdominal Pain: A Survey of Pediatric Emergency Physicians and Pediatric Surgeons
Kim MK, Galustyan S, Sato TT, et al (Med College of Wisconsin, Milwaukee; Bronx-Lebanon Med Ctr, NY)
Pediatrics 112:1122-1126, 2003   9–39

Introduction.—Analgesia is sometimes withheld from patients with acute abdominal pain because of concern that masking symptoms might delay diagnosis and treatment of a surgical condition. Current consensus statements, however, recommend judicious use of analgesia soon after an initial assessment. A survey sent to pediatric emergency physicians (PEMs) and pediatric surgeons (PSs) sought to evaluate current opinion and practice regarding the use of opioid analgesia in children with acute abdominal pain during evaluation in the ED.

Methods.—The 1-page survey to be answered anonymously was sent to board-eligible or board-certified PEMs, PSs certified by the American Board of Surgery or Royal College of Surgeons, and to physicians whose practice included children. Included in the survey were demographic data and questions related to practice and opinions regarding analgesia for acute nontraumatic abdominal pain in children.

Results.—A total of 1441 surveys were sent to 875 PEMs and 566 PSs, and 702 were returned. Exclusion of responses from ineligible physicians yielded 385 PEM and 189 PS surveys eligible for analysis. Those in the PEM group were more willing to provide analgesia before a definitive diagnosis. However, when PEMs and PSs with fewer than 10 years' experience were analyzed separately, the 2 groups did not differ in willingness to provide analgesia. Among more experienced physicians, PSs were much less likely than PEMs to provide analgesia. Both groups favored morphine as the opiate of choice (70.4% of PSs and 63.7% of PEMs). Most ((86%)) PEMs who completed an optional comment section cited disapproval by PSs as the main reason for withholding analgesia.

Conclusion.—Recent studies indicate that opioid analgesia can be used safely, without affecting diagnostic accuracy, in the initial evaluation of patients with acute abdominal pain. But for children with acute abdominal pain, disapproval of analgesia use by more experienced PSs has led to undertreatment of pain in children.

▶ This article explored the quintessential issue of providing analgesia for children with acute abdominal pain. The results are not surprising. There is still a strong belief that analgesia could change physical findings, delay diagnosis and treatment of a surgical abdomen. PEMs were more willing to give morphine, the most commonly used analgesic agent, than PSs before there was a definitive diagnosis. This disparity was more evident among PSs with greater than 10 years of experience. The most commonly cited reasons for withholding or providing analgesia were level of discomfort, pain relief, masked examination, and diagnosis delay.

There have been several articles that provide evidence to give analgesia early in acute abdominal pain without any deleterious effects. Thomas et al[1] performed a prospective, double-blind clinical trial in adult, nonpregnant patients with acute abdominal pain that showed that there was no difference between control (no morphine) versus morphine groups with respect to physical or diagnostic accuracy. The overall likelihood of complete disappearance of abdominal tenderness due to morphine was not statistically significant. A parallel study in children (5-18 years old) also determined that there was no significant change in the areas of abdominal tenderness in the group receiving morphine versus the control subjects.[2] There was no statistical difference in the diagnostic accuracy between PEMs and PSs.

Dr Kim's survey suggests that PEMs' practice of providing analgesic agents for acute abdomen is strongly influenced by the PSs' attitudes and availability within each institution. It is unfortunate that these beliefs are still engrained, despite the plethora of evidence-based articles that disprove the myth.

E. C. Quintana, MD, MPH

References

1. Thomas SH, Silen W, Cheema F, et al: Effects of morphine analgesia on diagnostic accuracy in emergency department patients with abdominal pain: A prospective, randomized trial. *J Am Coll Surg* 196:18-31, 2003.
2. Kim MK, Strait RT, Sato TT, et al: A randomized clinical trial of analgesia in children with acute abdominal pain. *Acad Emerg Med* 9:281-287, 2002.

Dating of Bruises in Children: An Assessment of Physician Accuracy
Bariciak ED, Plint AC, Gaboury I, et al (Univ of Ottawa, Ontario, Canada; Childrens' Hosp of Eastern Ontario, Ottawa, Canada)
Pediatrics 112:804-807, 2003   9–40

Introduction.—Pediatricians continue to provide expert witness testimony in child protection investigations, partially by estimating the age of a

TABLE 1.—Accuracy of Different Physician Groups in Estimating Age of Accidental Bruising

	Emergency Pediatricians (n/N, %)†	Other Physicians* (n/N, %)	Trainees (n/N, %)
Accurate within 24 h	20/42 (47.6)	5/17 (29.4)	14/38 (36.8)
Accurate within categories‡			
Overall	32/42 (76.2)	9/17 (52.9)	20/38 (52.6)
Fresh bruises	17/22 (77.3)	5/8 (62.5)	8/18 (44.4)
Intermediate bruises	10/13 (76.9)	3/5 (60.0)	9/15 (60.0)
Old bruises	5/7 (71.4)	1/4 (25.5)	3/6 (50.0)

*Includes nonemergency-trained physicians and family physicians working in the emergency department.
†Number of accurate age estimates/total number of bruises observed.
‡Fresh bruise < 48 hours old, intermediate bruises, 48 hours to 7 days old, and old bruises > 7 days.
(Courtesy of Bariciak ED, Plint AC, Gaboury I, et al: Dating of bruises in children: An assessment of physician accuracy. *Pediatrics* 112:804-807, 2003. Copyright 2003. Reproduced with permission.)

suspected inflicted injury in an attempt to identify the perpetrator(s). Recent debate has concerned whether the use of photographs to estimate the age of a bruise based on color alone is accurate or specific enough to provide useful information in a child abuse investigation. Children seen in the ED of a children's hospital with accidental bruises of known age and origin were evaluated to determine whether physicians could estimate the age of an accidental bruise on direct physical examination.

Methods.—All children had documented demographic data and information concerning their injuries. Emergency pediatricians, other physicians, and trainees (ie, fellows, residents, and medical students) who were unaware of the patient's history independently evaluated the bruised area and documented injury characteristics and age estimation. They ranked characteristics that influenced their estimation.

Results.—Fifty children with accidental bruises were enrolled. The accuracy of the emergency physicians for age estimation within 24 hours of actual age was 47.6% (Table 1). Individual physician accuracy ranged from 0% to 100%, and interobserver reliability was poor (κ, −0.03). The accuracy within 24 hours of the actual age was 29.4% for other physicians, and 36.8% for trainees, which are rates similar to those of emergency pediatricians. Observers reported using the color mainly to estimate the age, followed by tenderness, then swelling. None of these characteristics were significantly correlated with accuracy.

Conclusion.—Physician estimates of a bruise's age are highly inaccurate within 24 hours of the actual age of the bruise. Large individual variability and poor interrater reliability also indicate that caution needs to be used when interpreting these estimates. These data support earlier findings that extreme caution is needed in estimating the age of a bruise, even when such estimates are based on direct examination of the injured area.

▶ Evaluation for physical abuse or trauma is a common presentation. It is not uncommon for physicians to be called as witnesses or experts in an attempt to estimate age of bruises, frequency of alleged assaults, and safety of children. This study's objective was to determine whether the age of a bruise could be more accurately dated by physical examination and whether other factors may influence this determination. Fifty percent of physicians used color alone, followed by 21.4% who used color and tenderness, and 7.1% who used color and swelling for determining the bruises' age. None of these factors had any statistical correlation with dating accuracy. There was a wide and poor interobserver accuracy on dating bruises. The dating accuracy of bruises within 24 hours was poor. These results support other studies that advise extreme caution in estimating bruise age even when direct examination of the area is available.

E. C. Quintana, MD, MPH

Effectiveness of Lidocaine Lubricant for Discomfort During Pediatric Urethral Catheterization
Gerard LL, Cooper CS, Duethman KS, et al (Univ of Iowa, Iowa City)
J Urol 170:564-567, 2003   9–41

Introduction.—Because urethral catheterization can be a painful and traumatic experience for children, clinicians may avoid the procedure to the detriment of optimal management. A sterile lubricant containing lidocaine is used as a topical anesthetic for adult patients and has been recommended for pediatric catheterization. The effectiveness of lidocaine for decreasing pain sensation with ureteral catheterization of children was assessed.

Methods.—In a prospective double-blind trial, 20 children (ages 4-11 years) were randomly selected to receive urethral lubricant with lidocaine or without (placebo) 10 minutes before urethral catheterization. The lidocaine and placebo groups each included 8 girls and 2 boys. There were no significant differences between groups in age, number of previous catheterizations, or distress with previous catheterizations. Children included in the trial were scheduled to have a urethral catheter inserted for a cystogram. Their perception of pain associated with the procedure was measured using the Oucher Pain Scale; a visual analog scale assessed preprocedure anxiety. A pediatric urology nurse and a child life therapist independently rated each child's behavioral distress on a 7-point scale.

Results.—Self-rated pain and observed-rated behavioral distress were significantly lower in the lidocaine group than in the placebo group. Adjustment for a possible confounding effect of preprocedure anxiety suggested that patient anxiety did not interfere with the main effects of lidocaine.

Conclusion.—Urinary catheterization is a particularly stressful procedure for children, some of whom will have to undergo repeated catheterizations because of chronic urinary tract problems. The use of topical lidocaine for pain reduction is recommended for all pediatric urethral catheterizations.

▶ Catheterization could be a painful and traumatic experience for anyone, especially those children with vesicoureteral reflux and frequent urinary tract infections requiring frequent catheterized urine specimens. It has been my experience that sterile viscous lidocaine helps in adult catheterization. Why not use it for children? This study evaluated the effectiveness of lidocaine in reducing anxiety and discomfort during urinary catheterization. Preoperative and postprocedure anxiety, pain and distress were measured using the Oucher Pain Scale. It found that the lidocaine lubricant-catheterized group had less pain and distress. Common sense would state that the use of lidocaine lubricant would also reduce pain and distress in children, just like this study showed. Other contributing factors that could ease urinary catheterization could be oral analgesia, and child distraction techniques (ie, child life). Should we use lidocaine during our catheterizations in children? Based on this study, why not?

E. C. Quintana, MD, MPH

Bispectral Index Monitoring Quantifies Depth of Sedation During Emergency Department Procedural Sedation and Analgesia in Children
Agrawal D, Feldman HA, Krauss B, et al (Harvard Med School, Boston)
Ann Emerg Med 43:247-255, 2004   9–42

Introduction.—Undersedation in children fails to relieve the anxiety and pain associated with procedures, whereas oversedation can result in serious adverse events and prolonged recovery times. An objective measure of sedation depth is needed to avoid these extremes. The ability of the bispectral index to monitor depth of nondissociative procedural sedation and analgesia was assessed in children undergoing nonelective procedures or diagnostic imaging in the ED.

Methods.—The study group included 14 boys and 6 girls with a median age of 4.6 years. Excluded were children for whom bispectral index scores might not be reliable because of deafness, acute or chronic alteration in mental status, or use of ketamine for sedation and analgesia. Fourteen patients received the combination of midazolam and fentanyl, and 6 received pentobarbital alone. The emergency physician administering procedural sedation selected the type, route, and total dose of medication. Paired bispectral index and Ramsay Sedation Scale scores were assigned every 5 minutes during sedation. A study investigator blinded to the bispectral index score assigned the Ramsay Sedation Scale scores.

Results.—A total of 217 paired bispectral index/Ramsay Sedation Scale measurements were obtained. The mean bispectral index score was 81.6, and the mean Ramsay Sedation Scale score was 3.3. The adjusted correlation between these measures was -0.67; the linear regression coefficient was estimated at between -5.7 and -12.7. Bispectral index scores between 60 and 90 were of moderate accuracy in predicting traditional clinical levels of sedation typically encountered in the study situation.

Conclusion.—The correlation between bispectral index monitoring and clinical sedation scores indicated that the index may be a useful, objective adjunct in quantifying depth of nondissociative procedure sedation and analgesia in children. The range of 60 to 90, which is wider than that recommended in adults (adult range, 65-85), better encompasses the sedation goals in the pediatric ED.

▶ Procedural sedation and analgesia are an essential aspect of our daily clinical practice, especially in children. The accurate assessment of sedation has been an area of continuous improvement and importance. This study used bispectral index monitors, which are commonly used in the operating rooms, and general anesthesia, as an adjunct, to determine its correlation with a clinical sedation scoring system. Even though this observational study had a small sample size, it showed that bispectral index monitoring could potentially have an increasing importance in the pediatric sedation assessment. It is an innovative way to more objectively titrate sedation in numerous procedural sedations. Clearly, more studies in this field are needed.

E. C. Quintana, MD, MPH

10 Emergency Medical Service Systems

EMS Systems

A Geographic Information System Simulation Model of EMS: Reducing Ambulance Response Time

Peleg K, Pliskin JS (Sheba Med Ctr, Tel-Hashomer, Israel; Ben-Gurion Univ of the Negev, Beer-Sheva, Israel; Harvard School of Public Health, Boston)
Am J Emerg Med 22:164-170, 2004   10–1

Background.—Among the many factors that determine the quality of EMS, response time is an important EMS benchmark. The importance of response time is reflected in the term the Golden Hour, which was derived from the observation that survival of patients who receive inhospital definitive treatment within 1 hour of surgery was much higher than of those who received it later. A number of national strategies have been developed for increasing the quality of EMS, especially the administration of life-saving procedures at the earliest time. The response by Israeli ambulances was modeled and model-derived strategies for improved deployment of ambulances to reduce response time were offered.

Methods.—A geographic information system (GIS) was used to conduct a retrospective review of computerized ambulance call and dispatch logs in 2 different regional districts, one large and urban and the other rural. The study included all calls that were pinpointed geographically by the GIS, and data for these calls were stratified by weekday and by daily shifts. Geographic areas of a maximum of 8 minutes' response time were simulated for each of these subgroups to maximize the timely response of calls.

Results.—Before the use of the GIS model, the mean response times in the 2 districts were 12.3 and 9.2 minutes, respectively, with 34% and 62% of calls, respectively, responded to within 8 minutes. When ambulances were positioned within the modeled geographic areas, more than 94% of calls met the 8-minute criterion.

Conclusions.—The GIS simulation model used in this study suggested that EMS could be more effective if a dynamic load-responsive ambulance deployment is used, as it showed potential to increase survival and cost effectiveness.

▶ The locations and staffing of EMS and fire units in the United States have traditionally been determined by parochial and political boundaries rather than county or area-wide analysis of demographics, call volumes, and response times. The result is often a less than optimal allocation of resources, especially in areas with many small townships with independent fire and EMS systems. This article is a nice demonstration of the potential for improvement in response times, survival, and cost effectiveness by using GIS or similar systems to determine unit placement and staffing rather than political boundaries.

S. L. Werner, MD

Community Influenza Outbreaks and Emergency Department Ambulance Diversion
Schull MJ, Mamdani MM, Fang J, et al (Univ of Toronto)
Ann Emerg Med 44:61-67, 2004   10–2

Background.—Several studies have identified an association of influenza with increased hospitalizations of elderly patients, but studies of influenza and ED visits have produced conflicting results in terms of the effect of outbreaks of influenza-related illnesses on ED crowding. The relationship between ED crowding and influenza outbreaks was investigated.

Methods.—A retrospective time series analysis was conducted in Toronto for 170 weeks, from January 1996 to April 1999. Data were obtained weekly for laboratory-confirmed influenza and other respiratory virus cases in the community, ED ambulance diversion, and visits to all 20 EDs in the city. The main outcome measure was ambulance diversion, as measured by the mean number of hours per week in which EDs were forced to divert all ambulances.

Results.—There was a mean of 10,936 ED visits weekly; the average age of the patients was 39.9 years and 51% of them were women. EDs diverted ambulances an average of 3.4 hours per week (range, 0.3-15 hours). There were 4 influenza seasons in the study period, each lasting from 18 to 30 weeks, with weekly influenza counts that ranged from 0 to 236. There were fewer than 10 cases per week in 119 of 170 weeks (70%). Time-series models showed that influenza was independently associated with ED diversion of the ambulance. For every 100 cases of influenza in a given week, ED ambulance diversion would be expected to increase by 2.5 hours per week at the average ED. During influenza seasons, 24.3% of observed weekly ambulance diversion was attributable to influenza.

Conclusions.—There is an increase in ED ambulance diversions in association with influenza seasons. The effect of these diversions is substantial but brief because there is little or no influenza activity during most of the year.

▶ The results of this study are not surprising. Every ED and EMS system needs a plan to deal with a severe flu season. The first part of this plan is vaccination of health care workers. Ill health care providers reduce the ability to provide care and violate the "do no harm" principle by spreading the disease. This seems like a no-brainer, but the vaccination rate of health care providers in previous years is absolutely abysmal, reported at only 35% by the CDC.[1] Secondly, for systems looking to enhance the role of paramedics as out-of-hospital providers, paramedic administered vaccination programs, mobile, or at fire stations, would be well-worth pursuing from a public health perspective.

S. L. Werner, MD

Reference

1. Bridges CB, Harper SA, Fududa K, et al: Prevention and control of influenza: Recommendations of the Advisory Committee on Immunization Practices. *MMWR Recomm Rep* 52:RR-8, 2003.

The Use of National Highway Traffic Safety Administration Uniform Prehospital Data Elements in State Emergency Medical Services Data Collection Systems

Mann NC, Dean JM, Mobasher H, et al (Univ of Utah, Salt Lake City; Univ of North Carolina, Chapel Hill)
Prehosp Emerg Care 8:29-33, 2004   10–3

Background.—For many persons needing medical treatment the EMS system is the point of entry into the health care system. The concept of EMS has been in existence for 3 decades, but there is little scientific evidence validating its effect on morbidity and mortality. The lack of reliable and uniform EMS data has been a significant barrier to the conduct of meaningful assessments of the effects of EMS in improving morbidity and mortality. The extent to which states incorporate the Uniform Prehospital EMS Data Elements into statewide EMS data collection systems was investigated.

Methods.—All state Emergency Medical Services for Children (EMS-C) directors or health departments having regulatory responsibilities for the oversight of state EMS and EMS-C activities (including the District of Columbia) were asked whether a statewide prehospital data collection system existed in their state. Coordinators in states in which such a system existed were asked to provide a data dictionary.

Results.—During the study period, 443 states with statewide EMS data collection systems captured an average of 79% of the Uniform Prehospital EMS Data Set. Variables thought to be essential to EMS evaluation were more likely collected (84%) than variables considered desirable (72%). Only 8 (10%) of the 81 uniform data elements are collected by all 43 participating states.

Conclusion.—Related EMS data variables are collected by most states across the country. The degree of similarity observed in this study can provide a foundation for the establishment of common fields that can be used to develop a national EMS registry.

▶ This is a nice summary of where we stand in the development of a national EMS database. Although not perfect, the report is encouraging. It appears that most states are collecting a significant amount of the Uniform Prehospital EMS Data Set. If the recommended next steps can be completed, it is possible that a powerful resource for EMS research will exist.

S. L. Werner, MD

Impact of a Triage Tool on Air Versus Ground Transport of Cardiac Patients to a Tertiary Center

Werman HA, Jaynes C, Blevins G (MedFlight, Columbus, Ohio)
Air Med J 23:40-47, 2004   10–4

Background.—The American College of Cardiology and the American Heart Association have developed guidelines for the optimal treatment of acute myocardial infarction. The guidelines range from prehospital response to rehabilitation and include the pharmacotherapeutic management of acute myocardial infarction. In addition, these guidelines address the role of adjunctive therapies such as cardiac catheterization, percutaneous transluminal coronary angioplasty, cardiac surgery, and hemodynamic monitoring and support. However, "24/7" availability of these specialized cardiac services in the rural or community hospital setting is often limited or absent.

In this setting, current practices include the transportation of eligible cardiac candidates to regional centers that perform high volumes of interventional and diagnostic cardiac procedures. The optimum method of transport for these patients is controversial. This study investigated the feasibility of a physician-developed triage scheme for appropriate use of air versus mobile ICUs in the transfer of cardiac patients. It also investigated the effect of this approach on the distribution of transport mode for cardiac patients in areas of personal characteristics and whether this approach would aid the decision-making process in referral of cardiac patients to tertiary centers.

Methods.—The intervention studied in this prospective, observational comparison was an educational program designed to teach a triage decision tool developed by a receiving cardiologist with input from the critical care transport team. Short-distance (less than 30 minutes) and long-distance transports were examined. A follow-up survey of referring hospitals was also performed.

Results.—There was excellent compliance with short-distance transports, with 41 of 42 patients being transported by mobile ICU. In addition, there was an increase in long-distance transports by mobile ICU from 55% to 65% during the study period. However, a third of the mobile ICU patients actually met air transport criteria. Long-distance patients transported by air had significantly higher transport costs, total hospital charges, and direct admission to the catheterization laboratory. Of 10 ED directors surveyed, 5 directors responded that they found the triage instrument useful in making transport decisions.

Conclusion.—A physician-developed triage instrument for selection of the appropriate transport mode for acute cardiac transfers was found to be effective. There is a need for further studies to validate the cardiac triage criteria against clinical outcome.

▶ This study is troubling for several reasons. First is the authors' conclusion that the triage tool was effectively applied. Their results suggest just the opposite for the group of patients presenting to EDs greater than 30 minutes from a tertiary care center. There was actually an increase in the number of patients transported by mobile ICU who actually met their triage criteria for air transport after implementation of the triage tool, suggesting serious problems with the triage tool itself or its implementation. While the triage tool is reported to be a "consensus" tool, it appears to have been developed without input from the transferring physicians who, as the authors point out, are ultimately responsible for the patients until they reach the tertiary care facility.

The study is also troubling in that it fails to address the main question, a theme common to EMS research: It would seem that before the usefulness of a transport triage tool can be determined, we need to know when air versus mobile ICU transport makes a difference in the clinical outcomes of cardiac patients. While the answer to this question is quite clear for patients meeting criteria for immediate percutaneous transluminal coronary angioplasty, there is no compelling evidence for air versus mobile ICU transport of other types of cardiac patients, and it is here that research efforts should be concentrated.

S. L. Werner, MD

Denial of Ambulance Reimbursement: Can Reviewers Determine What Is an Emergency?
Hauswald M, Jambrosic M (Univ of New Mexico, Albuquerque; Bernalillo County Health Care Corp/Albuquerque Ambulance Service, NM)
Prehosp Emerg Care 8:162-165, 2004   10–5

Introduction.—Third-party payers are motivated to deny payment for ambulance transport when used for nonemergency or routine illnesses. The criteria applied for denial of payment are not clear, however. Hospital records of patients for whom ambulance claims were denied were reviewed for appropriateness of ambulance transport and whether the denial was justified.

Methods.—A total of 146 consecutive ambulance run forms were obtained from claims rejected by Medicare providers at the study institution. The corresponding ED charts were reviewed for evaluation of medical risk. The appropriateness of ambulance transport was determined by extracting the final diagnosis and the most serious written diagnosis in the differential.

Transport was defined as appropriate if either diagnosis could benefit from treatment in an ambulance or by rapid transport to a hospital.

Results.—The ED charts were available for 104 patients, including 3 who were assigned via triage to the obstetric unit. Sixty-three (61%) of these transports were determined to have at least 1 diagnosis that made ambulance transport medically necessary; risk was described as high in 38 cases. Among the serious final diagnoses for patients whose ambulance transport payment was denied were ruptured ectopic pregnancy, pneumonia in a patient with AIDS, closed head injury with loss of consciousness, and hypoglycemia with insulin overdose.

Conclusion.—A large proportion of cases in which payment for ambulance transport was denied proved to be serious emergencies requiring prompt medical care. Because there is no agreed-upon standard for ambulance utilization, payers can develop arbitrary criteria for payment.

▶ This article illustrates one of the reasons it is so important that we develop a consensus on criteria defining medical necessity for EMS dispatch and transport. In the absence of uniform criteria from the emergency medical community, patients and EMS systems financed to any degree by reimbursements will continue to be at the mercy of government's and third-party payers' various methodologies and criteria for determining reimbursements. The development of standard criteria for medical necessity, a process begun at the Neely conference (see Abstract 10–6), would not only help provide a standard for appropriate EMS response and transport, but it would also serve as a useful tool for the emergency medicine community in responding to the current ambulance reimbursement practices of governmental entities and third-party payers.

S. L. Werner, MD

Defining Research Criteria to Characterize Medical Necessity in Emergency Medical Services: A Consensus Among Experts at the Neely Conference
Mann NC, Schmidt TA, Cone DC (Univ of Utah, Salt Lake City; Oregon Health & Science Univ, Portland; Yale Univ, New Haven, Conn)
Prehosp Emerg Care 8:138-153, 2004   10–6

Introduction.—The goal of the 2003 Neely Conference was to bring together experts in the field of EMS to define a set of criteria applicable to the evaluation of dispatch triage and field triage systems. Previous studies in this area are difficult to assess because protocols and outcome criteria have varied considerably.

Methods.—During the opening session of the Neely Conference, participants completed a multistage survey to evaluate the strength of published evidence regarding dispatch triage and field triage applications. At closing sessions, the use of specific triage criteria and outcome measures for assess-

TABLE 3.—Presenting Complaints, Prehospital Interventions, and Other Outcomes Considered Important When Defining the Need for an EMS Response or When Judging the "Correctness" of a Decision to Provide (or Not Provide) an EMS Response

Dispatch Triage Criteria	Outcome Measures
Presenting complaints:	*Prehospital interventions:*
Chest pain	Airway Interventions
Respiratory difficulty	*Other outcome measures:*
Altered mental status	Emergent surgery
Syncope	Emergency department diagnosis
Focal neurologic deficit/	Procedures in the
cerebrovascular accident	emergency department
Gastrointestinal bleed	
Difficulty in pregnancy	

(Courtesy of Mann NC, Schmidt TA, Cone DC: Defining research criteria to characterize medical necessity in emergency medical services: A consensus among experts at the Neely Conference. *Prehosp Emerg Care* 8:138-153, 2004. Hanley & Belfus, Philadelphia, 215-546-4995, www.hanleyandbelfus.com.)

ing EMS medical necessity were evaluated. Agreement among responses was assessed with the use of consensus theory.

Results.—Thirty-one experts attended the symposium and completed the surveys. Attendees included emergency physicians (61%), emergency medical technicians/paramedics (13%), EMS administrators (7%), and research scientists (8%). Seventy percent of participants had an MD degree and 55% were involved in the area of field triage protocols addressing medical necessity. Participants judged current evidence regarding the utility of EMS triage criteria to be weak, yet they agreed on a set of research criteria that could define the need for an EMS response or EMS transport. Field triage criteria were judged more plausible than dispatch criteria.

In an examination of presenting complaints (Table 3), only airway interventions were considered adequate outcome measures when assessing dispatch triage criteria. The ED assessment and the need for immediate surgery were considered valid outcome criteria for determining the effectiveness of triage protocols. Hospital admission, final diagnosis, and expert opinion were not judged to be adequate outcome measures.

Conclusion.—There is a consensus among EMS experts that prehospital triage criteria founded on medical necessity can and should be determined. Available evidence from the literature, however, was considered "weakly supportive" of such criteria. The identification of a core set of criteria would increase the comparability of published studies.

▶ Financial and legal pressures are increasingly forcing EMS systems to attempt to allocate prehospital resources based on "medical need." Over the past 10 to 15 years, many systems have adopted priority or criteria based emergency medical dispatch programs and field triage protocols in order to more appropriately allocate resources. While there have been a number of research efforts to examine the safety and effectiveness of triage protocols, this area of study suffers from the same problems as much other EMS research: the absence of uniform data collection and outcome measures.

While the findings of this article are limited to the determination that a consensus was reached, I have included it in the YEAR BOOK because it marks a significant first step toward what will be some of the most important changes in EMS. As financial and system pressures increase, EMS will need to think beyond the provision of prehospital care and toward providing out-of-hospital care, including triaging patients to the appropriate type of facility by the appropriate means and at the appropriate time. A solid body of research, based on uniform criteria and outcomes measures, will be necessary to ensure these changes are both cost effective and meet our patients' needs.

S. L. Werner, MD

The Effect of Emergency Department Crowding on Paramedic Ambulance Availability
Eckstein M, Chan LS (Univ of Southern California, Los Angeles; Los Angeles Fire Dept)
Ann Emerg Med 43:100-105, 2004   10–7

Background.—When paramedics transport a patient to a crowded ED, they may be confronted with a lack of gurney availability. In that case, they must wait with their patient until an empty gurney becomes available. During this time, the ambulance is incapable of responding to further emergency calls. This prospective study examines the effect of ED crowding on EMS services in Los Angeles from April 2001 through March 2002.

Study Design.—During the study period, each incident in which an ambulance was out of service for more than 15 minutes because of the lack of an open ED gurney was prospectively captured in the dispatch computer system. Data collected included the total time out of service, the time of year, and the hospital involved.

Findings.—There were 21,240 incidents in which ambulances were out of service for more than 15 minutes while waiting to transfer their patients to an open gurney. These incidents occurred during 1 out of every 8 transports during the study period. Of these incidents, 8.4% exceeded 1 hour in duration. The median waiting time per incident was 27 minutes. These incidents were more common during the winter (January through March).

Conclusion.—Los Angeles paramedic ambulances are often out of service while waiting to transfer their patients to overcrowded EDs. This problem may significantly impact the ability of the EMS to provide timely response.

▶ This study is a nice start in looking at the effects of overcrowding on prehospital care, but it falls short of demonstrating the impact of having ambulances out of service for extended periods. If the effect is simply that the medics are sitting at the hospital rather than at the firehouse or designated location, can we really say to the public and the policy makers that ED overcrowding has an impact on the delivery of prehospital care? A better study would examine the correlation between the length of time to transfer patients to ED beds and response times, transport times, rate of nonresponse, and mortality rates.

S. L. Werner, MD

The Effect of Simple Interventions on Paramedic Aspirin Administration Rates
Snider JB, Moreno R, Fuller DJ, et al (American Med Response Northwest, Portland, Ore; Oregon Health & Science Univ, Portland; Ctr for Policy and Research in Emergency Medicine, Portland, Ore)
Prehosp Emerg Care 8:41-45, 2004   10–8

Background.—Aspirin has been demonstrated to be beneficial to patients with acute coronary syndromes, but it is underutilized. The baseline rate of aspirin administration by paramedics in Multnomah County, Oregon (1 of 3 counties that compose the Portland metropolitan area) was assessed, and the effects of 2 interventions on the rate of administration were assessed.

Study Design.—Adult patients seen with a suspected cardiac event were retrospectively selected from the medical transport provider's database. Data from 1999 (period 1) were used to establish the baseline of aspirin use by paramedics for suspected cardiac events. January 2000 to December 2001 (period 2) was the period after the protocol change intervention. January to June 2002 (period 3) was the period after the educational intervention. Use of aspirin by paramedics was compared over these 3 periods.

Findings.—During period 1 (baseline), 15.1% of patients with a possible cardiac event received aspirin. During period 2, 26.8% of these patients received aspirin, while during period 3, 37% of these patients received aspirin. When period 1 (baseline) was compared to period 3 (after both interventions) there was a 22% absolute improvement in aspirin administration by paramedics.

Conclusion.—Aspirin appears to be underutilized before hospital transport by paramedics treating patients with suspected acute cardiac events. A protocol change and educational intervention increased aspirin usage in this setting, although use of aspirin remained low. Further research is needed to determine how to increase aspirin use by paramedics in the prehospital setting.

▶ Good to know that the rate of prehospital aspirin administration can be improved. But the real question here is why the rate was so low in the first place. It's a simple intervention that doesn't even require IV access. There is mounting evidence that early aspirin administration improves outcomes. Several recent studies have shown early aspirin improves outcomes, including Barbash's 2002 study in cardiology which found that prehospital administration of aspirin in acute myocardial infarction was an independent determinant of survival.[1]

Hopefully, the low rate of aspirin administration found in this system is not typical. However, this study, combined with the increasing evidence that early aspirin administration improves outcomes, should prompt every EMS medical director to evaluate their chest pain protocols for aspirin inclusion and to do some quality assurance to ensure that their system is doing better than this. EMS should be a leader, not a laggard, in carrying out this simple, effective intervention.

S. L. Werner, MD

Reference

1. Barbash IM: Outcome of myocardial infarction in patients treated with aspirin is enhanced by prehospital administration. *Cardiology* 98:141-147, 2002.

Human Resources

Are Emergency Medical Technician–Basics Able to Use a Selective Immobilization of the Cervical Spine Protocol? A Preliminary Report
Dunn TM, Dalton A, Dorfman T, et al (Univ of Northern Colorado, Greeley; Pridemark Paramedic Services, Boulder, Colo; Boulder Community Hosp, Colo; et al)
Prehosp Emerg Care 8:207-211, 2004   10–9

Introduction.—Protocols for selective immobilization of the cervical spine allow EMS providers to identify patients who have sustained high-mechanism trauma but do not require spinal precautions. Paramedics appear to be as reliable as emergency medicine physicians in using selective protocols, but the ability of an emergency medical technician (EMT)–Basic to use such protocols has not been determined. A prospective scenario-based study examined the ability of EMT-Basics to effectively use a selective spinal immobilization protocol.

Methods.—The 95 participants were drawn from 11 EMS agencies in 3 counties and a non-EMS college class. Most of the paramedics were from advanced life support transport agencies that had an existing selective spinal immobilization protocol. Participants from other agencies and college students attended a 1-hour lecture regarding applying the protocol. All participants evaluated 6 patients in written scenarios and were asked to determine when spinal precautions were necessary.

Results.—Thirty-nine participants were EMT-Basics with a mean of 6.3 years of EMS experience. There were 26 paramedics with a mean of 11.6 years of EMS experience and 30 college students who served as a non-EMS comparison group. Decisions made by EMT-Basics were essentially the same as those made by paramedics, and in no case did an EMT-Basic fail to immobilize a patient when spinal precautions were indicated. Non-EMS college students who received a modified lecture were also successful in reaching the correct decision regarding spinal immobilization.

Conclusion.—The protocol for selective immobilization of the cervical spine was simple and straightforward, thus allowing even non-EMS college students with minimal training to make the correct decision when presented with a written scenario. Adoption of these protocols would reduce the number of patients needlessly placed in spinal immobilization. Errors made by EMT-Basics were conservative ones, and all patients who would require the intervention were identified.

▶ While this study is small and very limited, it is a good first step in the right direction: development and implementation of selective cervical spine (c-spine) immobilization protocols for all EMS providers. Although there is continued discussion of the relative merits of the Canadian c-spine rule versus the NEXUS (National Emergency X-Radiography Utilization Study) criteria, both studies have shown us that clinical criteria can be safely used to clear c-spines. Stroh and Braude previously demonstrated that advanced life support providers can safely apply a c-spine clearance protocol and avoid unnecessary spinal immobilization.[1] Since the vast majority of EMS responses are provided by basic EMTs, it only makes sense to pursue development of selective immobilization protocols adaptable to all levels of EMS providers.

S. L. Werner, MD

Reference

1. Stroh G, Braude, D: Can an out-of-hospital cervical spine clearance protocol identify all patients with injuries? An argument for selective immobilization. *Ann Emerg Med* 37:609-615, 2001.

Incidence of Transient Hypoxia and Pulse Rate Reactivity During Paramedic Rapid Sequence Intubation
Dunford JV, Davis DP, Ochs M, et al (Univ of California, San Diego)
Ann Emerg Med 42:721-728, 2003   10–10

Background.—Outcomes from severe closed head injury are related to the nature of the primary and secondary injury. The CNS has a high rate of oxygen consumption, and no alternate energy reserves are available to the system. The presence of hypoxia and hypotension has been associated with worsened outcomes, and the preservation of cerebral perfusion and oxygenation is essential. Rapid sequence intubation has been recommended as the preferred method for securing the airways in combative patients with closed head injury; however, the role of rapid sequence intubation in out-of-hospital airway management has been a subject of debate. The incidence of desaturation and pulse rate reactivity was determined during out-of-hospital rapid sequence intubation of patients with severe head injuries (Glasgow Coma Scale score ≤ 8).

Methods.—The study was conducted among adult patients with severe head injuries who were treated by 12 EMS in the San Diego area. All the patients had recording oximeter-capnometers applied before rapid sequence intubation. Desaturation was defined as a reduction in oxygen saturation (SpO_2) to less than 90% from an initial SpO_2 of 90% or greater, or a decrease from a baseline of less than 90%. EMS run sheets and debriefing reports were used to analyze event records.

Results.—Of the 54 patients studied, 31 (57%) demonstrated desaturation during rapid sequence intubation. Of these 31 events, 26 (84%) occurred in patients whose initial SpO_2 values with basic airway skills were 90% or greater. The median duration of desaturation was 160 seconds, and the median decrease in SpO_2 was 22%. Significant bradycardia occurred in 6 patients (19%) during desaturation events. The paramedics reported that rapid sequence intubation was "easy" in 26 (84%) of the 31 patients with desaturation.

Conclusions.—Out-of-hospital rapid sequence intubation by paramedics was complicated by a troublesome incidence of desaturation and bradycardia. The presence of these derangements was not reflected in the paramedic reports. Most of the patients had acceptable SpO_2 values before rapid sequence intubation. An effective strategy for preoxygenation is necessary before it can be determined that rapid sequence intubation is valuable in the out-of-hospital treatment of patients with serious closed head injury.

▶ This article may help explain, at least in part, the increase in mortality and morbidity reported last year by Davis et al[1] in head-injured patients intubated by paramedics using rapid sequence intubation (RSI). The average length of hypoxia (nearly 3 minutes), combined with paramedics' perceptions of many of the intubations with prolonged hypoxia and bradycardia as "easy," is quite concerning. Also concerning is that complete data were collected on only one half of the patients intubated with RSI. It is possible that the incidence of hypoxemia and bradycardia may have been significantly higher than recorded. The authors note that adequate preoxygenation with an oxygen saturation of greater than 90% was achieved before intubation in the majority of patients. While there may be some validity to their argument that preoxygenation was not adequate, the prolonged and deep hypoxia suggests that either basic bag-valve-mask ventilation between intubation attempts was inadequate, or that paramedics significantly exceeded the 30 seconds allowed per attempt by protocol.

The authors conclude that "an effective out-of-hospital preoxygenation strategy is needed before it can be concluded that RSI is of value in head injured patients." Although we cannot directly link the findings of prolonged hypoxia in this study with the previous evidence that out-of-hospital RSI increases mortality, it certainly suggests that far more than an effective preoxygenation strategy may be needed before further evaluation of the effectiveness of out-of-hospital RSI can be pursued. While some authors have called for a randomized controlled study of out-of-hospital RSI, I would suggest that an evaluation of RSI training, protocols, and practices to determine and mitigate the factors contributing to this potentially serious problem may be in order before further investigation of the value of out-of-hospital RSI in head-injured patients is conducted.

S. L. Werner, MD

Reference

1. Davis DP, Hoyt DM, Ochs M, et al: The effect of paramedic rapid sequence intubation on outcome in patients with severe traumatic brain injury. *J Trauma* 54:444-453, 2003.

Endotracheal Intubation and Esophageal Tracheal Combitube Insertion by Regular Ambulance Attendants: A Comparative Trial
Rumball C, Macdonald D, Barber P, et al (Univ of British Columbia, Vancouver, Canada; British Columbia Ambulance Service, Vancouver, Canada; Angiotech Industries, Vancouver, British Columbia, Canada)
Prehosp Emerg Care 8:15-22, 2004   10–11

Background.—The optimal method for basic ambulance attendants to protect a patient's airway and provide ventilation in cases of cardiac or respiratory arrest has not been established. Studies in this area have so far provided conflicting results. Recent guidelines for cardiac arrest resuscitation have recommended the esophageal tracheal Combitube (ETC) as an advanced airway management alternative for persons who do not frequently perform endotracheal intubation (ETI). The basic ambulance attendant success rates at ETI and ETC insertion, as well as their continuing skill competency over time, were analyzed. Whether ongoing practice on mannequins can improve skill performance was also determined.

Methods.—The study group was composed of 357 adult patients in cardiorespiratory arrest who were treated by 81 basic ambulance attendants. The study design involved the analysis of 2 treatment options in 3 patient groups: ETC insertion, ETI insertion with mannequin practice (ETI-MP), and ETI insertion without mannequin practice (ETI-NMP). The main outcome measures were successful insertion and ventilation with ETC or ETI, as assessed by receiving physicians; and differences in successful insertion/ventilation between the MP and NMP groups. Analysis of the outcomes was by intention to treat.

Results.—Successful insertion was obtained in 63% of patients in the ETI-NMP group; in 76% of patients in the ETI-MP group; in 62% of the ETC-NMP group; and in 68% of the ETC-MP group. ETI success appeared to improve with continuing mannequin practice (75% for MP vs 61% for NMP).

Conclusions.—Rates of successful insertion and ventilation were similar with the ETC and ETI. ETI was less successful without mannequin practice. However, the erosion of ETI skills was partially mitigated by additional field experience.

▶ More evidence that an ideal airway intervention suitable for basic emergency medical technicians (EMTs) does not yet exist. Also more evidence that increased frequency of training and field performance increases the success rate for a given procedure. This study argues for continued emphasis on good basic airway management—2-person bag-valve-mask with oropharyngeal or nasopharyngeal airways for most EMTs and advanced airway management, ideally with endotracheal tube intubation, reserved for a subset of providers for whom the system can provide the necessary ongoing practice and sufficiently frequent field performance of the procedure to ensure skill maintenance.

S. L. Werner, MD

Accuracy of Arrhythmia Recognition in Paramedic Treatment of Paroxysmal Supraventricular Tachycardia: A Ten-Year Review
Goebel PJ, Daya MR, Gunnels MD (Oregon Health & Science Univ, Portland; Tualatin Valley Fire & Rescue, Aloha, Ore)
Prehosp Emerg Care 8:166-170, 2004   10–12

Background.—One of the most common rhythm disturbances encountered in the clinical setting is paroxysmal supraventricular tachycardia (PSVT). Adenosine has been shown to be a very safe and effective therapy for PSVT and is widely used in EMS settings. Recently, there was a report of 2 EMS deaths that were temporally associated with the inappropriate use of adenosine. In both cases, the patients had dyspnea resulting from underlying pulmonary conditions and had associated rapid atrial fibrillation that was misidentified. Trends in paramedic use of adenosine for presumed PSVT during a 10-year period were examined, as well as trends in paramedic rhythm misidentification rates.

Methods.—A retrospective analysis was conducted of all cases in which paramedics treated presumed PSVT with adenosine from 1993 to 2002. Rhythm strips were categorized as narrow or wide complex and regular or irregular. Appropriate use of adenosine was defined as narrow-complex regular tachycardia with no visible P waves and a rate greater than 140 beats/min.

Results.—A total of 224 patients were studied. The patients had a mean age of 60 years (range, 15-94 years); most of the patients (70%) were women and predominantly white. The majority of patients (54%) had initial heart rates of 161 to 200 beats/min, and 49% of the patients had a history of PSVT. The inappropriate use of adenosine occurred in 45 cases (20%). The misidentification rates per year ranged from 9% to 31%, with the lowest occurring after a targeted education program on tachydysrhythmias. An initial heart rate of less than 160 beats/min and the absence of a history of either a fast heart rate or palpitations were associated with inappropriate use of adenosine.

Conclusions.—Paramedics in the EMS system are more likely to use adenosine appropriately for patients with initial heart rates of greater than 160 beats/min and a history of rapid heart rate or palpitations. Additional studies are needed to identify factors associated with rhythm interpretation errors in the prehospital setting and to evaluate error reduction strategies.

▶ Notable about this 10-year retrospective study of the prehospital use of adenosine in 224 patients is that all the adverse reactions that occurred resolved spontaneously and that there was not a statistically significant association with adverse reactions and the inappropriate use of adenosine. The article does suggest that protocols calling for the use of adenosine only in patients with a heart rate greater than 160 would eliminate a large portion of its improper use. Overall, this study seems to indicate that with appropriate training, adenosine can be used effectively in the prehospital environment.

S. L. Werner, MD

Albuterol Sulfate Administration by EMT-Basics: Results of a Demonstration Project
Markenson D, Foltin G, Tunik M, et al (Columbia Univ, New York; NYU School of Medicine, New York)
Prehosp Emerg Care 8:34-40, 2004   10–13

Background.—Asthma is a major cause of morbidity in both adults and children, accounting for 1.5 million visits to the ED and 5000 deaths annually. The incidence of and mortality from asthma are increasing in both children and adults. Children arriving by ambulance are 4 times as likely to be admitted as those who access the ED by other means. Albuterol inhalation therapy has been demonstrated to be effective in reversing bronchospasm. This study assessed the ability to train emergency medical technicians–basic (EMT-Bs) to accurately identify bronchospasm and, on the basis of a treatment protocol, to administer albuterol sulfate via nebulization as a standing order and to measure the improvement in patient conditions after treatment.

Methods.—EMS agencies were enrolled in the study, and EMT-Bs were trained with the use of a 4-hour curriculum. For each patient, a prehospital data collection form was completed that included identifying data for the EMT-B, patient assessment, and history information. Pretreatment and posttreatment assessments and a hospital data collection form were completed, including the diagnosis of the ED physician, assessment of bronchospasm, number of albuterol treatments received in the ED, and final disposition of the patient.

Results.—During the year-long study, EMT-Bs treated 190 patients. Across all values, patients showed a clinical improvement as a result of the therapy. Concurrence in the assessment of bronchospasm by the EMT-B with an ED physician was found in 87.4% of patients. The accuracy rate increased to more than 94% when allergic reaction, anaphylaxis, bronchiolitis, and chronic obstructive pulmonary disease were included in the diagnosis list of bronchospasm.

Conclusion.—This study found that EMT-Bs were very successful in the evaluation of bronchospasm. It is safe for EMT-Bs, based on their assessment, to administer albuterol via nebulizer for bronchospasm.

▶ With the introduction of assisting patients with the self-administration of albuterol and epi-pens into the EMT-B curriculum, it was only a matter of time before the question of EMT-Bs administering these medications was raised. This small study suggests that albuterol can be safely administered by EMT-Bs. While perhaps not appropriate for all EMS systems, the timely administration of albuterol can be life saving, and its administration by EMT-Bs should certainly be considered by systems without rapid advanced life support response. EMT-B administration of epi-pens and possibly atropine/pralidoxime in prefilled, pen-type syringes should also be investigated.

S. L. Werner, MD

Emergency Physician–Verified Out-of-Hospital Intubation: Miss Rates by Paramedics
Jones JH, Murphy MP, Dickson RL, et al (Indiana Univ, Indianapolis)
Acad Emerg Med 11:707-709, 2004   10–14

Background.—Endotracheal intubation in the out-of-hospital setting is a standard intervention for an unstable patient in need of definitive airway management. It is believed that the use of endotracheal intubation is associated with improved outcomes. The consequences of an unrecognized misplaced endotracheal tube (ETT) included increased patient morbidity and mortality. Previous studies have reported the out-of-hospital miss rate for endotracheal intubation to range from 1% to 4%. In these studies, the verification of placement for all these studies was performed in the ED arrival, and a variety of techniques were used to verify ETT placement. However, a recent study found a much higher miss rate of 25% in a setting in which verification of ETT placement was performed by emergency physicians. The number of unrecognized missed out-of-hospital intubation by ground paramedics using emergency physician verification as the criterion for verification of ETT placement was prospectively quantified.

Methods.—This observational, prospective study included consecutive intubated patients arriving by ground emergency medical service transport to 2 urban teaching hospitals. Placement of the ETT was verified by emergency physicians and evaluated by the use of a combination of direct visualization, esophageal detector device (EDD), colorimetric end-tidal carbon dioxide (ETCO2), and physical examination.

Results.—In the 6-month study period, 208 out-of-hospital intubations were performed, including 160 (76.9%) medical patients and 48 (23.1%) trauma patients. There were 12 (5.8%) ETTs misplaced outside the trachea in 10 medical patients and 2 trauma patients. Of these 12 misplaced ETTs, a verification device (ETCO2 or EDD) was used in 3 cases (25%) and was not used in 9 cases (75%).

Conclusions.—This study in 2 urban, midwestern teaching hospitals found a rate of unrecognized misplaced out-of-hospital intubation of 5.8%. This finding is consistent with the results of previous studies but discordant with a study that used only emergency physician verification performed on arrival at the ED.

▶ This is the first study of verification of prehospital intubation by emergency physicians since the study by Katz and Falk[1] that found an alarming rate of 24 percent of missed field intubations. Although the results of this study seem encouraging, a miss rate of 6% for this critical intervention is still unacceptably high. In addition, this study differs significantly from the Katz and Falk study in that three quarters of the intubations were conducted by paramedics from a single EMS system, all of whom had received a fairly high level of initial training (requiring at least 10 in hospital intubations) and ongoing training, and who, on average, perform approximately 60 intubations annually, standards unlikely to occur in many EMS systems.

Also of note is the lack of secondary verification of tube placement by either EDD or ETCO2 in more than half of the field intubations. No means of secondary confirmation was used in 9 of the 12 missed intubations. Although this was not statistically significant for the relatively few number of missed intubations in this study, it does raise the question of the possibility of improved miss rates through the use of secondary confirmation.

S. L. Werner, MD

Reference

1. Katz SH, Falk JL: Misplaced endotracheal tubes by paramedics in an urban emergency medical services system. *Acad Emerg Med* 37:32-37, 2001.

Basic Cardiac Life Support Providers Checking the Carotid Pulse: Performance, Degree of Conviction, and Influencing Factors

Lapostolle F, Le Toumelin P, Agostinucci JM, et al (Hôpital Avicenne, Bobigny, France; Croix Rouge Française, Paris)
Acad Emerg Med 11:878-880, 2004   10–15

Background.—Because of concerns that inaccuracy could delay the start of CPR, the American Heart Association and the European Resuscitation Council recently recommended lay people stop checking the carotid pulse in unconscious persons. Whether health care providers are any better at accurately assessing the carotid pulse in unresponsive persons was evaluated with the use of a mannequin model.

Methods.—Participants were 64 health care providers (55% men; median age, 22 years) who had been trained in basic cardiac life support for a median of 3 years. Each participant checked the carotid pulse on a computerized mannequin for 10 or 30 seconds with the pulse absent, weak, or strong. Seven test conditions were examined, and the order of the conditions was randomized. After each simulation, participants were asked whether they felt a pulse and how certain they were of their answer (graded on a 100-mm visual analogue scale).

Results.—When the pulse was absent, 58% of participants responded correctly during each of the two 10-second examinations, and 50% responded correctly when checking the pulse for 30 seconds. A weak pulse was tested only in the 10-second condition, and 83% of participants gave the correct answer. When the pulse was strong, 92% and 84% of participants responded correctly during the 10-second examination (performed twice), and 84% responded correctly when checking the pulse for 30 seconds. The accuracy of the answer increased significantly as the pulse strength increased. Participants were 100% convinced their answer was accurate, except in 2 conditions: when checking an absent pulse for 10 seconds and for 30 seconds, the median degrees of conviction were only 66% and 83%, respectively. Also, the degree of conviction participants felt about the accuracy of their response increased significantly as the accuracy of the answer increased and as the pulse strength increased.

Conclusion.—Even these experienced health care providers often inaccurately assessed the strength of the carotid pulse, and they had less faith in the accuracy of their answer when the pulse was absent. These data suggest that health care providers, like lay people, should forego checking the carotid pulse before initiating CPR.

▶ This article confirms some of my suspicions about our accuracy in determining the presence of a pulse during evaluation of an unresponsive, apneic, hypotensive patient. I am probably not the only one who has received 3 simultaneous responses—"yes," "no," and "I'm not sure,"—to the inquiry of the presence of a palpable pulse during a resuscitation. This study does show that a strong pulse can usually be detected by health care providers, so I do not advocate abandoning the pulse check altogether. But, if the findings regarding our ability to detect weaker pulses in mannequins are replicated in humans, it raises a number of questions regarding the potential harm or benefit of performing chest compressions on patients with some level of perfusion.

S. L. Werner, MD

Clinical Variables Associated With Mortality in Out-of-Hospital Patients With Hemodynamically Significant Bradycardia
Schwartz B, Vermeulen MJ, Idestrup C, et al (Sunnybrook and Women's College Health Sciences Centre, Toronto; Univ of Toronto)
Acad Emerg Med 11:656-661, 2004   10–16

Background.—Hemodynamically unstable bradycardia is characterized by a heart rate below 60 bpm, low systolic blood pressure, and other symptoms such as change in mental status, angina, or pulmonary edema. There have been few studies of the clinical course, treatment, or longer-term outcomes of patients with hemodynamically unstable bradycardia in the out-of-hospital setting. Such studies would provide important baseline data for the evaluation of new therapies for this disorder. Mortality rates were estimated and clinical variables associated with mortality among patients with hemodynamically unstable bradycardia in an urban EMS system were identified.

Methods.—This retrospective study was conducted in a large urban EMS system and included all adult noncardiac arrest patients transported by advanced life support paramedics from March 1996 to February 1997 with a heart rate of 60 bpm or less and systolic blood pressure 90 mm Hg or less. Transcutaneous pacing was not available. Patients were excluded if they were under 18 years of age or pregnant or presented without vital signs. Multivariate analysis was conducted of the association of patient characteristics with 30-day mortality.

Results.—There were 247 patients in the study, of whom 133 (53.9%) received a final bolus, 37 (15%) were treated with atropine, and 17 (6.9%) received dopamine. There were 51 deaths (20.7%) in the 19-month follow-up period, including death on the same day in 10.5% of patients and death within 1 year in 17.8% of patients. Variables associated with 30-day mortality included wide QRS complex, use of heart rate–lowering calcium channel blockers, and paramedic assessment of lack of patient improvement over the course of the call.

Conclusions.—The mortality rate among out-of-hospital patients with hemodynamically unstable bradycardia is high. A wide QRS complex and the use of heart rate–lowering calcium channel blockers were associated with 30-day mortality.

▶ Fair warning. Take symptomatic bradycardia in the out-of-hospital setting seriously. This study provides background and demonstrates the need for investigation of therapies aimed at improving outcomes in bradycardic patients, including fluid, the use of atropine and vasoactive medications, as well as transcutaneous pacing.

S. L. Werner, MD

Air Medical Transport of Severely Head-Injured Patients Undergoing Paramedic Rapid Sequence Intubation
Poste JC, Davis DP, Ochs M, et al (UCSD Emergency Medicine, San Diego, Calif)
Air Med J 23:36-40, 2004   10–17

Background.—Traumatic brain injury is responsible for a significant amount of morbidity and mortality, and numerous studies have documented an association between hypoxia and increased mortality. As a result of these findings, aggressive prehospital airway protocols have been developed for severely head-injured patients, including the use of rapid sequence intubation (RSI) by flight nurses and some paramedic agencies. One study, the San Diego Paramedic RSI Trial, documented an increase in mortality in association with paramedic RSI of severely head-injured patients when compared with nonintubated historical control subjects from the same prehospital system. The effect of air medical transport of trial patients on outcome was investigated.

Methods.—This prospective study enrolled adult trauma victims with severe traumatic brain injury and a Glasgow Coma Scale (GCS) score of 3 to 8. Paramedics performed RSI using midazolam and succinylcholine. Air medical crews were available at the discretion of ground paramedics, generally for lengthy transports. The patients were matched to historical controls using the parameters of age, gender, mechanism, severity of injury score, and abbreviated injury scale scores for each body system. The patients transported by air and ground were compared with regard to demographics, clinical parameters, vital signs, arterial blood gas data, and outcome.

Results.—A total of 336 patients were included in the study, including 79 air medical transports and 257 ground transports. There were no significant differences between the groups in terms of demographic, clinical, vital sign, and arterial blood gas data. Air medical patients had decreased mortality versus matched controls (28% vs 31%) and ground patients had increased mortality versus matched controls (33% vs 22%). Discordant group analysis demonstrated a statistically significant effect of transport personnel on outcome. The improved outcomes were not explained by the use of advanced procedures or the use of mannitol. Capnometry was used by air medical crews to guide ventilation in all study patients.

Conclusions.—Air medical transport of patients with severe head injuries undergoing paramedic RSI was associated with improved outcomes. A portion of these improved outcomes may be attributable to improved ventilation by capnometry.

▶ This study has a number of problems. First, the methodology is troublesome. Rather than a randomized controlled study of air transport versus ground transport of intubated trauma patients, the authors compared intubated patients transported by air versus ground to nonintubated historical controls with similar injury patterns. In addition, the transport method was determined by ground crew, not randomization. Controls were matched for multiple factors but there may be some inherent difference in intubated versus nonintubated patients regardless of injury score and GCS. Second, there is a substantial, unexplained difference in mortality between the 2 control groups—21% in the ground transport control group versus 31% in the air transport group, which is not addressed. From the limited data provided, it appears that the control groups were very similar in demographics and injury scores so the significantly lower mortality in the ground transport control group warrants investigation. Lastly, the authors cite improved ventilation management by air transport crews as a possible cause of decreased mortality in air transport patients, yet their data show no difference in pO_2 or pCO_2 of the air versus ground transport patients.

S. L. Werner, MD

Against All Advice: An Analysis of Out-of-Hospital Refusals of Care

Knight S, Olson LM, Cook LJ, et al (Univ of Utah, Salt Lake City)
Ann Emerg Med 42:689-696, 2003   10–18

Background.—Among the many unique patient care issues that EMS providers face is the treatment of patients who refuse care or transport by ambulance to a hospital. The rate of refusal of out-of-hospital care has been reported to be as high as 30% of all EMS calls, but most studies have reported refusal rates between 5% and 10%. Most research on refusal of out-of-hospital care has focused on the adult population, and thus little is known of the out-of-hospital incidents that result in refusal of care for extreme age groups such as children or the elderly. To identify the characteristics of out-of-hospital incidents that result in refusal of care by the age of the patient and to determine the rate of subsequent out-of-hospital care, ED visits, inpatient stays, and deaths for patients involved in a refusal of out-of-hospital care were the goals.

Methods.—State wide EMS data for Utah identifying incidents of refusal of care were probabilistically linked to data on Utah statewide inpatient, ED, and death certificate data within 7 days of the initial EMS refusals for 1996 to 1998. A refusal of care was defined as an incident in which field treatment or transport was refused and did not include incidents in which EMS providers decided that the patient did not require care or transport.

Results.—Of the 277,244 EMS incidents in Utah in the study period, there were 14,109 (5.1%) refusals of care. Dispatches for motor vehicle accidents resulted in the highest rate of refusal of care for all age groups, ranging from 8% to 11.7%. Just over 3% of patients involved in a refusal of care incident were involved in a subsequent EMS dispatch within 1 week. One fifth of the patients involved in EMS refusals of care had a subsequent visit to the ED. The rate of hospitalization for patients who refused EMS care was less than 2%, with hospitalization highest among children younger than 3 years and adults older than 64 years. There were 25 deaths among adults within 1 week of refusing EMS care, with 19 of these deaths (76%) among persons older than 64 years.

Conclusions.—This statewide study found that refusal of care incidents are representative of only a small proportion of all EMS incidents. There are many reasons for refusals of care, and the risk for missed intervention would appear to be minimal.

▶ This ambitious study provides reassurance that the risk of refusal of care appears to be minimal. However, it did find that patients at the extremes of age were at risk for recurrent hospital visits and older patients were at higher risk of death. This finding is similar to that of Moss et al[1] who examined AMA refusals and found that older patients were more likely to have repeat EMS calls after AMA refusals. Whether the data from this study can be extrapolated to other populations is unclear. It is also unclear as to the protocols followed by EMS providers in Utah with regard to patients who are allowed to refuse care and transport. In addition, it would be interesting to see this data stratified by AMA versus "appropriate" refusals in a future study.

S. L. Werner, MD

Reference

1. Moss ST, Chan TC, Buchanan J, et al: Outcome study of prehospital patients signed out against medical advice by field paramedics. *Ann Emerg Med* 31:247-250, 1998.

Ultrasound Image Quality Comparison Between an Inexpensive Hand-held Emergency Department (ED) Ultrasound Machine and a Large Mo-bile ED Ultrasound System
Blaivas M, Brannam L, Theodoro D (Med College of Georgia, Augusta; North Shore Univ, Manhasset, NY)
Acad Emerg Med 11:778-781, 2004
10–19

Background.—The use of emergency US has been expanded as a result of the development of smaller and less expensive US equipment. These portable US machines have been found to be well suited to use in the small rooms and tight corridors of many EDs and to the budget constraints under which most EDs operate. However, questions have been raised about the image quality provided by portable US machines. Whether a difference exists between images obtained with a common portable US machine and those obtained with a larger, more expensive US machine when comparing typical views used by emergency physicians was investigated.

Methods.—A cross-sectional blinded comparison was performed of images from similar sonographic windows obtained from healthy models with an inexpensive handheld US device and a large mobile US machine. The images obtained included typical abdominal and vascular applications with the use of the abdominal and linear transducers on each machine. All of the images were printed on identical high-resolution printers and then digitized, cropped, masked, and placed in random order for comparing each view per model. Each image pair was rated by 3 credentialed emergency physician radiologists for resolution, detail, and total image quality according to a 10-point Likert scale. A score of 10 was the best rating for each category.

Results.—A total of 49 image pairs were evaluated. The mean resolution, detail, and image quality scores for the large mobile machine were 6.8, 6.8, and 6.6, respectively. Corresponding means for the portable handheld machine were 6.3, 6.3, and 6.0, respectively. The difference in detail scores between the 2 US systems was not statistically significant. However, there were small but statistically significant differences for resolution and total image quality between the 2 machines (Fig 1).

Conclusion.—The small handheld US machine and larger mobile US system were found to be comparable in terms of image detail in ED applications. There were small but statistically significant differences between the 2 systems in terms of resolution and overall image quality, but the clinical implications of this finding have not been determined.

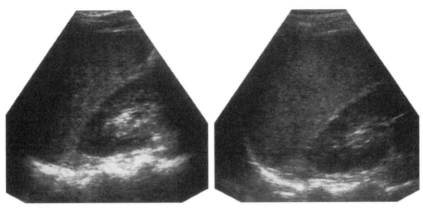

FIGURE 1.—A comparison of a Morison's pouch image from the same model obtained in the same orientation. The left shows the SonoSite 180 Plus image and the right shows the GE 400 Pro image. (Courtesy of Blaivas M, Brannam L, Theodoro D: Ultrasound image quality comparison between an inexpensive handheld emergency department (ED) ultrasound machine and a large mobile ED ultrasound system. *Acad Emerg Med* 11:778-781, 2004.)

▶ This is important information as the use of bedside US by emergency physicians increases and more emergency physician groups and hospitals are purchasing US equipment for use in the ED. In addition to mobility and overall image quality, other important factors to consider before investing in US equipment include the user friendliness of the machine and the options for image acquisition and storage.

US machines vary in the number of settings that are preset or bundled by the manufacturer. Bundled presets increase ease of use but allow the user less flexibility in fine-tuning image quality. Machines with many settings that require individual manual adjustment by the user allow fine-tuning of image quality but may require significantly more user knowledge/training to operate. How the images are acquired and will ultimately be stored in the medical record (PAX vs hard copy vs CD/video) should also be considered in the determination of the appropriate US machine for a group or ED.

S. L. Werner, MD

12-Lead Electrocardiograms During Basic Life Support Care
Provo TA, Frascone RJ (Advanced Circulatory Systems Inc, Eden Prairie, Minn; Regions Hosp Emergency Med Services, St Paul, Minn)
Prehosp Emerg Care 8:212-216, 2004   10–20

Background.—Prehospital 12-lead ECGs (PTLs) are vital to the diagnosis of myocardial ischemia. Twelve-lead ECGs were moved out of the hospital several years ago in an effort to determine whether PTLs would be of diagnostic quality and would provide earlier detection of acute myocardial infarctions. They have been performed successfully by paramedics for several years, but emergency medical technicians (EMTs) have not typically performed PTLs. It was determined (1) whether the acquisition of PTLs by basic life support (BLS) EMTs prolongs scene times, (2) whether EMTs can make appropriate decisions regarding which patients would be likely candidates for PTL assessment, and (3) what value physicians place on PTLs performed by BLS personnel.

Methods.—A prospective evaluation was performed of PTL performance in 4 BLS agencies. EMTs in these agencies provided standard care to patients on even days, while on odd days, the EMTs also performed a PTL. The scene times for 77 patients receiving a PTL were compared with scene times for 100 patients who did not receive a PTL.

Results.—The mean scene time for patients who did not receive a PTL was 11.9 minutes, whereas the mean scene time for patients who did receive a PTL was 16.9 minutes. Physician feedback was received on 63 of the 77 PTLs. The receiving physicians were in agreement with the EMTs regarding the need for PTL in 93.6% of patients and found them moderately helpful.

Conclusions.—The scene time was increased by approximately 5 minutes when PTLs were performed by EMTs. Most of the physicians agreed on the need for the PTLs. PTL acquisition by EMTs is feasible but is associated with slightly increased scene times. However, evaluation in other BLS agencies is necessary for validation of these findings.

▶ Acquiring a 12-lead ECG is a skill that with the appropriate training and repetition should be easily performed by BLS providers. The real question is how the information obtained by the 12-lead will be used. If BLS providers are acquiring ECGs that are not being transmitted to the receiving ED physician or being reviewed immediately on arrival to the ED, the on-scene delay probably is not justified. On the other hand, if BLS PTLs are used as part of the initial evaluation of chest pain patients, there is no reason to think that their performance by basic providers should be any less useful than performance of 12-leads by paramedics. Indeed, it could be argued that in rural, BLS-only systems, a PTL transmitted to medical command could be extremely useful in expediting the care and even in determining the appropriate destination facility for patients meeting criteria for primary percutaneous transluminal coronary angioplasty or thrombolysis.

S. L. Werner, MD

Evaluation of an End-Tidal Portable ETCO$_2$ Colorimetric Breath Indicator (COLIBRI)

Rabitsch W, Nikolic A, Schellongowski P, et al (Univ of Vienna)
Am J Emerg Med 22:4-9, 2004   10–21

Background.—Endotracheal intubation has become a routine procedure for the provision of oxygenation, ventilation, airway protection, or delivery of medication. Endotracheal intubation is considered a simple procedure, but it can have serious adverse consequences. Outcome studies during the past 30 years have consistently reported endotracheal intubation as a leading cause of injury in anesthetic practice. Thus, evaluation of the position of the endotracheal tube is important after in-hospital and prehospital emergency intubation. Colorimetric breath indicators have been developed to provide immediate control of the tube positioning by showing a color change according to end-tidal CO_2 (ETCO$_2$) concentrations. It was hypothesized that colorimetric breath indicators can provide reliable confirmation of endotracheal tube positioning.

Methods.—The effectiveness and safety of a new colorimetric breath indicator (Colibri; ICOR AB, Bromma, Sweden) were evaluated in 147 patients during general anesthesia, in critically ill patients, during transport to in-hospital interventions, and in a study design after insertion of a second tube into the esophagus in patients receiving long-term ventilation. The indicator was attached between the respective airway and ventilatory tubing.

Results.—The Colibri indicator functioned well in all the groups and demonstrated no false results in the group with tubes inserted into the trachea and esophagus.

Conclusions.—The Colibri colorimetric breath indicator may be a valuable tool for the evaluation and control of endotracheal tube position. This indicator is small and portable and independent of a power supply or electronic equipment, which means it is available for immediate use.

Accuracy of Portable Quantitative Capnometers and Capnographs Under Prehospital Conditions

Biedler AE, Wilhelm W, Kreuer S, et al (Universitätskliniken des Saarlandes, Homburg/Saar, Germany; Klinikum Leverkusen, Germany; Klinik für Anaesthesiologie und Operative Intensivemedizin, Krankenanstalten Gilead, Bielefeld, Germany)
Am J Emerg Med 21:520-524, 2003   10–22

Background.—The application of capnometry and capnography was for many years limited to the operating room. Under preclinical conditions outside the hospital, ventilated patients were excluded from routine quantitative carbon dioxide monitoring. Most of the reasons for this exclusion were technical restrictions, in that formerly available devices did not meet the requirements for routine use in emergency medicine. In the last few years, several capnometers and some capnographs have been introduced to meet those needs. However, only a few investigations have reported on the accuracy of carbon dioxide measurement of portable devices. None of these studies have considered the special ambient conditions when capnometers are operated outside the hospital. Of particular concern are changes in ambient temperature in cold conditions. The CO_2 accuracy of portable mainstream and sidestream capnometers with respect to international standards and preclinical emergency medical conditions was assessed.

Methods.—Measurements were performed under temperature conditions of $+22°C$ and $-20°C$ by using dry gas mixtures with different CO_2 concentrations (standard temperature pressure dry [STPD] conditions), and in patients ventilated with pure oxygen (body temperature pressure saturated [BTPS] conditions).

Results.—The accuracy was between $+1\%$ and $+12\%$ for STPD conditions and -0.4% and $+11\%$ for BTPS conditions. The measurements were affected by low ambient temperature only in the NPB-75 device ($+15\%$).

Conclusion.—Portable quantitative capnometers have the capability to meet the accuracy requirements mandated by international standards but are affected by changes in ambient temperatures.

▶ Continuous end-tidal CO_2 ($ETCO_2$) monitoring has long been accepted by anesthesiologists as standard of care for confirming endotracheal intubation. However, continuous $ETCO_2$ monitoring equipment is often expensive and previously had not been shown to be suited to the prehospital environment. While some EMS systems and EDs are using disposable colorimetric $ETCO_2$ devices to make the initial confirmation of tube placement, these have not been shown to be reliable for continuous monitoring during transport, and are often removed from the endotracheal tube after the initial confirmation. Given Katz and Falk's recent study[1] demonstrating that significantly more prehospital intubations may be misplaced on arrival in the ED than previously thought, consideration of continuous $ETCO_2$ monitoring in the prehospital environment is certainly warranted. In addition, further research of prehospital intubations with continuous $ETCO_2$ monitoring may help answer one of the questions raised by Falk and Katz' study—whether their findings demonstrate a high rate of initial endotracheal tube misplacement or a high incidence of postintubation displacement in prehospital intubations.

S. L. Werner, MD

Reference

1. Katz SH, Falk JL: Misplaced endotracheal tubes by paramedics in an urban emergency medical services system. *Ann Emerg Med* 37:32-37, 2001.

The Feasibility of Pain Assessment in the Prehospital Setting
McLean SA, Domeier RM, DeVore HK, et al (Univ of Michigan, Ann Arbor)
Prehosp Emerg Care 8:155-161, 2004   10–23

Background.—The alleviation of pain and discomfort is important for prehospital patients. Pain in this population, as in other patient populations, appears to be undertreated. There is an urgent need for research examining the effectiveness of EMS interventions for common conditions, and the identification of pain as an important prehospital outcome, but there have been no studies of the feasibility of pain measurement in prehospital patients in the United States. Among patients aged 13 years and older, the feasibility of prehospital pain measurement with a verbal and numeric rating scale was determined, as well as the distribution of pain severity present in this population.

Methods.—A retrospective cross-sectional study was performed of EMS run sheets after implementation of a universal prehospital pain assessment protocol. The assessment used a 4-item scale for the verbal rating scale, with pain rated as "none," "mild," "severe," and "unable to respond." For the numeric rating scale, the paramedics were asked to complete an additional column on the run sheet. In this column, pain was rated from 0 to 100 on the basis of the patient's response to a request to rate the pain on this basis. Demographic, location, and call information was also included.

Results.—A total of 1227 run sheets were reviewed; 582 (47%) of the patients were male, and 452 (36%) were aged 65 years or older. Three quarters of the patients were nontrauma transports, and 2% were unconscious. Among the conscious patients, pain was assessed with the protocol in 1002 (84%) of 1200 patients. Among those who reported pain, 104 (20%) of 518 patients completed a verbal rating scale but not a numeric rating scale. The greatest risk factor for no pain assessment was altered mental status; 39% of patients were not assessed for pain for this reason. Among the patients with altered mental status who reported pain, 48% completed a verbal rating scale only. Moderate or severe pain was reported by 31% of patients in the sample.

Conclusions.—The prehospital assessment of pain with a verbal rating scale and a numeric rating scale is feasible. Additional studies are necessary to confirm this finding in other settings. Moderate or severe pain was present in about 31% of the patients.

▶ This is the first study addressing the EMS Outcomes Project (EMSOP) IV goal of determining the feasibility of assessing pain in the out-of-hospital setting. Given the widespread use of previously validated pain scales by health care providers at all levels, it comes as no surprise to me that they can be used by prehospital providers. I would hope that we can rapidly move on and direct research in this area toward determining effective strategies for pain management in the prehospital setting.

S. L. Werner, MD

The Location and Incidence of Out-of-Hospital Cardiac Arrest in Georgia: Implications for Placement of Automated External Defibrillators

Malcom GE III, Thompson TM, Coule PL (Med College of Georgia, Augusta; Wake Forest Univ, Winston-Salem, NC; Mountain Area Health Education Ctr, Asheville, NC)
Prehosp Emerg Care 8:10-14, 2004   10–24

Background.—Access to defibrillation has been demonstrated to increase survival from out-of-hospital cardiac arrest (OOHCA). The relationship between population density and incidence and location of OOHCAs in the state of Georgia was examined.

Study Design.—Data from 6530 Georgia state EMS patient care reports of OOHCA for the year 2000 were divided into 159 counties of incidence.

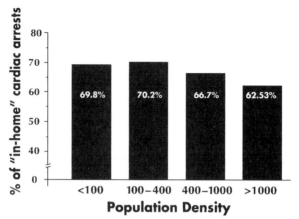

FIGURE 1.—Percentage of "in home" cardiac arrests by population density. (Courtesy of Malcom GE III, Thompson TM, Coule PL: The location and incidence of out-of-hospital cardiac arrest in Georgia: Implications for placement of automated external defibrillators. *Prehosp Emerg Care* 8:10-14, 2004. Hanley & Belfus, Philadelphia, 215-546-4995, www.hanleyandbelfus.com.)

Counties were subdivided by population density. The incidence of OOHCAs for each location type was calculated by population density.

Findings.—The less-than-100-people-per-square-mile density group had only 21.77% of the state's population but 30.96% of the cardiac arrests. The more-than-1000-people-per-square-mile density group had 35.46% of the population but only 23.55% of the cardiac arrests (Fig 1). The majority of OOHCAs occurred in the home in all population density groups (Fig 2).

Conclusion.—In the state of Georgia, there are significant differences in OOHCA incidence based on population density. These differences should be considered when automated external defibrillator (AED) placement strategies are being developed.

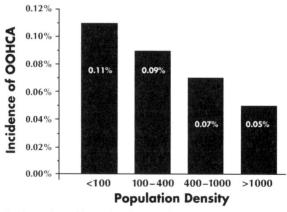

FIGURE 2.—Incidence of out-of-hospital cardiac arrest by population density. (Courtesy of Malcom GE III, Thompson TM, Coule PL: The location and incidence of out-of-hospital cardiac arrest in Georgia: Implications for placement of automated external defibrillators. *Prehosp Emerg Care* 8:10-14, 2004. Hanley & Belfus, Philadelphia, 215-546-4995, www.hanleyandbelfus.com.)

▶ This article demonstrates the importance of incorporating demographic information and area-specific patterns of OOHCAs in the development of AED placement and public access defibrillation strategies. Of note is the finding that in all of the different population density location types, the large majority of OOHCAs occurred in the home. Except for residential institutions, only a small percentage of OOHCAs occurred at each of the other location types. In addition, there was a significantly higher overall incidence of OOHCAs in rural areas. Unfortunately, the authors did not stratify the data by age or other demographic information, which would likely be useful in explaining this finding.

A similar study of the locations of OOHCAs in an urban setting (Pittsburgh) by R. L. Frank also found that the majority of OOHCAS over the 3-year study period occurred in the home and failed to identify any high-risk location types for nonresidential OOHCAs except dialysis centers and nursing homes.[1] These studies reinforce the need for states and communities to use demographic data and analysis of OOHCA locations in determining optimal resource allocation for AED placement and in developing public access defibrillation programs.

We may not quite be ready for over-the-counter defibrillators, as recently suggested by Matt Eisenberg,[2] but, with the continued AED price reductions, additional strategies to place AEDs out into the communities where arrests are most likely to occur may be worth exploring, especially in those locations where fire/EMS response times are long. Of course, these strategies would necessarily include a commitment to community cardiopulmonary resuscitation programs—with AED training.

S. L. Werner, MD

References

1. Frank RL, Rausch MA, Menegazzi JJ, et al: The locations of nonresidential out-of-hospital cardiac arrests in the city of Pittsburg over a three-year period: Implications for automated eternal defibrillator placement. *Prehosp Emerg Care* 5:247-251, 2001.
2. Eisenberg MS: Is it time for over-the-counter defibrillators. *JAMA* 284:1435-1438, 2000.

Evacuation Priorities in Mass Casualty Terror-Related Events: Implications for Contingency Planning
Einav S, Feigenberg Z, Weissman C, et al (Hadassah Hebrew Univ, Jerusalem; Magen David Adom Israeli Natl Emergency Med Services, Jerusalem)
Ann Surg 239:304-310, 2004   10–25

Introduction.—Civilian mass casualty events are becoming an increasingly important security issue worldwide. The recent onslaught of terror-associated mass casualty incidents (MCIs) in Israel has forced a change in the way rescue teams manage critically ill patients. During a mass casualty with multiple and severe civilian injuries, evacuating all critically injured patients to a level I trauma center may not be appropriate because treatment of a patient population must take priority over treatment of individuals. Evacuation priorities during terror-related MCIs and their implications for hospital organizations/contingency planning were examined.

Methods.—A retrospective analysis was performed of emergency medical evacuations from terror related MCIs by the rescue teams of the Israel Magen David Adom Israeli National Emergency Medical Services (MDA) organization that occurred between September 29, 2000, and September 31, 2002. MCIs were considered to be terrorist attacks of a large enough scale to recruit most of the rescue teams and security force resources within a defined region, regardless of the actual number of casualties. The MDA records were screened to exclude poor quality or inadequate data.

Results.—During the evaluation period, 1116 terror-related incidents occurred in Israel. Of these, 45 were mass casualty incidents. Thirty-three MCIs provided data adequate on 1156 casualties. Five hundred and six of the 1123 (57%) available and mobilized ambulances were needed to perform 612 evaluations. Rescue teams arrived on the scene in less than 5 minutes and evacuated the last urgent casualties within 15 to 20 minutes. Most nonurgent and urgent patients were transferred to medical centers close to the attack. Fewer than half of the urgent casualties were evacuated to more distant trauma centers. Independent variables predicting evacuation to a trauma center were it being the hospital closest to the attack (odds ratio [OR], 249.2; $P < .001$), evacuation in fewer than 10 minutes of the attack (OR, 9.3; $P = .003$), and an urgent patient in the ambulance (OR, 5.6; $P < .001$).

Conclusion.—Hospitals near terror-induced MCIs have an important role in trauma patient care. All hospitals should be included in contingency plans for MCIs. The challenges posed by terror-induced MCIs necessitates the consideration of a paradigm shift in trauma care.

▶ This article reviews evacuation from civilian MCIs in Israel from 2000 to 2002.

In these events, medics did not have the luxury to transport all critically injured trauma patients to level I trauma centers as they would have in typical civilian trauma. Instead, the demands of the MCIs appear to be well managed by large-scale "scoop and run" to the nearest hospital. The nearest hospital (whether level I trauma facility or not) then serves as a civilian equivalent to an evacuation hospital, where further triage, major stabilization, and damage control surgery are performed; patients are later transferred to other hospitals. The remaining, less critically injured patients would then be transported to other hospitals away from the casualty site to minimize overwhelming any one hospital.

The success of this transport scheme relies on rapid on-scene triage, multiperson transport, central command and communication for all medics, and preparation of all hospitals to serve as evacuation hospitals. These infrastructural elements may not be easily recreated in other settings, whether because of a lack of organization or the investment of time and money. Intensive care, surgical (ICS) may manage the communication and command in any casualty, however, in the setting of multiple paramedic services and competing hospitals (absent any memoranda of understanding that would make the system less likely to work). This may be a call for the organization of multiple small systems into larger regional systems.

N. B. Handly, MD, MSc, MS

Mass Casualty Terrorist Bombings: A Comparison of Outcomes by Bombing Type
Arnold JL, Halpern P, Tsai M-C, et al (Tufts Univ, Springfield, Mass; Tel-Aviv Sourasky Med Ctr, Israel; Natl Cheng-Kung Univ, Taiwan, Republic of China)
Ann Emerg Med 43:263-273, 2004   10–26

Introduction.—Between 1991 and 2000, 88% of the 93 reported worldwide terrorist attacks that caused more than 30 casualties involved explosions. These attacks resulted in significant death and destruction and challenged emergency medical care systems in 27 countries. Mass casualty terrorist bombings were examined for outcomes, with comparisons between those causing immediate structural collapse, those occurring in open air, and those conducted within a confined space.

Methods.—English language articles reporting epidemiologic outcomes of terrorist bombings were identified in a MEDLINE search from 1966 through September 2002. Studies eligible for analysis reported terrorist bombings causing 30 or more casualties. Excluded were bombings that occurred after evacuation of the building had started, those in confined spaces in which the majority of victims were outside the space, and bombings that occurred in flying aircraft. Pooled and median rates of mortality, number of survivors among the immediately injured, ED use, and number of hospitalizations according to specific injury types were determined for each bombing type.

Results.—Thirty-five of 76 articles that reported epidemiologic outcomes of terrorist bombing met inclusion criteria. The 2001 World Trade Center attack was excluded because of a lack of sufficient outcome data during the study period, the evacuations that occurred before the second tower was attacked, and the mixed bombing type. The 29 terrorist bombings analyzed collectively produced 8364 casualties, 903 immediate deaths, and 7461 immediately surviving injured. Pooled immediate mortality rates were structural collapse, 25%; confined space, 8%; and open air, 4%. Pooled hospitalization rates for these bombing types were, respectively, 25%, 36%, and 15%.

Penetrating soft tissue injuries were the injuries most frequently seen in EDs after structural collapse and open air bombings. In addition to penetrating soft tissue injuries, victims of bombings in confined spaces were likely to also have fractures, burns, tympanic membrane rupture, and pulmonary blast.

Conclusion.—Deaths and injuries in terrorist bombing reflected multiple factors, including the explosion magnitude, composition, environment, and location; each bombing type produced unique patterns of mortality and injury rates in survivors. Structural collapse bombing caused the most immediate deaths, whereas hospitalization rates tended to be higher in confined space bombings.

▶ Preparation for sudden onset disasters is difficult, beyond drills, without epidemiologic guidance. Drs Arnold et al reviewed reports of mass casualties (greater than 30 casualties) from terrorist bombings and found distinct injury patterns and mortality, depending on whether the bombings occurred with immediate structural collapse, within confined space, or in open air.

Any bombings where evacuations occurred prior to the explosion were excluded, as it would be harder to define the bombing type and injuries according to the 3 scenarios. A number of limitations were acknowledged by the authors including that their analysis did not include characteristics of the explosive device, locations of the victims relative to the explosive, the density of victims, structural characteristics, sequelae including fires, and the prehospital and ED resources available.

The value of this work is that we may be able to better provide resources for care with knowledge of the setting of bombings. Additionally, it will offer guides to gathering data more carefully with each successive event.

N. B. Handly, MD, MSc, MS

11 Toxicology

Natural Toxins and Envenomation

Evidence of Myocardial Ischaemia in Severe Scorpion Envenomation: Myocardial Perfusion Scintigraphy Study

Bahloul M, Hamida CB, Chtourou K, et al (CHU Habib Bourguiba, Tunisia)
Intensive Care Med 30:461-467, 2004   11–1

Introduction.—Cardiorespiratory manifestations, primarily cardiogenic shock and pulmonary edema, are the principal causes of death after scorpion envenomation. The myocardial perfusion by thallium-201 scintigraphy was examined in patients with evidence of myocardial damage after scorpion envenomation in a 1-year prospective investigation.

Methods.—Six nonconsecutive patients admitted to an ICU for severe scorpion envenomation were evaluated. Evidence of myocardial damage was verified via ECG and echocardiography in all 6 patients. Myocardial perfusion scintigraphy (^{201}T1 scintigraphy) along with radionuclide ventriculography (^{99m}Tc) was performed in all participants at an average of 32 hours (range, 12-72 hours) after the sting.

Results.—Radionuclide ventriculography was abnormal in all patients. Abnormalities were similar to those seen on echocardiography. ^{201}T1 scintigraphy demonstrated evidence of myocardial hypoperfusion in all participants. The myocardial hypoperfusion grade and localization were more striking in the abnormal localization demonstrated by echocardiography and ECG, compared with the normal wall. Repeated studies, performed in 2 patients within 6 and 15 days, respectively, revealed considerable, yet not complete, improvement of wall motion and myocardial perfusion. Segments with improved perfusion demonstrated markedly improved regional wall motion. The mean ICU stay was 5.3 days (range, 3-8 days).

Conclusion.—Myocardial hypoperfusion was observed after severe scorpion envenomation in the 6 patients evaluated. The mechanisms of the myocardial hypoperfusion have yet to be determined. The great improvement in wall motion and myocardial perfusion in 2 patients defines the presence of a hypoperfused, yet viable myocardium.

▶ This article represents good evidence for the cardiotoxic effects of scorpion venom, and evidence is building that it is a catecholamine-related effect, rather than a venom effect. I suspect that the partial reversal of the myocardial injury in these patients had much to do with their relative youth and lack of pre-existing cardiac disease. Others are not so lucky.

R. J. Hamilton, MD

Suction for Venomous Snakebite: A Study of "Mock Venom" Extraction in a Human Model

Alberts MB, Shalit M, LoGalbo F (Univ of California, San Francisco–Fresno; Community Med Ctr of Central California, Fresno)
Ann Emerg Med 43:181-186, 2004   11–2

Background.—First aid for a venomous snakebite remains controversial. This prospective human trial determined the percentage of "mock venom" recovered by the Sawyer Extractor pump in a simulated snakebite model.

Study Design.—Radioactively labeled mock venom was injected with a curved 16-gauge needle 1 cm into the right lateral lower leg of 8 adult male volunteers. After 3 minutes, the Sawyer Extractor pump was applied, and the blood removed was collected after 15 minutes. The radioactive counts extracted and remaining were calculated.

Findings.—The envenomation load injected was 89,895 counts per minute. The average radioactivity in the extracted blood was 38.5 counts per minute. The postextraction leg count was 1832 counts lower than the envenomation load, which yields a 2% decrease in the total body venom load after extraction.

Conclusions.—The Sawyer Extractor pump removed bloody fluid from simulated snakebite wounds, but it removed virtually none of the simulated venom. This suggests that this device, and suction in general, is not effective in reducing the amount of total body venom after a snakebite.

▶ This well-designed study adds a nice piece of data to our understanding of the field management of snakebites: leave the suction device at home. It just doesn't work!

R. J. Hamilton, MD

Initial Experience With Crotalidae Polyvalent Immune Fab (Ovine) Antivenom in the Treatment of Copperhead Snakebite

Lavonas EJ, Gerardo CJ, O'Malley G, et al (Carolinas Med Ctr, Charlotte, NC; Duke Univ, Durham, NC; Albert Einstein Med Ctr, Philadelphia; et al)
Ann Emerg Med 43:200-206, 2004   11–3

Background.—Crotalidae polyvalent immune Fab (ovine) (CroFab or FabAV) is effective for the treatment of rattlesnake bites. The effect of FabAV on copperhead snakebites was reported.

Study Design.—A retrospective chart review was performed for all copperhead snakebites reported to the Carolinas Poison Control Center. Symptom progression, coagulopathy, and adverse effects, as well as the use of FabAV, were recorded.

Findings.—Of the 400 copperhead snakebites reported during this 2-year period, 32 received FabAV. The median time to administration of FabAV was 4 hours. The median time to achieve initial control was 1 hour, and the median dose was 4 vials of FabAV. A rapid response occurred in 28, but 4 were considered treatment failures. Swelling recurred in 6 cases. Swelling was not reduced by repeated doses of antivenom. Late-onset coagulopathy developed in 1 patient. One minor allergic reaction occurred.

Conclusions.—In most cases, local effects of envenomation by copperheads were rapidly stopped by FabAV treatment. Some treatment failures occurred. A swelling recurrence and coagulopathy also developed in some patients. A controlled clinical trial with long-term follow-up is required to define the role of FabAV in the treatment of copperhead bites.

▶ A copperhead snakebite is a crotalidae envenomation that is less likely to cause serious or systemic effects than many others. The use of CroFab does not cause serious side effects, and the authors investigated whether the use of this antivenom was of benefit to patients. It appears that it was beneficial in only two thirds of the patients; the remainder experienced recurrent swelling or no response. The numbers in this study are revealing, as less than 10% of all copperhead envenomations required therapy. This study suggests a rather limited role for CroFab in these patients, and I would continue to reserve its use for the more severe cases.

R. J. Hamilton, MD

A Canine Study of Immunotherapy in Scorpion Envenomation
Abroug F, Nouira S, El Atrous S, et al (CHU F Bourguiba, Monastir, Tunisia; CHU, Paris; Unité de Recherche, Monastir, Tunisia)
Intensive Care Med 29:2266-2276, 2003   11–4

Introduction.—Most scorpion stings produce only localized or unpleasant systemic manifestations. Severely envenomated patients usually have acute heart failure with pulmonary edema and circulatory compromise. Reports on experimental scorpion envenomation have had conflicting results. The hemodynamic and humoral effects of various doses of scorpion antivenom (SAV) administered at various times after scorpion envenomation were examined with a dog model in a prospective controlled investigation.

Methods.—Twenty-nine anesthetized and ventilated dogs received either venom alone (0.05 mg/kg), simultaneous administration of venom plus 10 mL SAV, 10 mL SAV 10 minutes after administration of venom, or 40 mL SAV 10 minutes after administration of venom. At baseline and 60 minutes after envenomation, hemodynamic measurements were obtained from a right heart catheter, plasma catecholamine levels were determined, and these tests were performed: neuropeptide Y assay, atrial natriuretic peptide radioimmunoassay, and endothelin-I assay.

Results.—In the group that received venom only at 5 minutes, there was a sharp rise in pulmonary artery occluded pressure from 2 mm Hg to 23 mm Hg, the mean arterial pressure rose from 125 mm Hg to 212 mm Hg, and systemic vascular resistance increased from 2450 dyn sec^{-1} m^5 to 5775 dyn sec^{-1} m^5 ($P < .05$ for all). The heart rate, cardiac output, and stroke volume dropped. There was a 40-fold increase in both epinephrine and norepinephrine plasma concentrations. Circulating neuropeptide Y and atrial natriuretic peptide dosages increased also. The pulmonary artery occlusion pressure and mean arterial pressure dropped thereafter to baseline levels. The concurrent administration of SAV with venom totally offset the hallmarks of scorpion envenomation. Delayed administration of SAV at any dose failed to change the features of scorpion envenomation.

Conclusion.—The simultaneous administration of SAV and scorpion venom is effective in preventing scorpion envenomation-associated manifestations, but delayed administration of SAV, either at standard or elevated dosages, did not modify any of the scorpion envenomation features.

▶ This is a very interesting animal study that shows that scorpion envenomation is resistant to immunotherapy given as soon as 10 minutes after the envenomation. This suggests that scorpion venom is a trigger for a cascade of neurohumoral signals that result in the classic envenomation syndrome, rather than a direct and prolonged venom effect. It opens some interesting areas of research and suggests to me that understanding the mechanism of how scorpion venom causes its toxicity may lead to great insights. It also suggests that immunotherapy may be of little value as a hospital-based treatment for this envenomation.

R. J. Hamilton, MD

Drugs of Abuse

Acute, Transient Urinary Retention From Combined Ecstasy and Methamphetamine Use

Delgado DJ, Caruso MJ, Waksman JC, et al (Denver Health Med Ctr; Rocky Mountain Poison and Drug Ctr, Denver; Univ of Colorado, Denver; et al)
J Emerg Med 26:173-175, 2004   11–5

Introduction.—As the popularity of abused drugs has grown, a better understanding of the adverse health effects associated with their use has emerged. A case of acute, transient urinary retention associated with methamphetamine and 3,4-methylenedioxymethamphetamine (MDMA or "ecstasy") use was reported.

> *Case Report.*—Man, 18, was seen in the ED for acute-onset urinary retention. He attended a party the previous evening where he consumed a large amount of alcohol. The next morning, he experienced lower abdominal pain and an inability to void. He had suprapubic tenderness on palpation and obvious bladder distention. About 1.6 L of clear, yellow urine was drained from the bladder upon

Foley catheter insertion. His discomfort improved markedly. He had normal renal function and leukocytosis (white blood cell count, 25,700/mL). Urinalysis revealed trace proteinuria and trace hematuria. There was no structural abnormality of the pelvis on CT scan. A urine radioimmunoassay screen was positive for amphetamines. The presence of MDMA was detected by thin-layer chromatography. The patient denied taking any illegal substances but did say that he had taken 2 Sudafed tablets (pseudoephedrine HCl, 30 mg) within the previous day. He conjectured that perhaps someone had spiked his drink. After 8 hours, the catheter was removed and he was able to void spontaneously. He returned the next day for follow-up, had no pain or hesitancy on urination, and had no further complaints.

Conclusion.—The use of MDMA and other amphetamine derivatives should be considered in the differential diagnosis of young persons with acute urinary retention in whom no structural abnormality of the genitourinary tract is evident.

▶ This case is another example of a sympathomimetic effect of amphetamines. It is not entirely clear whether the effect can be attributed to the MDMA per se. In my mind, the combination of the pseudoephedrine and MDMA were the most likely culprits.

R. J. Hamilton, MD

The Effects of Ecstacy (MDMA) on Rat Liver Bioenergetics
Rusyniak DE, Tandy SL, Kamendulis LM, et al (Indiana Univ, Indianapolis; Ohio Northern Univ, Ada)
Acad Emerg Med 11:723-729, 2004   11–6

Introduction.—The drug ecstasy (3,4-methylenedioxymethamphetamine [MDMA]) can cause life-threatening hyperthermia. Agents that uncouple mitochondrial oxidative phosphorylation have been shown to produce severe hyperthermia. The pharmacodynamic profile of MDMA on mitochondrial bioenergetics was characterized by studying the in vitro and ex vivo effects of MDMA on oxygen consumption. This was accomplished by using isolated rat liver mitochondria and a rat cell line as models for evaluating mitochondrial function.

Methods.—The in vivo experiments consisted of measuring the effects of MDMA (0.1-5.0 mmol/L) on states of respiration in isolated rat liver mitochondria and on mitochondrial membrane potential in a rat liver cell line. In ex vivo experiments, mitochondrial rates of respiration were determined in the livers of rats 1 hour after MDMA (40 mg/kg subcutaneously) treatment.

Results.—Only concentrations of 5 mmol/L MDMA showed evidence of uncoupling with the in vitro mitochondrial preparations. There was a slight increase in state 4 respiration and a corresponding reduction in the respiratory control index. MDMA (0.1-5.0 mmol/L) did not reduce the mitochondrial membrane potential in 3,3-dihexyloxacarbocyanide iodine–stained WB-344 cells after either 1 or 24 hours of incubation. Ex vivo rates of respiration acquired from the livers of rats 1 hour after treatment with MDMA (40 mg/kg subcutaneously) revealed no evidence of mitochondrial uncoupling.

Conclusion.—High concentrations of MDMA have some mild uncoupling effects in isolated mitochondria, but these effects do not translate to cell culture or ex vivo studies in treated animals. These data do not support the hypothesis that hyperthermia induced by MDMA is from a direct effect on mitochondrial oxidative phosphorylation.

▶ This animal experiment suggests an uncoupling effect for MDMA in rats, but does not fully explain the cause of the severe rise in temperature that MDMA causes. Uncoupling is generally associated with a temperature rise that is independent of the activity of the patient, and my clinical experience is that MDMA causes a great deal of increased motor activity—some voluntary and some involuntary. For now, it looks like the common theory is correct—the hyperthermia from MDMA has more to do with the social phenomenom that it either encourages or is associated with (eg, dancing for hours in a hot room).

R. J. Hamilton, MD

Determinants of Overdose Incidents Among Illicit Opioid Users in 5 Canadian Cities

Fischer B, Brissette S, Brochu S, et al (Univ of Toronto; Université de Montréal; Foothills Hosp, Calgary, Alta, Canada; et al)
Can Med Assoc J 171:235-239, 2004   11–7

Introduction.—Drug overdose is an important cause of death and illness in illicit drug users. Earlier reports have indicated that most illicit drug users have nonfatal overdoses, and have suggested various factors linked with the risk of overdose. The incidence of, and factors associated with, nonfatal overdose were examined in a Canadian sample of illicit opioid users not enrolled in treatment at the time of trial recruitment.

Methods.—A standard questionnaire was used to obtain data regarding sociodemographic characteristics, drug use, health and health care, experience in the criminal justice system, and treatment for drug problems. Standard evaluations for mental health and infectious disease were also conducted. The correlation between overdose and sociodemographic and drug-use factors was calculated.

Results.—Of 679 persons interviewed, 651 provided answers adequate for analysis. A total of 112 (17.2%) of respondents reported an overdose episode within the prior 6 months. After adjusting for sociodemographic factors, logistic regression analysis revealed that homelessness, noninjection use of hydromorphone in the past 30 days, and involvement in drug treatment in the past 12 months were predictive of overdose ($P < .05$).

Conclusion.—A diverse and complex combination of factors was linked with overdose episodes. Efforts at prevention may be more effective if directed to specific causal factors.

▶ This study is flawed by its design. The data rely on self-reporting of overdoses of a preenrolled cohort of opioid users, something which may be sufficient for clinical decision making, but is less than perfect for characterizing overdoses for study.

R. J. Hamilton, MD

Antidotes and Treatment

Home Syrup of Ipecac Use Does Not Reduce Emergency Department Use or Improve Outcome
Bond GR (Cincinnati Children's Hosp, Ohio)
Pediatrics 112:1061-1064, 2003   11–8

Introduction.—The usefulness of syrup of ipecac as a home treatment for poisoning is under increasing debate. Many poison centers do not recommend that syrup of ipecac be used for any reason. The American Association of Poison Control Centers' Toxic Exposure Surveillance System Database was searched to determine whether the use of ipecac in children at home is linked with decreased utilization of ED resources or improved outcomes after unintended exposure to a pharmaceutical.

Methods.—Masked data for each of the United States poison centers was documented and included the ED referral recommendation rate, the actual rate of ED use, actual home use of syrup of ipecac, and outcomes. These data were obtained from cases in 2000 and 2001 involving children younger than 6 years who unintentionally ingested a pharmaceutical agent and in which the call to a poison center came from home (752,602 children). The primary outcome measure was the correlation between the rate of home use of syrup of ipecac and the rate of recommendation for ED referral. Secondary measures included the rate of adverse outcomes and the actual ED use and home syrup of ipecac use rates from 7 specific centers. These data were compared with the published rates for the same centers from 1990 data to determine the trend in practice for this subgroup.

Results.—The mean home rate of referral to the ED was 9% (range, 3%-18%), and the mean home use of syrup of ipecac rate was 1.8% (range, 0.2%-14%). The increased home use of syrup of ipecac was not linked with referral to the ED ($r = 0.18$; 95% CI of r, –0.06-0.41). The incidence of adverse outcomes was 0.6% (range, 0.2%-2.1%). No significant differences were found in the referral rate or adverse outcomes rate between 2 groups of 32 centers divided by relative use of syrup of ipecac. In 7 centers, the ED use diminished from a mean of 13.5% in 1990 to a mean of 8.1% in 2000-2001. Ipecac use dropped from a mean of 8.65% to 2.1%.

Conclusion.—There is no decrease in resource utilization or improvement in patient outcomes from the use of syrup of ipecac at home. These data cannot exclude a benefit in a very limited set of poisonings; nonetheless, any benefit remains to be proven.

▶ This study showed that ipecac, when used at home, will not improve the outcome or decrease the visits to the ED of children with accidental inges- tions. This finding challenges the current practices of anticipatory guidance during routine pediatric office visits that advocate the use of ipecac as a home decontaminant. With the current toxicologic knowledge in all the poison con- trol centers, the number of children that would meet the criteria to use ipecac is very small. Moreover, after reviewing current evidence, AAP no longer be- lieves that ipecac should be used routinely in homes.[1]

Unfortunately, the ingested substance and its respective dose of the sub- group of those children who visited the ED after ipecac use at home were not identified. If ipecac doesn't play a significant role in helping poison control cen- ters in reducing ED visits, then why use it or recommend it at all?

E. C. Quintana, MD, MPH

Reference

1. American Academy of Pediatrics Policy Statement. Committee on Injury, Violence and Prevention. *Pediatrics* 112:1182-1185, 2003.

Hexafluorine vs Standard Decontamination to Reduce Systemic Toxicity After Dermal Exposure to Hydrofluoric Acid
Hultén P, Höjer J, Ludwigs U, et al (Karolinska Hosp, Stockholm)
Clin Toxicol 42:355-361, 2004   11–9

Introduction.—Hydrofluoric acid (HF) is one of the most corrosive in- organic acids known and can cause both severe burns and systemic toxicity. The immediate rinsing with water followed by topical application of cal- cium is currently widely accepted as first aid treatment after skin exposure to HF. Hexafluorine (Prevor, France) is marketed as an emergency decon- tamination fluid for skin and eye exposure to HF. Its precise content and molecular structure have not been revealed, and there is inadequate and contradictory scientific documentation in peer-reviewed journals. Yet, many industries in several countries include Hexafluorine in their safety plans. The capacity of Hexafluorine to decrease HF-induced systemic tox- icity was examined by using a rat model.

Methods.—Sprague Dawley rats were anesthetized, the left femoral artery was catheterized, and the back was shaved. A filter paper (3.5 × 6 cm) was soaked in 50% HF and applied on the back of every rat for 3 minutes. At 30 seconds after removal of the paper, a 3-minute rinsing was performed with either 500 mL of Hexafluorine (group H), 500 mL of water (group W), or 500 mL of water followed by a single application of 2.5% calcium gluconate (group Ca). Blood samples were analyzed for ionized calcium and potassium levels before injury and 1, 2, 3, and 4 hours after injury, and ionized fluoride levels were also determined at 1, 2, and 4 hours after injury.

Results.—All animals developed hypocalcemia, hyperkalemia, and hyperfluoridemia after HP exposure. The only significant difference seen between groups was in serum potassium levels at 1 hour between group Ca and group W. There was a consistent trend toward milder hypocalcemia and less pronounced hyperkalemia in group Ca versus the other groups. There were no differences observed in the electrolyte disturbances between the Hexafluorine-treated rats and those treated with water only. Five of 39 animals died before experiment completion because of HF exposure: 1 from group Ca, 2 from group W, and 2 from group H.

Conclusion.—Decontamination with Hexafluorine was not more effective than rinsing with water in diminishing electrolyte disturbances caused by dermal exposure to HF.

▶ The authors conclude appropriately that water is the decontaminating agent of choice after HF exposure. The efficacy of water might improve when high volumes for longer periods are employed. One of the benefits of water decontamination is that it is so readily available and can be used in great quantities for virtually unlimited time!

R. J. Hamilton, MD

Ecgonine Methyl Ester Protects Against Cocaine Lethality in Mice
Hoffman RS, Kaplan JL, Hung OL, et al (New York Univ)
Clin Toxicol 42:349-354, 2004   11–10

Introduction.—Plasma cholinesterase (PChE) metabolizes cocaine to ecgonine methyl ester (EME), a mild vasodilator. Exogenous PChE protects against cocaine-induced seizures and lethality, perhaps resulting from enhanced degradation of cocaine, loss of active metabolites (benzoylecgonine, norcocaine), or production of a beneficial metabolite (EME). The pharmacologic effects of EME were examined in mice.

Methods.—Female ICR Swiss albino mice weighing 20 to 30 g were acclimated to 12-hour alternating light-dark cycles and were given food and water ad libitum. With the use of a randomized, blinded protocol, 80 mice were pretreated with intraperitoneal EME (50 mg/kg) in a 0.9% sodium chloride solution or an equal volume of 0.9% sodium chloride solution. All mice received 126 mg/kg of cocaine intraperitoneally 5 minutes later and were observed for seizures and death.

Results.—Pretreatment with EME increased survival after cocaine administration (9/40 vs 2/40 for EME vs control, respectively; $P < .05$). The median time to seizure was 2.0 minutes for EME versus 1.5 minutes for controls ($P > .05$). The median time to death was 4.5 minutes for EME and 4.6 minutes for controls ($P > .05$).

Conclusion.—In this murine model, EME was protective against cocaine lethality. The effect was consistent with that of previously described vasodilatory effects of EME. Further investigation is needed to determine whether the increase in EME produced by exogenous PChE administration contributes to the benefits that occur when PChE is administered to cocaine-poisoned animals.

▶ Predicting which patients will exhibit the toxic effects of cocaine, or why some patients appear to manifest more toxicity than others at a particular dose has been a difficult question to answer. Some authors speculate that the decreased activity of pseudocholinesterase present in subpopulations of cocaine users accounts for this problem. Pseudocholinesterase metabolizes cocaine to EME, a metabolite that has vasodilator properties. This investigation attempts to determine whether this metabolite is protective or merely the product of a metabolism that produces less of the most toxic metabolite, benzoylecgonine. The authors observed a small but statistically significant difference in death in the EME pretreated group, and conclude that EME is protective against cardiovascular toxicity but not seizures. Since EME does not cross the blood-brain barrier, the lack of effect on seizures is expected. One other observation that I would make is that the EME's small protective effect on death suggests the larger role that cocaine's CNS toxicity plays in fatal outcomes.

R. J. Hamilton, MD

Anticonvulsant Hypersensitivity Syndrome: Treatment With Corticosteroids and Intravenous Immunoglobulin
Mostella J, Pieroni R, Jones R, et al (Univ of Alabama, Tuscaloosa)
South Med J 97:319-321, 2004   11–11

Introduction.—Anticonvulsant hypersensitivity syndrome (AHS) is a rare, yet potentially lethal adverse reaction to treatment with the aromatic anticonvulsant drugs phenytoin, phenobarbital, primidone, and carbamazepine. The case of a patient in whom AHS developed during treatment with phenytoin and progressed when therapy was changed to phenobarbital was reported.

Case Report.—Woman, 43, with a history of mental retardation secondary to static encephalopathy was admitted to the hospital with fever, cough, facial and lower extremity swelling for about 1 week, and a rash for about 4 weeks. She was started on phenytoin, 300 mg/d, 2 months earlier to treat a possible seizure disorder. Four days before admission, she was seen in the ED with similar complaints. On physical examination she had a temperature of 39°C, erythematous tonsils, anterior bilateral cervical lymphadenopathy, pharyngitis, and an erythematous maculopapular rash of her face, neck, trunk, arms, and legs. Pharyngitis and a possible drug-induced rash were diagnosed, and she received ceftriaxone (1 g), diphenhydramine (25 mg every 6 hours as needed), acetaminophen (1000 mg), and amoxicillin (500 mg 3 times per day). She was discharged and followed up 2 days later by her primary care physician, who discontinued phenytoin and started phenobarbital therapy (60 mg/d). She returned to the ED within 2 days, was admitted to the hospital, and was diagnosed with acute AHS, along with concurrent urinary tract infection and vaginal trichomoniasis. Phenobarbital was discontinued on hospital day 1, and hydroxyzine (25-50 mg) was given for pruritis; acetaminophen (650 mg every 4 hours) was administered for fever. Her dermatitis and peripheral edema worsened, and mucosal lesions developed. By day 6, significant laboratory values were as follows: alkaline phosphatase, 183 U/L; aspartate aminotransferase, 1162 IU/L; alanine aminotransferase, 676 IU/L; total bilirubin, 10.2 mg/dL; serum creatinine, 3.6 mg/dL; potassium, 6.8 mmol/L; and ammonia, 93 µmol/L. She had shortness of breath, and chest radiography showed left basilar subsegmental atelectasis and a large right basilar opacity; pneumonia could not be excluded. She was admitted to the ICU. Acetaminophen was discontinued because of elevated liver transaminase values. She was given IV methylprednisolone, 125 mg every 6 hours, and was treated for hyperkalemia. On day 7, she was given 30 g (0.41 g/kg) of IV immunoglobulin, and her clinical status quickly improved. By day 11, she was started on a steroid-tapering regimen, and oral prednisone was started at 15 mg/d on day 14. She was discharged with a 2-day prednisone taper among her other discharge medications. At 3 days after discharge and 1 day after ceasing prednisone, she was readmitted with increasing facial and lower extremity swelling, erythema, and fever. Prednisone, 40 mg/d, was administered. After 9 days of treatment, she showed overall clinical improvement and was discharged on a very gradual steroid taper. After hospitalization, she experienced severe exfoliation, particularly of the hands and soles. At 4-month follow-up, the rash, edema, eosinophilia, and atypical lymphocytes were resolved, and renal and hepatic function were normal.

Conclusion.—Information is limited and controversial concerning the use of steroids and IV immunoglobulin for treatment of AHS, but these options should be considered when supportive care is exhausted.

▶ This is a nice case report to review the clinical course of this entity. I think the rebound of symptoms after stopping the prednisone supports the theory that the real therapeutic agent was the steroids. Nonetheless, the patient's most dramatic improvement occurred chronologically after the administration of IV immunoglobulin.

R. J. Hamilton, MD

Successful Treatment With Enoximone for Severe Poisoning With Atenolol and Verapamil: A Case Report

Sandroni C, Cavallaro F, Addario C, et al (Catholic Univ, Rome; Ospedale Maggiore della Cartià, Novara, Italy)

Acta Anaesthesiol Scand 48:790-792, 2004   11–12

Introduction.—Combined poisoning with calcium channel blockers and β-blockers usually causes severe hypotension and heart failure. Even at high doses, adrenergic agonists may be inadequate treatment because of β-receptor blockade, making it necessary to use β-independent inotropes such as glucagon. A case of severe atenolol and verapamil poisoning that was successfully treated with enoximone, a phosphodiesterase III inhibitor, was reported.

Case Report.—Man, 57, was admitted to the ED 1 hour after suicidal ingestion of twenty-eight 100-mg atenolol tablets (2800 mg total; recommended daily dose, 300 mg) and twenty 80-mg verapamil tablets (1600 mg total; minimum reported lethal dose, 1400 mg). His serum verapamil level at the time of admission was 857 ng mL^{-1} (therapeutic range, 125-400 ng mL^{-1}; minimum reported lethal level, 690 ng mL^{-1}). He had a history of a major depressive disorder and 2 previous acute myocardial infarctions. On admission, his Glasgow Coma Scale was 7, he had no palpable peripheral pulses, his blood pressure was 80/50 mm Hg, and heart rate was 40 beats/min. The ECG revealed sinus bradycardia with first-degree heart block. Chest radiography identified interstitial pulmonary edema. After intubation, he received 100% oxygen and positive end-expiratory pressure of 5 cm H$_2$O. He underwent gastric lavage and received 1 g kg^{-1} of activated carbon. The plasma calcium level was normal. He received 5 consecutive slow injections of calcium chloride 2.5 mmol (1.0 g) until his Ca^{++} level was increased up to 1.75 mmol L^{-1} (7.02 mg dL^{-1}), which produced only a transient increase in blood pressure that persisted for a few minutes. Dopamine was administered at 10 µg kg^{-1} min^{-1}, with no effect. Addition of epinephrine infusion at 4 µg kg^{-1} min^{-1} produced a slight increase in heart rate and blood pressure (65 beats/min and 90/60 mm Hg, respectively). Data from the pulmonary artery catheter (Fig 1) revealed pump failure with increased peripheral resistance. The cardiac index was 1.021 min^{-1} m^{-2}, pulmonary capillary wedge pressure was 18 mm Hg, and systemic vascular resistance index was 2536 dyne*s cm^{-5}m^{-2}. Progressive increases in dopamine and epinephrine infusions produced no improvements. At 4 hours after admission, his condition deteriorated, at which time a bolus of enoximone 1 mg kg^{-1} was administered and followed by a continuous infusion at 0.5 µg kg^{-1} min^{-1}. This produced progressive hemodynamic improvement to the extent that epinephrine was reduced and discontinued 6 hours later, and dopamine was reduced and discontinued 20 hours later. The enoxi-

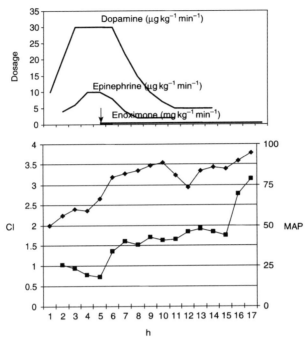

FIGURE 1.—Clinical and hemodynamic effect of dopamine, epinephrine, and enoximone infusion. Trends of cardiac index (CI) (L min^{-1} m^{-2}), mean arterial pressure (MAP; mm Hg) from the 1st to the 17th hour after admission. Infusion rates for dopamine, epinephrine, and enoximone are reported at the **top of the graph**. Note the improvement in MAP and CI after the enoximone infusion was started (*arrow*). (Courtesy of Sandroni C, Cavallaro F, Addario C, et al: Successful treatment with enoximone for severe poisoning with atenolol and verapamil: A case report. *Acta Anaesthesiol Scand* 48:790-792, 2004.)

mone infusion was maintained at the same rate for 5 days. The patient recovered consciousness and was weaned from mechanical ventilation and extubated on day 5. He was discharged to a medical ward on day 15 and later discharged.

Conclusion.—The administration of enoximone can be useful in the presence of a combined β-blocker and calcium channel blocker overdose when initial treatment with high-dose adrenergic agonists is not adequate and produces an excessive increase in peripheral vascular resistances.

▶ This is an encouraging case report. Phosphodiesterase inhibitors have always been considered a logical choice in calcium channel blocker or β-blocker overdose because they effectively bypass the calcium channel and the β-receptor. Note, the hemodynamic parameters reported for this patient are not typical of all overdoses of this type and may be more indicative of the patient's ischemic heart disease. Perhaps that is why enoximone had a beneficial effect. Still, glucagon may have had the same result as the enoximone. I think this case report does argue for aggressive critical monitoring of these overdoses and pharmacologic choices specifically tailored to the patient's cardiac index, systemic vascular resistance, wedge pressure, etc.

R. J. Hamilton, MD

Administration of Aerosolized Terbutaline and Budesonide Reduces Chlorine Gas–Induced Acute Lung Injury
Wang J, Zhang L, Walther SM (Univ of Linköping, Sweden)
J Trauma 56:850-862, 2004   11–13

Background.—The pathophysiology and treatment of chlorine gas–induced acute lung injury have not been well documented. Furthermore, what is known is based on anecdotal evidence. The effects of aerosolized β_2-adrenergic agonist and corticosteroid therapy on chlorine gas–induced lung injury were assessed in a pig model.

Methods.—Anesthetized, ventilated pigs were exposed to chlorine gas, 400 ppm, for 20 minutes. Thirty minutes later, the pigs received aerosolized terbutaline, budesonide, terbutaline followed by budesonide, or placebo by random assignment. Each group contained 6 pigs. For the next 5 hours, hemodynamics, gas exchange, and lung mechanics were assessed.

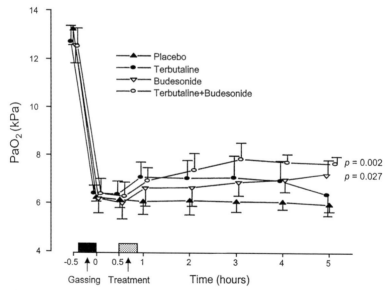

FIGURE 1.—Arterial oxygen tension (Pa_{O_2}) in pigs with chlorine gas injury expressed as mean ± standard deviation (n = 6). The *P* values denote the statistical significance of differences within groups 0 to 5 hours after gassing. Overall differences in 0 to 5 hours between the nebulized saline (PLA) group and the other groups were significant: PLA group vs nebulized terbutaline (TERB) group ($P < .001$), PLA group vs nebulized budesonide (BUD) group ($P < .001$), and PLA group vs nebulized terbutaline followed by nebulized budesonide (TERB + BUD) group ($P < .001$). (Courtesy of Wang J, Zhang L, Walther SM: Administration of aerosolized terbutaline and budesonide reduces chlorine gas–induced acute lung injury. *J Trauma* 56[4]:850-862, 2004.)

Findings.—All pigs had an immediate increase in airway and pulmonary artery pressure and marked declines in arterial oxygen tension (PaO_2) and lung compliance (C_L). The pigs receiving terbutaline plus budesonide had the greatest recovery of PaO_2 and C_L. However, treatment with terbutaline alone and budesonide alone also was correlated with a significantly improved PaO_2 and C_L, compared with placebo (Fig 1).

Conclusions.—Aerosolized terbutaline treatment followed by aerosolized budesonide improved lung function in this pig model of acute chlorine gas lung injury. The combination of these agents was more effective than either one alone.

▶ It might be a bit surprising to see that chlorine-induced lung injury would respond so well to inhaled steroids, since it is classically thought of as a directly toxic effect. However, the combined therapeutic effect of budenoside and terbutaline demonstrates that regardless of the cause, the lung's response to injury is often bronchospasm and edema. The response to these 2 therapies in animal models supports their use in humans.

R. J. Hamilton, MD

Mitigation of Pennyroyal Oil Hepatotoxicity in the Mouse
Sztajnkrycer MD, Otten EJ, Bond GR, et al (Univ of Cincinnati, Ohio)
Acad Emerg Med 10:1024-1028, 2003   11–14

Background.—Ingesting pennyroyal oil can result in severe hepatotoxicity and death. The main constituent is R-$(+)$-pulegone, which is metabolized through hepatic cytochrome P450 to toxic intermediates. The ability of the specific cytochrome P450 inhibitors disulfiram and cimetidine to mitigate hepatotoxicity in mice exposed to toxic levels of R-$(+)$-pulegone was assessed.

Methods.—Female BALB/c mice weighing 20 g were pretreated with cimetidine, 150 mg/kg intraperitoneally, or disulfiram, 100 mg/kg intraperitoneally, or both. One hour later, the mice were given 300 mg/kg of pulegone intraperitoneally. At 24 hours, the mice were killed for examination.

Findings.—Compared with the R-$(+)$-pulegone group, a tendency for reduced serum glutamate pyruvate transaminase was noted in the disulfiram and cimetidine groups, with significant differences for the cimetidine as well as the combined disulfram and cimetidine groups (Table 1). Pretreatment with combined disulfiram and cimetidine mitigated against R-$(+)$-pulegone–induced hepatotoxicity most effectively.

Conclusions.—In this animal model, cimetidine and disulfiram combined significantly mitigated the effects of pennyroyal toxicity. The combination of these 2 agents was more effective than either agent alone. Metabolism of R-$(+)$-pulegone through CYP1A2 appears to be more important in hepatotoxic metabolite development than metabolism through CYP2E1.

TABLE 1.—Mean Serum Glutamate Pyruvate Transaminase (*SGPT*) and 95% Confidence Intervals (*95% CIs*) of the Mean SGPT for the Control and Experimental Groups

Group	n	Mean SGPT (IU/L)	±SEM	95% CI
Negative control groups				
No treatment	5	27.0	2.3	20.73, 33.27*
Dimethyl sulfoxide	5	25.2	3.1	16.71, 33.69*
Corn oil	5	17.0	1.8	11.96, 22.04*
Positive control group				
R-(+)-pulegone	9	182	50.7	65.17, 298.83
Experimental groups				
Disulfiram & R-(+)-pulegone	11	93.3	18.9	51.27, 135.27
Cimetidine & R-(+)-pulegone	10	71.2	5.6	58.65, 83.75*
Cimetidine & disulfiram & R-(+)-pulegone	10	64.0	7.3	47.45, 80.55*

*Significant differences from the positive control group, defined by $P < .05$.
(Courtesy of Sztajnkrycer MD, Otten EJ, Bond GR, et al: Mitigation of pennyroyal oil hepatotoxicity in the mouse. *Acad Emerg Med* 10:1024-1028, 2003.)

▶ A nicely designed study that demonstrates the roles of cytochrome P2E1 and P1A2 in generating the toxic metabolites of pulegone. I am not certain what role this suggests for cimetidine or disulfiram in treating pennyroyal hepatotoxicity, but there would seem to be no real harm in starting cimetidine, at least, shortly after a pennyroyal ingestion. This might mitigate the toxicity of the ingestion.

R. J. Hamilton, MD

Preparing for Chemical Terrorism: Stability of Injectable Atropine Sulfate
Schier JG, Ravikumar PR, Nelson LS, et al (NYC Poison Control Ctr, New York; Bureau of Laboratories, New York; Saint John's Univ, Jamaica, NY)
Acad Emerg Med 11:329-334, 2004   11–15

Introduction.—Current hospital stockpiles of in-date antidotes for chemical terrorism may not be sufficient to deal with a mass casualty event. Expired atropine sulfate may still contain substantial amounts of active drug. Since dosing is based on clinical effect, the potential benefit of using an expired drug in a crisis situation should be explored. The stability of premixed injectable atropine sulfate samples with varying expiration dates was examined, along with the presence of tropine as a marker of atropine degradation in current and expired drugs.

Methods.—An in vitro investigation was conducted with the use of gas chromatography and mass spectrometry (GC/MS). Four solutions of atropine (labeled concentration, 400 µg/mL) that ranged from "in date" to 12 years past expiration (exp), and a sample of atropine sulfate (labeled concentration, 2000 µg/mL) obtained from a World War II era autoinjector were assayed for atropine stability. Standards of atropine sulfate and tropine were prepared and quantified by GC/MS. Samples were prepared by adding a buffer solution to free the base, extracting with an isopropanol/methylene chloride mixture and followed by evaporating the organic layer to dryness.

TABLE 1.—Measured Atropine Concentration, 95% Confidence Intervals (CIs) and Measured pH

Sample	Manufacturer	Labeled Concentration (µg/mL)	Measured Concentration (µg/mL)	Calculated 95% CI = (µg/mL)	pH Value
In date	American Pharmaceutical Partners, Inc.	400	252	(235, 268)	3.88
Exp 2001	Elkins-Sinn, Inc.	400	290	(272, 308)	3.93
Exp 1999	Elkins-Sinn, Inc.	400	314	(295, 333)	3.82
Exp 1990	Elkins-Sinn, Inc.	400	398	(375, 420)	4.02
WWII	Strong, Cobb & Co. Inc.	2,000	1,475	(1,385, 1,565)	4.85

(Courtesy of Schier JG, Ravikumar PR, Nelson LS, et al: Preparing for chemical terrorism: Stability of injectable atropine sulfate. *Acad Emerg Med* 11:329-334, 2004.)

Pentafluoropropionic anhydride and pentafluoropropanol were used as derivatization reagents. Samples were heated, derivatization reagents were evaporated, and the remaining compound was reconstituted in ethyl acetate for injection into the GC/MS.

Results.—All solutions were both clear and colorless. Atropine concentrations were as follows: in date, 252 µg/mL; 2001 exp, 290 µg/mL; 1999 exp, 314 µg/mL; 1990 exp, 398 µg/mL; and World War II sample, 1475 µg/mL (Table 1). Tropine was detected in concentrations of less than 10 µg/mL in all samples.

Conclusion.—Significant amounts of atropine were detected in all samples. All samples were clear and colorless, with no substantial amount of tropine in any sample. Further investigation is needed to determine clinical effect.

▶ The authors suggest that we ought to stockpile "expired" atropine as a resource for nerve agent exposures. Another example of how an expired drug is better than no drug available at all and a brilliant idea!

R. J. Hamilton, MD

Effect of Whole Bowel Irrigation on the Pharmacokinetics of an Acetaminophen Formulation and Progression of Radiopaque Markers Through the Gastrointestinal Tract

Ly BT, Schneir AB, Clark RF (Univ of California, San Diego)
Ann Emerg Med 43:189-195, 2004 11–16

Background.—Whole bowel irrigation is used to treat poisoning, but its clinical efficacy has not been well studied. Whole bowel irrigation's effect on the pharmacokinetics of delayed release acetaminophen and on the progression of radiopaque markers through the gastrointestinal tract was investigated in healthy volunteers.

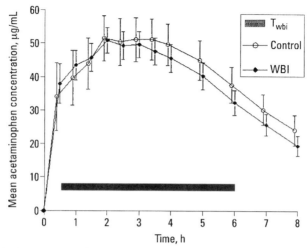

FIGURE 4.—Mean acetaminophen concentration versus time curves. *Abbreviation: WBI,* Whole bowel irrigation. (Courtesy of Ly BT, Schneir AB, Clark RF: Effect of whole bowel irrigation on the pharmacokinetics of an acetaminophen formulation and progression of radiopaque markers through the gastrointestinal tract. *Ann Emerg Med* 43:189-195, 2004.)

Study Design.—The study group consisted of 10 healthy adult volunteers who participated in this prospective, randomized, 2-armed crossover study. Participants fasted for 8 hours before randomization. Participants were administered 75 mg/kg of delayed release acetaminophen caplets orally, along with a Sitzmarks capsule containing 24 radiopaque polyvinyl chloride markers. Whole bowel irrigation was initiated 30 minutes later until rectal effluent was clear of stool. Serial abdominal radiography was performed to track the radiopaque markers. Adverse effects were recorded. The duration of irrigation, the volume of irrigation, and the volume of rectal output were also recorded. The control arm was performed without whole bowel irrigation. Blood samples were obtained for serial serum acetaminophen analysis. The area under the acetaminophen concentration versus time curve (AUC) was calculated and compared between control and experimental arms.

Findings.—Whole bowel irrigation was associated with an 11.5% reduction in the AUC, and the bulk of the effect occurred during the delayed-release portion of the curve (Fig 4); however, this reduction was not statistically significant. Radiographs obtained at the end of whole bowel irrigation showed the radiopaque markers in the right hemicolon in 8 of the 10 study participants. No marker position pattern was seen in the control arm (without irrigation).

Conclusions.—Whole bowel irrigation did not appear to significantly reduce the AUC for delayed release acetaminophen. An effect on radiopaque markers was seen, but the clinical significance of this finding is unknown.

▶ A number of studies have shown that delayed release acetaminophen has trivial pharmacologic differences from immediate release acetaminophen.[1] Thus, it makes a poor subject for a test of the efficacy of whole bowel irrigation. In fact, this study did not demonstrate an impact on the AUC for acetaminophen. However, this should not dissuade the reader from initiating this therapy for true sustained release preparations because this study does not disprove that whole bowel irrigation has a benefit in those cases.

R. J. Hamilton, MD

Reference

1. Stork CM, Rees S, Howland MA, et al: Pharmacokinetics of extended relief vs. regular release Tylenol in simulated human overdose. *J Toxicol Clin Toxicol* 34:157-162, 1996.

Miscellaneous

The Effect of Calcium Chloride in Treating Hyperkalemia Due to Acute Digoxin Toxicity in a Porcine Model#

Hack JB, Woody JH, Lewis DE, et al (East Carolina Univ, Greenville, NC)
Clin Toxicol 42:337-342, 2004   11–17

Introduction.—The administration of IV calcium in the treatment of hyperkalemia resulting from digoxin poisoning is regarded as potentially dangerous, based on earlier literature that reported increased cardiac glycoside toxicity with calcium administration (increased arrhythmias and a higher death rate). The effect of calcium administration in the setting of hyperkalemia induced by acute digoxin toxicity was evaluated in a porcine model.

Methods.—Digoxin IV at 0.25 mg/kg was established as appropriately toxic. When arrhythmias consistent with hyperkalemia occurred, pigs were given either an IV calcium chloride bolus (10 mg/kg; group 1, n = 6) or normal saline volume equivalent (group 2, n = 6). Three time intervals were observed. Interval 1 was the time interval from digoxin administration to when ECG changes consistent with hyperkalemia developed (at which point calcium chloride or placebo was administered). Interval 2 was the time interval from the development of ECG changes consistent with hyperkalemia to asystole. Interval 3 was the time interval from digoxin administration to asystole. Both groups were followed up for changes in heart rhythms, serum potassium levels, and time to asystole.

Results.—The IV digoxin dose of 0.25 mg/kg induced hyperkalemia, arrhythmias, and death about 1 hour after administration in all animals. In group 1, interval 1 averaged 18.75 minutes; interval 2, 16.75 minutes; and interval 3, 35.5 minutes. In group 2, interval 1 averaged 24.8 minutes; interval 2, 19.5 minutes; and interval 3, 44.3 minutes. There were no significant between-group differences at any time interval ($P = .43$, interval 1; $P = .65$, interval 2; and $P = .40$, interval 3). Serum potassium levels did not vary throughout the evaluation period.

Conclusion.—The administration of IV calcium chloride in the setting of hyperkalemia from acute digoxin toxicity did not impact mortality or time to death at the dose administered.

▶ This is a great study, and fortunately will start to clear up the concept of "stone heart"—that is, the heart that ceases to beat because of severe intracellular hypercalcemia caused by combined cardiac glycoside and calcium toxicity. One clear outcome of this study was that calcium had no beneficial effect on hyperkalemia. Thus, if calcium is used inadvertently to treat hyperkalemia in a digoxin-poisoned patient, we ought not to expect any untoward effects. However, we ought not to expect any beneficial effects as well.

R. J. Hamilton, MD

What Is the Rate of Adverse Events After Oral N-Acetylcysteine Administered by the Intravenous Route to Patients With Suspected Acetaminophen Poisoning?

Kao LW, Kirk MA, Furbee RB, et al (Indiana Univ, Indianapolis; Univ of Virginia, Charlottesville)
Ann Emerg Med 42:741-750, 2003   11–18

Introduction.—Acetaminophen poisoning accounted for 108,066 exposures and 156 deaths in 2000, according to the American Association of Poison Control Centers. N-acetylcysteine, the recommended treatment of acetaminophen poisoning, has several beneficial effects, including generation of glutathione, enhancing nontoxic routes of acetaminophen metabolism, detoxifying N-acetyl-p-benzoquinonimine, and free radical scavenging. The rate of adverse events (anaphylactoid and cardiorespiratory) associated with the use of oral N-acetylcysteine by the IV route for the treatment of suspected acetaminophen poisoning was examined.

Methods.—A retrospective medical record review was performed by using explicit criteria. All patients who received oral N-acetylcysteine by the IV route between September 1995 and September 2001 were evaluated. Three databases were used to crossmatch patients. Adverse events were placed in cutaneous, systemic, and life-threatening categories. Interrater reliability of 5 reviewers was determined.

Results.—Seven adverse events were observed in 187 patients (3.7%; 95% confidence interval, 1.0%-6.5%). Six of the adverse events were cutaneous; in these, there was a quick response to antihistamines. One life-threatening event was not clearly associated with N-acetylcysteine (Table 1). A high rate of antihistamine exposure (53%) was seen before administration of N-acetylcysteine. The interrater agreement was greater than 95%.

Conclusion.—IV administration of an oral solution of N-acetylcysteine is associated with a low rate of adverse events and should be considered in selected patients with suspected acetaminophen poisoning (Fig 1).

TABLE 1.—Adverse Events Associated With Intravenous Administration of Oral N-Acetylcysteine for Suspected Acetaminophen Poisoning

Patient, Age, y	Clinical Scenario	Asthma Present	Oral N-acetyl-cysteine Use	Antihistamine Exposure	APAP Level µg/mL	Timing of Adverse Event	Type of Adverse Event	Description of Adverse Event	N-acetylcysteine Continued?
17, WF	2 d after acute overdose	N	Y	N	5	1 h after loading dose	Cutaneous	Rash and urticaria on face and trunk, which resolved after antihistamine use	Changed to oral
47, WF	Chronic use	N	N	Y	30.4	Loading dose	Cutaneous	Rash on face and neck, which resolved after antihistamine use	Stopped; patient refused oral N-acetylcysteine
15, WF	Acute overdose	N	Y	Undetermined; outside hospital record missing	115	Loading dose	Cutaneous	Rash on arms, neck, and chest, which resolved after antihistamine use	Continued
14, WF	Acute overdose	N	N	N	268	Loading dose	Cutaneous	Rash on shoulders, which resolved after antihistamine use	Continued
17, WF	Acute overdose	N	N	N	158	1.5 h after loading dose	Cutaneous	Itchy scalp and palms, which resolved after antihistamine use	Continued
19, WF	Acute overdose	N	N	Y	277	9 h into mainte-nance infusion	Cutaneous	Lacy rash over face and neck while asleep, resolved after antihistamine use	Continued
37, WM	History of chronic APAP use with elevated trans-aminase levels	N	N	Y	80	1 h after loading dose	Life-threatening	Apnea and bradycardia; see text	Continued

Abbreviations: APAP, Acetaminophen; WF, white female; WM, white male; N, no; Y, yes.

(Courtesy of Kao LW, Kirk MA, Furbee RB, et al: What is the rate of adverse events after oral N-acetylcysteine administered by the intravenous route to patients with suspected acetaminophen poisoning? *Ann Emerg Med* 42:741-750, 2003.)

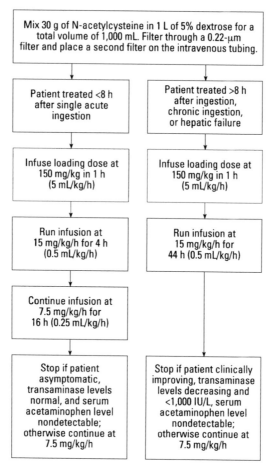

Mix 30 g of N-acetylcysteine in 1 L of 5% dextrose for a total volume of 1,000 mL. Filter through a 0.22-μm filter and place a second filter on the intravenous tubing.

Patient treated <8 h after single acute ingestion

Patient treated >8 h after ingestion, chronic ingestion, or hepatic failure

Infuse loading dose at 150 mg/kg in 1 h (5 mL/kg/h)

Infuse loading dose at 150 mg/kg in 1 h (5 mL/kg/h)

Run infusion at 15 mg/kg/h for 4 h (0.5 mL/kg/h)

Run infusion at 15 mg/kg/h for 44 h (0.5 mL/kg/h)

Continue infusion at 7.5 mg/kg/h for 16 h (0.25 mL/kg/h)

Stop if patient asymptomatic, transaminase levels normal, and serum acetaminophen level nondetectable; otherwise continue at 7.5 mg/kg/h

Stop if patient clinically improving, transaminase levels decreasing and <1,000 IU/L, serum acetaminophen level nondetectable; otherwise continue at 7.5 mg/kg/h

FIGURE 1.—Protocol for administration of oral N-acetylcysteine by the intravenous route. (Courtesy of Kao LW, Kirk MA, Furbee RB, et al: What is the rate of adverse events after oral N-acetylcysteine administered by the intravenous route to patients with suspected acetaminophen poisoning? *Ann Emerg Med* 42:741-750, 2003.)

▶ The 72-hour oral N-acetylcysteine (NAC) protocol has been in use for nearly 20 years and is the only approved protocol for acetaminophen poisoning. Now with the availability of Acetadote (IV NAC), we can use shortened IV protocols (already in use in Europe and Canada) such as the one used in this study to target the most sustained treatment for the patients who require it. This study will help guide the implementation of the IV formulation as well as its anticipated side effects. Despite the advent of the commercially prepared version, the method for preparation of oral NAC for IV use should remain an acceptable one for hospitals that are cost conscious.

R. J. Hamilton, MD

Acute Oral Selenium Intoxication With Ten Times the Lethal Dose Resulting in Deep Gastric Ulcer

Kise Y, Yoshimura S, Akieda K, et al (Tokai Univ, Isehara, Japan)
J Emerg Med 26:183-187, 2004   11–19

Introduction.—Selenium is an essential trace element and an important component of the antioxidant glutathione peroxidase. It has been used to improve the nutritional status of the digestive tract and enhance immune function in patients with cancer. Excessive doses can result in intoxication, characterized by gastrointestinal irritation, vomiting, and diarrhea. A patient with schizophrenia who took 2000 mg of selenium orally was described. With effective early treatment, she was discharged in good health.

Case Report.—Woman, 48, was seen 2 hours after attempted suicide via ingestion of one bottle of glass blue (used for stained glass manufacture), which contained 2000 mg of selenium dioxide. She had mildly altered consciousness and hematemesis. Her vital signs were stable. She vomited garlicky smelling blood a couple of times and complained of epigastric pain. She also had a garlic-smelling respiration. Endoscopy revealed erosion and oozing of the oral cavity, esophagus, and stomach (Fig 1). The gastric angulus was mostly replaced by necrotic tissue that formed a deep ulcer, classified as grade 3 corrosive gastritis. There was no perforation, and the duodenum was totally intact. No mucosal damage was detected on bronchoscopy. Intubation was performed to avoid aspiration pneumonia. Gastric lavage was performed to extract the residual toxic agent. Hemodialysis was performed. She was extubated on the following day after she was stabilized. Her serum selenium level was the highest before hemodialysis, then gradually diminished. The serum glutathione peroxidase activities were continuously higher than the normal range and did not parallel selenium levels (Fig 2). Repeat endoscopy revealed improvement, and oral feeding was initiated on day 7. She had evidence of liver dysfunction on day 5. She was treated conservatively and discharged uneventfully on day 16. At 3-month follow-up, the ulcerative lesion had become scar. At 1-year follow-up, there was no further mucosal damage, and she had no abnormalities of fingernails or alopecia.

Conclusion.—There are currently no known antidotes for selenium toxicity. The main treatment strategy is cessation of selenium intake and symptomatic care. This patient will require endoscopic follow-up for 6 years because grade 3 corrosive gastritis can lead to late complications, including gastric stenosis.

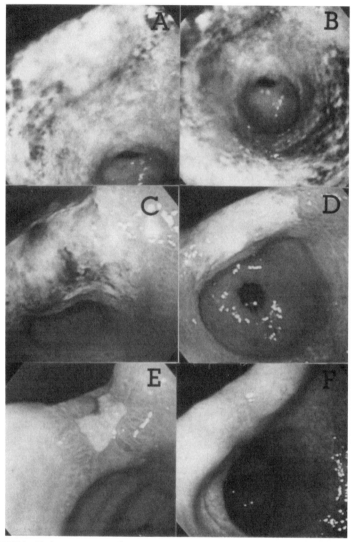

FIGURE 1.—Endoscopic images of gastric corrosive damage caused by acute selenium intoxication. **A,** Corrosive change at gastric angulus replaced by necrotic back tissues at transfer to the present hospital. **B,** This corrosive change causing erosion and oozing was found throughout the stomach. This change was extending from oral cavity and esophagus, but duodenum was intact. **C,** Gastric angulus is still corrosive and the other regions are still edematous on the 7th day. **D,** Corrosive change became localized at the angulus, covered by white coat, surrounded by regenerative tissues. But the other regions are still edematous on the 16th day. **E,** Mucosal damage became more localized to form an A2 stage ulcer at angulus 6 weeks later. **F,** The ulcerative lesion became scar and the other regions became normal mucosa 3 months later. (Reprinted from Kise Y, Yoshimura S, Akieda K, et al: Acute oral selenium intoxication with ten times the lethal dose resulting in deep gastric ulcer. *J Emerg Med* 26:183-187, 2004. Copyright 2004, with permission from Elsevier Science.)

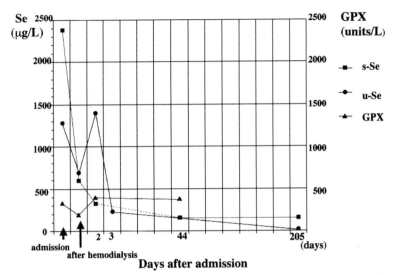

FIGURE 2.—Serum and urinary selenium level of the patient during the course as well as serum glutathi-one peroxidase activity. *Abbreviations: Se*, Selenium; *GPX*, glutathione peroxidase; *s-SE*, serum selenium level; *u-Se*, urinary selenium level. (Reprinted from Kise Y, Yoshimura S, Akieda K, et al: Acute oral selenium intoxication with ten times the lethal dose resulting in deep gastric ulcer. *J Emerg Med* 26:183-187, 2004. Copyright 2004, with permission from Elsevier Science.)

▶ A rare and interesting case report. Although hemodialysis lowered the serum selenium level, its role in the resolution of toxicity is unclear. What is clear is that glass blue (selenium dioxide) is extremely corrosive to the gastrointestinal tract, especially the stomach, and can cause permanent injury and sequelae.

R. J. Hamilton, MD

Chinese Red Rice–Induced Myopathy
Smith DJ, Olive KE (East Tennessee State Univ, Johnson City)
South Med J 96:1265-1267, 2003   11–20

Introduction.—Chinese red rice, initially used to make rice wine and as a food preservative during the Tang Dynasty in AD 800, is used to improve blood circulation and reduce cholesterol and triglycerides. The main active ingredients are hydroxymethylglutaryl coenzyme reductase inhibitors, primarily lovastatin (also known as *monacolin K* or *mevinolin*). A case of symptomatic myopathy associated with the use of Chinese red rice was reported.

Case Report.—Man, 50, was seen by his primary care physician for joint pain and muscle weakness. He was well until 2 months previously when he developed pain in his left wrist and muscle discomfort in his left forearm. The muscle discomfort progressed to involve the right upper extremity. He complained of diffuse body aching, upper extremity weakness, and stiffness of the lower back. He had hypertension, hypercholesterolemia, and anxiety, and he used tobacco and occasionally used alcohol. Current medications were quinapril, clonazepam, rofecoxib, paroxetine, ginseng, and Chinese red rice. The former 2 medications he had been taking for years, rofecoxib for about 1 month, and the herbal supplements for 3 months. He had minimal edema of the metacarpophalangeal joint of the first digit of his left hand. He had difficulty extending his upper extremities on range-of-motion evaluation. The muscle strength in his hands was reduced to 4/5 bilaterally. He had crepitus in his knees bilaterally with extension. All laboratory testing was normal except for a creatine kinase (CPK) level of 358 IU/L (normal range, 30-160 IU/L). He was instructed to cease taking ginseng and Chinese red rice. At 3-week follow-up, his muscle weakness and joint pain had resolved completely. The CPK was 179 IU/L. At 8-month follow-up, the patient had resumed Chinese red rice, and his CPK was 212 IU/L.

Conclusion.—Physicians need to be aware that Chinese red rice can produce a clinically significant myopathy. Physicians need to be aware of all substances their patients are using.

▶ Chinese red rice toxicity will probably surface again as patients with hypercholesterolemia seeking herbal remedies realize that it contains lovastatin. Like other HMG coenzyme reductase inhibitors, it can cause a myopathy. The evidence that this drug caused the problem is the resolution upon its withdrawal, and the elevation of CPK when it was restarted. I would have liked to have known the patient's cholesterol to see if the Chinese red rice was actually working!

R. J. Hamilton, MD

Catastrophic Brain Injury After Nicotine Insecticide Ingestion
Rogers AJ, Denk LD, Wax PM (Emory Univ, Atlanta, Ga; Univ of Rochester, NY; Good Samaritan Reg Med Ctr, Phoenix, Ariz)
J Emerg Med 26:169-172, 2004   11–21

Introduction.—Nicotine ingestion can be an immediate life-threatening event. A case of severe acute nicotine toxicity in an adolescent that resulted in hypoxic brain injury was reported.

Case Report.—Boy, 15 years, was seen in the ED after cardiopulmonary arrest at home. He reportedly had a seizure, then stopped breathing. CPR was initiated by his father. EMS administered 2 mg of naloxone and 2 mg of atropine; there was no demonstrable effect. The patient was intubated, and 100% oxygen was administered. His initial Glasgow Coma Scale score was 4, rectal temperature was

33.8°C, his heart rate was 157 beats/min, blood pressure was 170/ 108 mm Hg, and spontaneous respiratory rate was 6 breaths/min. Mechanical ventilation was initiated. Neurologic examination showed midline fixed pupils, right slightly larger than left, with weak corneal reflexes. He was globally hypotonic, with decerebrate posturing to painful stimuli. His blood glucose was 334 mg/dL, sodium was 142 mEq/L, potassium was 3.8 mEq/L, chloride was 106 mEq/L, CO_2 was 19 mEq/L, BUN was 14 mg/dL, creatinine was 0.8 mg/dL, calcium was 8.1 mg/dL, and magnesium was 1.4 mEq/L. His white blood cell count was 10.1 THOU/μL, hemoglobin was 13.9 g/dL, and platelet count was 252 THOU/μL. Initial arterial blood gas values while receiving 100% oxygen were a pH of 7.33, PCO_2 of 41 mm Hg, and PO_2 of 511 mm Hg. A CT scan of the brain was normal, and ECG identified sinus tachycardia with a rate of 144 beats/min, with multiple atrial premature contractions. The patient had a history of depression and smoked cigarettes and marijuana. He was currently taking trazadone and sertraline. Comprehensive urine drug screening was positive for caffeine, nicotine, and cotinine (a nicotine metabolite). MRI on day 1 of hospitalization revealed severe hypoxic-ischemic encephalopathy with multiple areas of cortical and basal ganglia infarction. A friend of the patient revealed that the patient kept a bottle of "poison" in his room. Upon recovery, it was found to contain an insecticide with the trade name of Black Leaf 40. It contained nicotine sulfate 40% as an active ingredient and 60% inert ingredients. The friend verified that a significant amount of the brown liquid was absent from the bottle. A presumptive diagnosis of nicotine ingestion was made. Laboratory analysis showed the bottle contained 357 mg of nicotine per milliliter of solution. Despite aggressive intensive care support, the patient had minimal improvement and was ultimately discharged to a long-term care facility. At 6-month follow-up, he remained neurologically devastated and was dependent on gastric tube feedings and full-time care providers.

▶ This article points out the classic toxic effects of nicotine, including status epilepticus, which probably resulted in this patient's hypoxic-ischemic encephalopathy. The only way the case was solved was through good, old-fashioned detective work at the patient's home and an alert toxicology laboratory technician.

R. J. Hamilton, MD

Baclofen Toxicity in an 8-Year-Old With an Intrathecal Baclofen Pump

Yeh RN, Nypaver MM, Deegan TJ, et al (Univ of Michigan, Ann Arbor)
J Emerg Med 26:163-167, 2004   11–22

Introduction.—With the increasing use of intrathecal baclofen pumps for treatment of spasticity of the spinal cord or cerebral origin, it is crucial that physicians become more familiar with the possible untoward effects of their use. Malfunction of the pump can cause intrathecal overdose of baclofen. A case of baclofen toxicity in a child with an intrathecal baclofen pump was reported.

> *Case Report.*—Boy, 8 years, with spastic diplegic cerebral palsy became unresponsive and bradycardic. He was airlifted from a community hospital to a tertiary care hospital. His rectal temperature at admission to the tertiary care hospital was 35°C, his pulse was in the high 50s to mid 60s, his blood pressure was 98/46 mm Hg, and pulse oximetry was 100% on 2 L of oxygen via nasal cannula. He was unresponsive and had minimal response to painful stimuli. He was flaccid and areflexic; his plantar responses were downgoing. He was able to protect his airway with a gag response and had minimal oral secretions. No abnormalities were detected at the pump or back incision sites. Radiographs at the community hospital had shown an intact pump-catheter system, with the tip at the T8 level. Findings at both hospitals suggested baclofen overdose. A test dose of physostigmine was administered. The patient had a short-lived response; he demonstrated eye-opening and coherent speech, and his heart rate briefly rose to the mid 80s before dropping to the mid 50s, concurrent with the relapse in clinical unresponsiveness. A pump programmer was not immediately available to stop pump action. Unsuccessful attempts were made to withdraw baclofen with a 23-gauge butterfly needle advanced through the palpable center of the pump. When a pump programmer, a laptop computer with specific software typically available only to the appropriate subspecialty service, was available for analysis, it identified the pump's identity, expected reservoir baclofen volume (4.6 mL), drug concentration (2000 μg/mL), and mode and rate of drug delivery (623.9 μg/d). The pump was programmed to a "stop" mode, and the pump's reservoir was aseptically and easily accessed; 3.5 mL of baclofen was withdrawn. The CSF drug load was reduced by removing 20 mL of fluid. The patient had signs of recovery within minutes of the reservoir tap and lumbar puncture. He was poorly responsive, and his heart rate steadily rose to the mid 90s. During the next 48 hours, he slowly recovered to his baseline state and had no medical complications. Saline was running in his pump at discharge, and he was given an oral baclofen-dosing schedule at his parents' request. He had repeated symptoms of withdrawal nightly until the catheter was replaced. Dysfunctional catheter positioning was considered the cause of malfunction.

Conclusion.—In emergency situations, when a pump programmer is unavailable, emptying the baclofen reservoir can stop the pump. Clinicians need to be aware of potential acute withdrawal symptoms.

▶ Baclofen pump problems are reported more often in the literature as their use increases. Most toxicity occurs shortly after the pump reservoir has been refilled. The authors demonstrate how difficult it can be to get assistance in managing these cases on an emergent basis. ED physicians who see patients with these pumps would do well to get an inservice on their use and potential causes of malfunction.

R. J. Hamilton, MD

Dose-Dependent Hemodynamic Effect of Digoxin Therapy in Severe Verapamil Toxicity
Bania TC, Chu J, Almond G, et al (Columbia Univ, New York; New York Med College)
Acad Emerg Med 11:221-227, 2004   11–23

Introduction.—Calcium chloride alone is not effective as an antidote in severe calcium channel antagonist overdoses. Digoxin has recently been investigated as a therapy that could increase the efficacy of calcium in large calcium channel antagonist overdoses. A controlled, unblinded investigation was performed in 8 adult male dogs to determine whether there is a dose-dependent hemodynamic effect of digoxin in the setting of verapamil toxicity treated with high-dose calcium chloride.

Methods.—Eight animals were instrumented to measure systolic and diastolic blood pressure, cardiac output, pulmonary artery pressures, and left ventricular pressures. Verapamil toxicity (50% reduction in mean arterial pressure) was induced via verapamil, 6 mg/kg/h, and maintained for 30 minutes by titrating the verapamil rate. After verapamil toxicity was achieved, all dogs received one dose of digoxin equivalent to 0, 1, 1.5, 2, 3, 4, 6, or 8 times the loading dose of digoxin (0.009 mg/kg). The verapamil dose was reduced to 4 mg/kg/h and continued for the next 5 hours. Calcium chloride boluses were administered (0.5 g immediately after verapamil toxicity and 1 g administered at 1, 2, and 3 hours). Measurements were compared with the loading dose of digoxin with the use of linear regression analysis.

Results.—Digoxin produced a dose-dependent increase in systolic blood pressure at 4 hours (10.23 mm Hg per loading dose of digoxin; 95% confidence interval [CI], 2.74-17.73), 4 hours 15 minutes (13.9 mm Hg per loading dose of digoxin; 95% CI, 8.75-19.01), and 5 hours (17.04 mm Hg per loading dose of digoxin; 95% CI, 1.76-32.32). Digoxin produced a dose-dependent increase in maximal ventricular pressure at the end of the third hour (8.55 mg Hg per loading dose of digoxin; 95% CI, 3.41-13.69), 3 hours 15 minutes (11.81 mm Hg per loading dose of digoxin; 95% CI, 4.89-18.73), hour 4 (8.26 mm Hg per loading dose of digoxin; 95% CI, 1.03-15.48), and 4 hours 15 minutes (9.74 mm Hg per loading dose of digoxin; 95% CI, 4.47-15.00). It was not possible to identify a dose-dependent increase in other parameters, including diastolic relaxation (diastolic change in pressure over time) and time to onset of death. There were no ventricular arrhythmias.

Conclusion.—A dose-dependent effect of digoxin on systolic blood pressure and maximal ventricular pressure occurs in the setting of severe verapamil toxicity treated with high-dose calcium chloride.

▶ The question of whether the treatment of a verapamil overdose is a combined overdose of digoxin and calcium remains unanswered by this study. However, the fact that some cardiovascular parameters increased (systolic blood pressure and maximal ventricular pressure), but that survival did not, suggests that this is probably not a fruitful venue of investigation for treating calcium channel blocker toxicity.

R. J. Hamilton, MD

A Picturesque Reversal of Antimuscarinic Delirium
Richardson WH III, Williams SR, Carstairs SD (Univ of California, San Diego; Naval Med Ctr, San Diego, Calif)
J Emerg Med 26:463, 2004   11–24

Introduction.—The impact of physostigmine administration is dramatically illustrated in a case report of an adolescent seen in the ED after ingestion of Tylenol PM.

> *Case Report.*—Boy, 16 years, was seen in the ED for confusion and mumbling speech. Physical examination revealed sinus tachycardia, large reactive pupils, hypoactive bowel sounds, and anhidrosis. He remained confused and picked at the buttons on the physician's coat several times. He was asked to draw the face of a clock (Fig 1). Among other abnormalities, he mistakenly wrote the words "beans" and "ham" in the 9 o'clock position. Five minutes after IV administration of physostigmine 0.5 mg, he was asked to repeat the drawing. An additional 0.5 mg physostigmine was given IV. His mental status normalized. He gave a history of Tylenol PM ingestion. He was discharged 3 days after an uncomplicated hospital course.

Discussion/Conclusion.—The antimuscarinic delirium caused by diphenhydramine was temporarily reversed. A potentially hepatotoxic acetaminophen ingestion was treated with N-acetylcysteine.

▶ The picture says it all, and the technique of having a patient draw a clock face is a time-honored and valuable approach to evaluating mental disorders of all sorts.

R. J. Hamilton, MD

Immediately before physostigmine administration

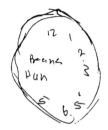

5 minutes after first physostigmine 0.5 mg IV dose

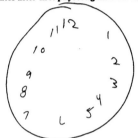

5 minutes after second dose of physostigmine 0.5 mg IV

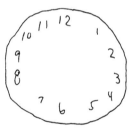

FIGURE 1.—Clock faces drawn before and after physostigmine administration. (Reprinted from Richardson WH III, Williams SR, Carstairs SD: A picturesque reversal of antimuscarinic delirium. *J Emerg Med* 26:463, 2004. Copyright 2004, with permission from Elsevier Science.)

Methylene 3, 4 Dioxymethamphetamine-Induced Acute Myocardial Infarction

Lai T-I, Hwang J-J, Fang C-C, et al (Natl Taiwan Univ, Taipei)
Ann Emerg Med 42:759-762, 2003   11–25

Introduction.—Only one case of acute myocardial infarction (AMI) resulting from methylene 3,4 dioxymethamphetamine (MDMA) has been reported. A case of AMI that occurred in a young man 3 hours after oral consumption of MDMA was reported.

Case Report.—Man, 27, was seen in the ED of a community hospital for a 3-hour history of chest discomfort and tightness, nausea, vomiting, and dizziness after drinking one bottle of whisky and one half of an MDMA pill. He claimed to have taken the drug orally 4 other times. He had a 2-year history of smoking 2 packs of cigarettes per day and of club hopping on a weekly basis, during which time he drank various amounts of liquor. An ECG revealed an ectopic atrial rhythm with ST elevation, Q wave, and T inversion over leads II, III, and aVF. His total creatine kinase level was 606 U/L, with a creatine kinase-MB level of 43 U/L and a troponin I level of 1.1 ng/mL. He was transferred to a university hospital after treatment with morphine, aspirin, and IV nitroglycerin for suspected AMI. His blood pressure was 104/49 mm Hg and pulse rate was 73 beats/min. He had a grade II/VI systolic murmur. Toxicology screening showed MDMA, morphine, and lidocaine metabolites (the latter from central venous catheter insertion). A V4R ST elevation was seen on right-sided EKG. At 6 hours after onset of chest pain, the creatine kinase level had increased to 857 U/L, the creatine kinase-MB was 85.6 U/L, and the troponin I level was 18.8 ng/mL. His cholesterol level was 189 mg/dL and triglyceride level was 36 mg/dL. Bedside US revealed left ventricular hypokinesia, particularly over the inferior and posterior wall of the heart. Emergency cardiac catheterization performed at 8 hours after onset of chest pain showed a substantial thrombus in the right coronary artery. Tirofiban was administered at an initial dose of 1.6 mg per 30 minutes and 0.4 mg/h thereafter. Heparin sodium 630 U/h, nitroglycerine 1 mg/h, oxygen, and aspirin were administered. He was admitted to the ICU for observation. The ST-segment elevation returned to normal, and he was free of symptoms by day 2 after the incident. Coronary angiography performed on day 5 showed a thrombus in the proximal part of the right coronary artery. An intracoronary injection of 300,000 units of urokinase was administered; heparinization was continued. At 10 days after the episode, repeat right coronary angiography showed a patent right coronary artery. He was discharged in stable condition.

Conclusion.—In young patients without apparent risk factors who present with acute coronary syndromes, drug abuse should be included in the differential diagnosis.

▶ This patient was successfully diagnosed and treated for AMI after MDMA overdose that caused a right coronary artery thrombosis at the age of 27. After the patient recovered, repeat catheterization showed a patent vessel. The immediate onset of his symptoms and the reversal of his condition would suggest vasospasm as the likely culprit for the formation of thrombus, an etiology in keeping with the sympathomimetic qualities of MDMA.

R. J. Hamilton, MD

Quetiapine Poisoning: A Case Series

Balit CR, Isbister GK, Hackett LP, et al (Children's Hosp at Westmead, Sydney, Australia; Univ of Newcastle, Callaghan, Australia; Newcastle Mater Misericordiae Hosp, Waratah, Australia; et al)
Ann Emerg Med 42:751-758, 2003
11–26

Introduction.—Quetiapine fumarate is a relatively new atypical antipsychotic drug used to treatment schizophrenia. Its antipsychotic actions are considered to be primarily mediated through the inhibition of serotonin receptors and dopamine receptors. It is rapidly absorbed orally; the median time to maximum observed plasma concentration is 1 to 2 hours. The first single-center case series of quetiapine overdose was reported. Factors predictive of ICU admission and length of stay (LOS) in excess of 24 hours that could assist in early patient discharge were evaluated.

Methods.—The quetiapine poisonings were identified from a prospective database of admissions to a regional toxicology service. Data were obtained concerning details of ingestion, clinical characteristics, diagnostic testing (including ECG), and other outcomes (LOS and ICU admission rate).

Results.—Of 45 cases of quetiapine overdose, 18 patients had quetiapine assay results. The median LOS was 35 hours (interquartile range [IQR], 14-42 hours) for the 18 patients, 9 of whom were admitted to the ICU. The median ingested dose was 3.5 g (IQR, 1.7-6.2 g). The reported ingested dose was highly associated with the estimated peak drug concentration ($P <$ .0001), which verified the patient-provided history of ingestion. Seizures were observed in 2 patients and delirium in 3 patients. Four patients required mechanical ventilation. There were no arrhythmias and no deaths. Six of the 18 patients ingested quetiapine alone (median LOS, 35 hours; 3 admitted to ICU). One patient who ingested 24 g experienced hypotension and seizures. Tachycardia occurred in 8 of 10 patients for whom ECGs were available and who had ingested no cardiotoxic drugs. For these 10 patients, the mean corrected QT (QTc) interval was increased at 487 milliseconds; the mean uncorrected QT interval was 349 milliseconds. The reported dose and peak quetiapine concentrations were significantly linked with ICU admission and LOS more than 24 hours. A reported dose of less than 3 g and a Glasgow Coma Score no lower than 15 predicted patients not needing ICU admission or LOS greater than 24 hours.

Conclusion.—Quetiapine overdose primarily produced CNS depression and sinus tachycardia. In large doses, patients may need intubation and ventilation for respiratory depression.

▶ I often get consults from concerned clinicians who are treating patients with prolonged QTc intervals after quetiapine overdoses. I've not seen that particular feature of toxicity portend any poor outcome. The authors attempt to project a useful cutoff of 3 g of quetiapine as a marker for severity. In fact, the patient's clinical condition determines the need for therapy, and this cutoff is of little value. There does seem to be a correlation between dose and toxicity, and so large overdoses are more likely to result in toxic effects.

R. J. Hamilton, MD

Acute Myocardial Infarction as a Complication of Clonidine Withdrawal

Simic J, Kishineff S, Goldberg R, et al (Saint Joseph Med Ctr, Burbank, Calif; USC Med Ctr, Los Angeles)

J Emerg Med 25:399-402, 2003   11–27

Introduction.—Acute clonidine withdrawal has been reported to produce a hyperdynamic state, sometimes within 24 hours of drug discontinuation. A case of acute clonidine withdrawal that caused myocardial infarction (MI), a rarely described complication, was reported.

Case Report.—Woman, 86, was seen in the ED with a 3-hour history of headache, nausea, vomiting, and severe precordial chest pain. She had a long history of hypertension and had been taking clonidine, 0.2 mg twice daily, until about 36 hours before admission; her physician advised her to discontinue the medication (reason unknown). She was also taking clonazepam. On admission, she was tremulous, profusely diaphoretic, and actively vomiting. Her blood pressure (BP) was 230/150 mm Hg, pulse rate was 140 beats/min, respiratory rate was 24 breaths/min, and oral temperature was 37.2°C. The precordium was hyperdynamic, and her heart tones were rapid and regular. An ECG showed evidence of an evolving anterolateral MI. Her white blood cell count was 16,200/mmq, hemoglobin was 13.4 g/dL, hematocrit was 39%, and glucose level was 202 mg/dL. Her troponin I level was 13.5 ng/mL (reference range, 0-0.5 ng/mL). Labetolol 20 mg and diazepam 7.5 mg were administered IV. Within 10 minutes of admission, her BP was 109/66 mm Hg, pulse rate was 103 beats/min, and her headache resolved. She was given clopidogrel 75 mg orally and heparin 5000 units IV. Cardiac catheterization performed about 2 hours after arrival showed that all coronary arteries were patent, and there was no evidence of narrowing. She had severe left ventricular dysfunction (left ejection fraction, about 25%). She had a stable hospital course. Clonidine was reinstituted and BP was well controlled. Serial troponin levels remained modestly elevated; the level peaked at 34 ng/mL at about 14 hours after admission. At 6-month follow-up, she was symptom-free and had no episodes of angina or congestive heart failure. Stress testing at 6-month follow-up was negative, and her ECG was normal except for the presence of first-degree atrioventricular block.

Conclusion.—Acute clonidine withdrawal should be considered in the differential diagnosis of patients who present with hyperadrenergic symptoms, particularly if the medical history is not readily available. Treatment in moderate to severe cases involves rapid restoration of hemodynamic stability, while instituting oral or transdermal clonidine replacement.

▶ Studies show that catecholamine levels begin to rise within 24 hours of cessation of clonidine intake. This case report demonstrates how serious that problem can become, why clonidine is such a poor choice in a noncompliant patient, and why it should never simply be stopped without a tapering dose.

R. J. Hamilton, MD

Acute Self-poisoning by Ingestion of Cadmium and Barium
Hung Y-M, Chung H-M (Kaohsiung Veterans Gen Hosp, Taiwan)
Nephrol Dial Transplant 19:1308-1309, 2004   11–28

Introduction.—Cadmium is a severe pulmonary and gastrointestinal irritant that can be fatal when inhaled or ingested. Acute poisoning from exposure to cadmium has increased in industrialized countries. A case of acute cadmium and barium self-poisoning was reported.

Case Report.—Man, 42, was seen in the ED with marked lethargy and fever. His blood pressure was 129/72 mm Hg, heart rate was 87 beats/min, respiratory rate was 16/min, and temperature was 38°C. He had diminished deep tendon reflexes of the lower limbs. Serum chemistry values were as follows: sodium, 142 mEq/L; potassium, 2.2 mEq/L; chloride, 112 mEq/L; serum urea nitrogen, 11 mg/dL; creatinine, 0.8 mg/dL; calcium, 9.5 mg/dL; and glucose, 144 mg/dL. His serum creatine kinase was 222 U/L, with the MB type 11 U/L. Room air arterial blood had a pH of 7.35; HCO_3, 19.4 mEq/L; PCO_2, 35.5 mm Hg; and PO_2, 105 mm Hg. His white blood cell count was 15,370 mm³. He had normal sinus rhythm on ECG. His wife stated he had been depressed and was taking sedatives for tension. He consumed about 50 mL of an industrial chemical solution about 1 hour before admission. About 20 minutes after ingestion, he experienced nausea, vomiting, abdominal pain, and profuse diarrhea. He had gradual onset of drowsiness about 20 minutes before admission. Barium intoxication was initially suspected. Half-normal saline was administered IV at a rate of 120 to 150 mL/h, along with potassium chloride, 40 mg every 8 hours. Contact with his workplace revealed that the industrial chemicals the patient consumed contained 2% to 15% of cadmium and barium stearate. His blood cadmium level on day 1 was 24.9 ng/mL (normal range, 0.2-6.0 ng/mL) and serum barium concentration was 34.1 µg/dL (normal range, 3.0-20.0 µg/dL). After stabilization on day 2, he was moved from the ICU to a medical ward. His diarrhea, vomiting, and abdominal pain subsided; weakness and myalgias persisted. On hospital day 3, his serum chloride was 111 mEq/L; sodium, 144 mEq/L; potassium, 4.2 mEq/L; and platelet count, 77,000/mm³. The platelet count returned to normal on day 7. The blood and urine cadmium concentrations diminished over time.

Conclusion.—Cadmium and barium intoxication should be suspected in the differential diagnosis of any patient with diffuse diarrhea, vomiting, and hypokalemia. A drug intake history is important for early diagnosis of a potentially fatal poisoning.

▶ The hypokalemia from barium ingestion can be profound and sustained, and occurs when the barium blocks the passive potassium efflux channel. This prevents potassium from effluxing from the cell, and allows serums levels to fall and intracellular levels to rise. Without potassium supplementation, the overdose can be fatal. Note that the soluble barium salts (in this case barium stearate) are the problem, not the insoluble salts such as those used for radiologic procedures.

R. J. Hamilton, MD

Natural Selection and Molecular Evolution in *PTC*, a Bitter-Taste Receptor Gene
Wooding S, Kim U, Bamshad MJ, et al (Univ of Utah, Salt Lake City; NIH, Rockville, Md)
Am J Hum Genet 74:637-646, 2004   11–29

Introduction.—The ability to taste phenylthiocarbamide (PTC) is a classic phenotype that varies in human populations; about 50% of humans are unable to taste PTC. This phenotype is of genetic, epidemiologic, and evolutionary interest since the ability to taste PTC is associated with the ability to taste other bitter substances, many of which are toxic. Variation in PTC perception may demonstrate variation in dietary preferences throughout human history and could correlate with susceptibility to diet-associated diseases in modern populations. The patterns of DNA sequence variation in the recently identified *PTC* gene, which is responsible for up to 85% of phenotypic variance in the trait, were examined to assess variability in PTC perception.

Methods.—The entire coding region of *PTC* (1002 base pairs) was analyzed in a sample of 330 chromosomes obtained from African (n = 62), Asian (n = 138), European (n = 110), and North American (n = 20) populations by using new statistical tests for natural selection that consider the potential confounding effects of human population growth.

Results.—Two intermediate-frequency haplotypes corresponding to "taster" and "nontaster" phenotypes were identified. These haplotypes had similar occurrences across Africa, Asia, and Europe. Genetic differentiation among the continental population samples was low ($F_{ST} = 0.056$), compared with estimates based on other genes. Tajima's D and Fu and Li's D and F statistics showed a significant deviation from neutrality because of an excess of intermediate-frequency variants when human population growth was considered (*P* < .01).

Conclusion.—These findings combine to suggest that balancing natural selection has acted to maintain "taster" and "nontaster" alleles at the *PTC* locus in humans.

▶ This article is for the emergency medicine/medical toxicologists out there. It doesn't have much of an impact on life and death in the ED. However, it explains why some people positively gag when they taste certain foods and others do not. The "gaggers" may be PTC tasters, and the "nongaggers" may be PTC nontasters. PTC is similar in structure to isothiocyanates and goitrin, both of which are bitter substances found in vegetables such as cabbage and broccoli. One wonders whether the correlation of PTC perception to the perception of other toxic bitter substances may be a potential paradigm for understanding how some people are symptomatic after exposure to substances at levels well below what others can tolerate without symptoms. All speculative at this point, but still fascinating.

R. J. Hamilton, MD

Exercise-Induced Syncope Associated With QT Prolongation and Ephedra-Free Xenadrine
Nasir JM, Durning SJ, Ferguson M, et al (Uniformed Services Univ of the Health Sciences, Bethesda, Md; Natl Naval Med Ctr, Bethesda, Md)
Mayo Clin Proc 79:1059-1062, 2004   11–30

Introduction.—Ephedra-containing substances used to promote weight loss and enhance athletic performance have been linked with several reports of arrhythmic events, sudden death, myocardial infarction, and death. After the Food and Drug Administration banned the use of these substances, formulations have emerged for weight loss and performance enhancement that are marketed as "ephedra free," yet contain other sympathomimetic substances for which safety has not been established. A case of exercise-induced syncope that occurred in a healthy woman 1 hour after she took Xenadrine EFX, an ephedra-free weight loss supplement, was reported.

Case Report.—Woman, 22, was seen in the ED after a syncopal event that occurred while running. She reported not running for a month before the event. She had been taking 1 Xenadrine EFX tablet for 1 year, stopped for 3 months, then restarted the dose the evening before the syncopal event. She had taken 1 Xenadrine EFX tablet 45 minutes before running, drank water, but did not eat breakfast before running. At 3.5 miles into the run, she had the syncopal episode. ECG showed a sinus tachycardia of 100 beats/min and prolongation of the QT interval (corrected QT, 516 milliseconds). This resolved in 24 hours. On admission, her serum potassium level was 4.1 mEq/L, calcium level was 8.8 mg/dL, anion gap acidosis level was 20 mEq/L, and glucose level was 225 mg/dL. On urinalysis, ketones were 40 mg/dL. With hydration, the anion gap acidosis and ketosis resolved quickly. Echocardiographic and exercise stress testing were normal. Nine months of monitoring with an implanted loop recorder showed no arrhythmias in the absence of Xenadrine EFX. The patient had no further episodes of syncope or presyncope, and ECGs remained normal.

Conclusion.—It was not clear whether the patient had an ion channel abnormality. It is possible that the combination of exercise and Xenadrine EFX is contraindicated in patients considered at risk for QT prolongation.

▶ Although I appreciate the authors' effort to point out the sympathomimetic drugs in the Xenadrine EFX (ephedra free), there is little evidence that this accounts for the patient's palpitations and syncope. In fact, the patient had an anion gap acidosis and a ketosis most consistent with starvation. While we stress the importance of obtaining a history of herbal and over-the-counter drug use in every patient, there is a chance that effort can also become a "red herring" in the patient's history.

R. J. Hamilton, MD

Co-worker Fatalities From Hydrogen Sulfide
Hendrickson RG, Chang A, Hamilton RJ (Oregon Health and Science Univ, Portland; Drexel Univ, Philadelphia)
Am J Ind Med 45:346-350, 2004   11–31

Background.—Hydrogen sulfide is a hazard in many industries and occupations. This colorless, odorless gas can cause rapid loss of consciousness and respiratory depression with no warning. Occupational hydrogen sulfide deaths occurring in the United States between 1993 and 1999 were analyzed.

Methods and Findings.—The US Bureau of Labor Statistics Census of Fatal Occupational Injuries were reviewed for occupational deaths related to hydrogen sulfide during the study period. In that 7-year period, 52 workers died of hydrogen sulfide toxicity. Eighty-five percent of the workers were white, and 98% were male. Forty-eight percent were in their first year of employment with the company. Industries commonly affected were waste management, petroleum, and natural gas. In 21% of the incidents, a coworker also died at the same time or in an attempt to save the afflicted worker.

Conclusions.—Hydrogen sulfide toxicity occurs uncommonly but can be deadly. Hydrogen sulfide–related deaths occur in new workers and coworkers. Adequate education on the warning signs of hydrogen sulfide toxicity may help decrease fatalities among workers.

▶ The nature of hydrogen sulfide and its knockdown effect is one of the important reasons that it is one of the toxins that produces mass casualties. The classic scene is a fatally poisoned worker and rescuer, and EMS workers and emergency physicians should be aware.

R. J. Hamilton, MD

Quinine-Induced Disseminated Intravascular Coagulation: Case Report and Review of the Literature
Knower MT, Bowton DL, Owen J, et al (Ochsner Clinic North Shore, Mandeville, La; Wake Forest Univ, Winston-Salem, NC)
Intensive Care Med 29:1007-1011, 2003   11–32

Background.—Quinine-induced disseminated intravascular coagulation (DIC) is a distinct clinical entity. Affected patients may be seen initially with unexplained thrombocytopenia, coagulopathy, or renal failure. The clinical course of quinine-induced DIC was reviewed.

Methods.—The MEDLINE database was searched for publications appearing between 1969 and 2000. All reported cases and reviews of quinine-induced thrombocytopenia, hemolytic-uremic syndrome, and DIC were analyzed. Fifteen patients reported in the literature met criteria for DIC temporally associated with recent quinine ingestion.

Discussion.—The immune response of susceptible patients to quinine may lead to the production of antiplatelet antibodies and antibodies against leukocytes, erythrocytes, and endothelial cells. The varying patterns and specificities of antibody production in individuals comprise a spectrum of clinical disease, ranging from mild, transient thrombocytopenia to overt intravascular hemolysis, renal failure, coagulopathy, and DIC. Recognizing quinine-induced DIC early is essential, as the prognosis of this condition is better than other adult forms of hemolytic-uremic syndrome or DIC.

▶ Severe toxin-induced thrombocytopenia is a rare event. This article adds an additional case report, as well as a nice review of the literature. It is notable that these cases present with features that may make it indistinguishable from other causes of thrombocytopenia; therefore, a high index of suspicion is necessary to make the diagnosis.

R. J. Hamilton, MD

A Case of Valproate-Associated Hepatotoxicity Treated With L-Carnitine
Romero-Falcón A, de la Santa-Belda E, García-Contreras R, et al (Hosp Universitario Virgen de Rocío, Sevilla, Spain)
Eur J Intern Med 14:338-340, 2003   11–33

Background.—Valproate, a major broad-spectrum antiepileptic, is effective against many epileptic seizure types. It is usually well tolerated, but this agent can produce serious side effects. One such effect, hepatotoxicity, is rare but often fatal. Long-term valproate may also result in a carnitine deficiency and nonspecific symptoms of hepatotoxicity and hyperammonemia.

One case of valproate-related hepatotoxicity treated with L-carnitine was reported.

> *Case Report.*—Boy, 16 years, was hospitalized after a 16-day history of apathy, lethargy, and progressive jaundice. He had been taking valproate, 1500 mg/d, for generalized epilepsy for 8 weeks until 5 days before his hospitalization. His serum valproate level was 65 μg/mL 4 weeks before admission, but it was only 10 μg/mL on admission. Four days later, the laboratory showed impairments in total bilirubin and aspartate aminotransferase. Thorough testing ruled out hepatitis A, B, and C; autoimmune disorders; other infectious causes; hemochromatosis; Wilson disease; and α_1-antitrypsin deficiency. IV L-carnitine, 2 g/d, was administered for 7 days. Gradually, the patient's condition improved. Within 2 weeks, his liver function tests normalized. Lamotrigine was substituted for valproate with a good neurologic response.

Conclusions.—Supplementation with L-carnitine may help prevent hepatotoxicity. This young patient with valproate-induced acute liver injury had a favorable course after L-carnitine therapy.

▶ This is another case report that supports the value of L-carnitine in valproate toxicity. The authors chose a 2-g daily dose IV. However, higher IV doses have been used. In addition, we know that oral doses can be given as a supplement in chronic valproate therapy to prevent hepatotoxicity. Oral carnitine (which is readily available and easy to administer) may also prove to be valuable as an antidote.

R. J. Hamilton, MD

Pilocarpine Toxicity and the Treatment of Xerostomia
Hendrickson RG, Morocco AP, Greenberg MI (Oregon Health and Sciences Univ, Portland; Guam Mem Hosp, Agana; Drexel Univ, Philadelphia)
J Emerg Med 26:429-432, 2004   11–34

Background.—Described is a case of muscarinic toxicity secondary to an accidental oral pilocarpine overdose as a result of a doctor–patient miscommunication.

> *Case Report.*—Woman, 46, with a history of Sjögren's syndrome, systemic lupus erythematosus, and Reynaud's syndrome, was seen at the ED complaining of abdominal pain. The previous day she had been instructed by her physician to take 4 pilocarpine tablets per day for treatment of xerostomia. She had ingested all 4 tablets (5 mg) 7 hours before arrival at the ED. Within 30 minutes of ingestion, she reported sweating and abdominal pain. Over the next 6 hours, she had excessive salivation, lacrimation, vomiting, anxiety, tremors,

and diarrhea develop. During her evaluation, her heart rate slowed to 38 beats/min, her blood pressure decreased to 102/42 mm Hg, and she complained of dyspnea and lightheadedness. IV atropine was administered. All symptoms resolved. She remained asymptomatic for the next 6 hours and was discharged. She was instructed to reinitiate the pilocarpine the next day beginning with 2.5 mg 3 times per day, slowly increasing the dose as tolerated.

Conclusions.—The case report describes clinically significant muscarinic symptoms after ingestion of oral pilocarpine tablets. Physicians should be aware of the possibility of this toxicity. This case also emphasizes the importance of physician–patient communication.

▶ We might think about adding pilocarpine to the list of medications we consider to have a narrow therapeutic window (eg, "deadly in a dose" for children). This concise report summarizes that nicely.

R. J. Hamilton, MD

Clinical Features and Management of Herb-Induced Aconitine Poisoning
Lin C-C, Chan TYK, Deng J-F (Chang Gung Mem Hosp, Taipei, Taiwan; Chinese Univ of Hong Kong; Natl Yang-Ming Univ, Taipei, Taiwan)
Ann Emerg Med 43:574-579, 2004   11–35

Background.—As interest continues in herbal medications, the possibility of herb-induced aconitine poisoning increases. This retrospective case series describes the clinical features and treatment of 17 patients with herb-induced aconitine poisoning.

Study Design.—The National Poison Center database of Taiwan was searched for patients with herb-induced aconitine poisoning from 1990 through 1999. The features of each case and its outcome were abstracted.

Findings.—During the 10-year period, 17 cases of herb-induced aconitine poisoning were reported (Table 2). All these patients were adults. Of these 17 patients, 13 ingested roots as a treatment for wounds or rheumatism, 2 patients were volunteers in a drug study, and 2 ingested roots accidentally. After 10 to 90 minutes, patients exhibited neurologic, cardiovascular, gastrointestinal, and other features of aconite poisoning. Four patients had ventricular tachycardia (Figure). All patients received supportive treatment, and those with tachycardia were also treated with charcoal hemoperfusion. All made a complete recovery.

Conclusions.—Life-threatening ventricular tachycardia can occur after ingestion of aconite roots. Inadequate processing or large dosages increase this risk.

▶ This is the largest case series of patients with aconitine poisoning in the literature. It provides some insights into the nature of the poison. The neurologic symptoms manifest as paresthesias in the limbs and face, and the car-

TABLE 2.—Seventeen Cases of Herb-Induced Aconitine Poisoning: Clinical Features and Treatment

Case	Latent Period*	Recovery Time	Cardiovascular Features†	Neurologic Features	Other Features	Treatment
1	Unknown	Unknown	Chest tightness, bradycardia	Sensory (limbs)‡	None	Supportive§
2	1 h	8 d	Palpitations, chest tightness, hypotension, bradycardia, ventricular tachycardia	Sensory (limbs)	Nausea, abdominal pain, hyperventilation	Lidocaine, direct current shock, temporary pacemaker, mechanical ventilation
3	1 h	2 d	Tachycardia, hypotension	Motor (limbs)	Dizziness	Supportive
4	1 h	7 d	Palpitations, chest tightness, hypotension, ventricular tachycardia	Sensory (limbs/face), motor (limbs)	Nausea, abdominal pain, dizziness	Hemoperfusion, lidocaine
5	1 h	9 d	Palpitations, chest tightness, hypotension, ventricular tachycardia, pulmonary edema	Sensory (limbs/face), motor (limbs)	Nausea, dizziness	Hemoperfusion, lidocaine, high-flow oxygen
6	1 h	2 d	None	Sensory (limbs/face)	None	Supportive
7	30 min	2 d	Palpitations	Sensory (limbs/face)	Dizziness	Supportive
8	1 h	2 d	Sinus tachycardia	Sensory (face), motor (limbs)	Nausea, dizziness	Supportive
9	Unknown	Unknown	Palpitations, chest tightness, sinus tachycardia	Motor (limbs)	Hyperventilation	Supportive
10	1.5 h	2 d	None	Sensory (limbs/face), motor (limbs)	Abdominal distention	Supportive
11	Unknown	2 d	Palpitations, chest tightness	Sensory (limbs)	Dizziness, hyperventilation	Supportive
12	30 min	2 d	Chest tightness, multifocal ventricular ectopics	Motor (limbs)	Nausea, dizziness, cold sweat, hyperventilation	Supportive
13	30 min	3 d	Chest tightness, hypotension	Sensory (limbs), motor (face)	Nausea, dizziness, cold sweat, abdominal pain, diarrhea	Supportive
14	20 min	2 d	Chest tightness, multifocal ventricular ectopics	Sensory (limbs)	Dizziness, hyperventilation	Lidocaine
15	20 min	2 d	Bradycardia, hypotension	Sensory (limbs/face)	Nausea, dizziness, cold sweat	Atropine
16	20 min	1.5 d	None	Sensory (limbs)	None	Supportive
17	10 min	7 d	Palpitations, chest tightness, hypotension, ventricular tachycardia	Sensory (limbs)/ motor (limbs)	Nausea, dizziness, cold sweat	Lidocaine

*The mean value of the latent period is 43.6 minutes.

†Hypotension: Systolic blood pressure decreased to <90 mm Hg with shock sign; lidocaine dosage: 1 mg/kg intravenously as a loading dose and then 4 mg/min as a maintenance dose; atropine dosage: 1 mg intravenously twice; dopamine dosage: 5 to 20 g/kg/min, adjusted according to patient's blood pressure.

‡Sensory (limbs) indicates paresthesia and numbness in 4 limbs; sensory (limbs/face) indicates paresthesia and numbness in 4 limbs, face, and perioral area; motor (limbs) indicates muscle weakness in 4 limbs.

§Supportive: Inotropic agents such as dopamine were used in patients with hypotension.

(Courtesy of Lin C-C, Chan TYK, Deng J-F: Clinical features and management of herb-induced aconitine poisoning. *Ann Emerg Med* 43:574-579, 2004.)

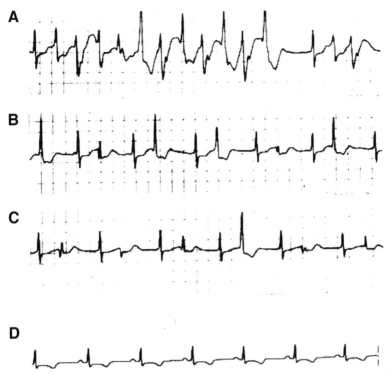

FIGURE.—**A,** Polymorphic multifocal ventricular ectopics after ingestion of an aconitine-containing herb 4 hours later. **B and C,** During charcoal hemoperfusion. **D,** Normal sinus rhythm after charcoal hemoperfusion. (Courtesy of Lin C-C, Chan TYK, Deng J-F: Clinical features and management of herb-induced aconitine poisoning. *Ann Emerg Med* 43:574-579, 2004.)

diovascular symptoms are life-threatening bradycardia and ventricular tachycardia. Because these cases are so rare, I would have enjoyed a detailed discussion of each patient's clinical course. Nonetheless, all the patients recovered with cardiorespiratory support. Two patients were treated with hemoperfusion, which is a therapy based on a few prior case reports. It appears that the sensory symptoms also resolved. The study lacks pharmacologic data, so only a few firm conclusions can be made.

R. J. Hamilton, MD

Successful Transplantation of Donor Organs From a Hemlock Poisoning Victim

Foster PF, McFadden R, Trevino R, et al (Texas Transplant Inst, San Antonio; Univ of Texas, Galveston; Auxilio Mutuo Hosp, San Juan, Puerto Rico)
Transplantation 76:874-876, 2003   11–36

Purpose.—This case report describes the successful use of donor organs from a patient who died of hemlock poisoning.

Case Report.—The donor was a previously healthy 14-year-old girl who ingested hemlock on a hike. She progressed to apnea and loss of consciousness. EMS personnel discovered her in respiratory arrest and bradycardia. An endotracheal tube was placed and cardiac function was restored. She was given IV fluids and was transported to a trauma center by helicopter. Plant samples were identified as hemlock (*Conium maculatum*). The patient was treated with gastric lavage and activated charcoal but remained comatose. Brain death was declared about 36 hours after hemlock ingestion. The family consented to organ donation. The medical examiner required that 1 kidney and 50 g of liver be retained for forensic testing. Prerecovery laboratory tests were normal. Standard multiorgan retrieval techniques were used and organ biopsies were normal. The autopsy was consistent with anoxic brain injury. Gas chromatographic/mass spectroscopic examination revealed that donor serum and tissue that had been removed for forensic testing were negative for coniine. The 3 organ recipients had immediate graft function without signs of toxicity. All are doing well more than 180 days after transplantation.

Conclusions.—Death as a result of hemlock ingestion is not a contraindication to donation of organs for transplantation. This may help to alleviate the critical shortage of organs for transplantation.

▶ This article demonstrates that patients who ingest poison hemlock (*Conium maculatum*) can be organ donors without harm to the recipient. A number of these articles have been reviewed by the YEAR BOOK over the years, and this adds to that database of important references.

R. J. Hamilton, MD

Unexpected Cardiovascular Deaths Are Rare With Therapeutic Doses of Droperidol

Mullins M, van Zwieten K, Blunt JR (Washington Univ, St Louis)
Am J Emerg Med 22:27-28, 2004   11–37

Background.—Droperidol has been in use for 31 years. In 2001, the US Food and Drug Administration added a "black box" warning based on Med Watch reports, which suggested that the use of this drug was associated with unexpected cardiovascular deaths, especially those involving QT prolongation. This association between droperidol and cardiovascular death was retrospectively examined.

Study Design.—MedWatch reports were obtained under the Freedom of Information Act. Summary data were obtained from 270 MedWatch reports, including 99 reports of death, submitted from November 1997 to January 2002. Primary MedWatch reports were obtained for all deaths and cardiovascular adverse events at doses of 10 mg or less. Outcomes, doses, symptoms, ages, sex, country of report, and other medications were abstracted from these reports. The association between droperidol and unexpected cardiovascular death was evaluated.

Findings.—The initial summary included reports of death in 89 patients. Of these, 74 were foreign. There were 66 reports that specified the dose. Among the 57 foreign reports with specified doses, 29 reported more than 50 mg, and 3 cases reported less than 2.5 mg. There were 9 death reports from the United States with specified doses. Of these, 5 cases reported less than 2.5 mg. The review of the primary MedWatch report forms describing low-dose deaths and cardiovascular adverse events described 33 patients and 20 deaths. All had confounding factors. Fifteen cases, including 8 of the death cases, were all reported on July 9, 2001 by Janssen-Cilag, the original manufacturer of droperidol. The interval from the event to the report for these cases was very long: the average was 7.4 years.

Conclusions.—Over a 15-month period, when 5 million vials of droperidol were sold by its largest supplier, there were approximately 200 adverse events, including 15 deaths, reported. This gives a spontaneous rate of voluntary death reports of approximately 3 deaths per million vials sold. Therefore, unexpected cardiovascular death in individuals receiving single therapeutic doses ($\leq$2.5 mg) of droperidol appear to be rare. Mandatory routine electrocardiographic screening for all patients does not appear to be necessary. Additional concern is warranted for patients with a family history of a prolonged QT interval or those taking concomitant medications that prolong the QT interval. Of interest, Janssen-Cilag has abandoned the sale of droperidol and has submitted a large backlog of old droperidol adverse event reports to the US Food and Drug Administration. Janssen is now marketing risperidone.

▶ The authors do a fine job of providing a much needed perspective on this problem—one that may be more influenced by the economic burden of product liability and the economic value of popularizing newer replacement pharmaceuticals.

R. J. Hamilton, MD

Out-of-Hospital Care of Critical Drug Overdoses Involving Cardiac Arrest
Paredes VL, Rea TD, Eisenberg MS, et al (Univ of Washington, Seattle; EMS Division, Seattle)
Acad Emerg Med 11:71-74, 2004   11–38

Background.—The role of EMS in a severe drug poisoning or overdose with cardiovascular collapse is not well characterized. The effect of EMS involvement and its potential benefit in averting mortality in cases of severe drug poisoning was investigated in this observational study.

Study Design.—All deaths caused by severe drug poisoning in King County (Seattle), Washington, for the year 2000 were studied. Death was defined as either a death or a successful resuscitation of an out-of-hospital cardiac arrest by EMS.

Findings.—During 2000 in King County, 234 people died of cardiac arrests caused by severe drug poisoning, and 11 were successfully resuscitated. EMS responded to 79.6%, attempted resuscitation in 34.7%, and achieved successful resuscitation in 4.5% of these poisonings. Opioids, cocaine, and alcohol were the most common drugs involved, and more than half the cases involved multiple drugs. Of the 11 successful resuscitations, 6 were achieved after cardiopulmonary resuscitation (CPR) only, 1 was achieved after CPR and defibrillation, and 4 were achieved after additional advanced life support.

Conclusions.—In King County, EMS was involved in the majority of severe drug poisonings with cardiovascular collapse in 2000. EMS intervention appeared to lower the total mortality rate from severe drug poisoning by 4.5%. Because resuscitation was achieved by CPR alone in some cases, the pathophysiologic process of cardiac arrest due to drug poisoning seems to be different from that caused by heart disease.

▶ This study provides some limited observational data about EMS involvement in drug overdoses. However, the lack of data specific to the type of overdoses and their particular outcomes makes it of limited interest. Follow-up research to identify scenarios in which EMS field interventions might affect outcomes could be interesting.

R. J. Hamilton, MD

Exposure to Extremely High Concentrations of Carbon Dioxide: A Clinical Description of a Mass Casualty Incident
Halpern P, Raskin Y, Sorkine P, et al (Tel Aviv Univ, Israel)
Ann Emerg Med 43:196-199, 2004   11–39

Purpose.—A mass casualty event caused by unintentional exposure to high concentrations of carbon dioxide is described.

Case Report.—A group of workers was exposed to high concentrations of carbon dioxide when the discharge valve of a truck containing liquid carbon dioxide was knocked open in an enclosed environment. Incapacitation occurred within seconds. Within 30 minutes, 25 casualties, including 2 rescue personnel, were transported to the ED. Symptoms included dyspnea, a headache, dizziness, coughing, and chest pain. Of these 25 patients, 3 had lost consciousness and 1 of these had convulsions. Five patients had tachycardia, and 1 had a systolic artery pressure of less than 100 mm Hg. ECG tracings were obtained for 15 patients: ischemic ST-segment changes were observed in 2, and atrial fibrillation was observed in 2, including 1 of the patients with ST-segment changes. Chest radiographs were obtained for 22 patients: 2 had pulmonary edema and 6 had pneumonitis. Arterial blood gases were obtained for 8 patients: 6 had respiratory acidosis and 1 had metabolic acidosis. Acute non–Q wave myocardial infarction was diagnosed in 1 patient. Eleven patients were admitted to the hospital for 1 to 8 days. All patients were treated with high oxygen concentrations. All recovered completely.

Conclusions.—The most important step for carbon dioxide intoxication is rapid removal of the victim from the contaminated environment followed by cardiorespiratory support until spontaneous recovery. Rescue workers must use airway protection to avoid injury.

▶ Carbon dioxide has been classified as a simple asphyxiant, in that it displaces oxygen from the ambient air and causes hypoxia. This unusual series points out that it can act as a "knockdown" agent (ie, a toxin that rapidly incapacitates) and has specific cardiopulmonary toxic effects such as hypotension, coronary ischemia, atrial fibrillation, pulmonary edema, and pneumonitis.

R. J. Hamilton, MD

Conventional and Diffusion-Weighted MRI in the Evaluation of Methanol Poisoning: A Case Report
Server A, Hovda KE, Nakstad PH, et al (Ullevål Univ Hosp, Oslo, Norway)
Acta Radiol 44:691-695, 2003   11–40

Background.—Methanol poisoning can be effectively treated. Unfortunately, the diagnosis is often delayed. MRI may be used in the late diagnosis of these patients. Conventional and diffusion-weighted MRI (DWI) of methanol poisoning is described.

Case Report.—Man, 42, was admitted because of dyspnea and blurred vision days after ingestion of a methanol–ethanol mixture. At admission, his serum methanol level was 32.5 mmol and serum formate level was 21 mmol. Bicarbonate and fomepizole were started immediately. Hemodialysis was begun after 2 hours and continued for 8 hours. Respiratory arrest occurred, and the patient was intubated. Conventional MRI revealed an extensive, symmetrical, bilateral increased signal in fluid attenuated-inversion recovery and T2-weighted images in the lentiform nuclei, as well as an increased signal in the hippocampus. Axial DWI corresponding with apparent diffusion coefficient maps was consistent with cytotoxic edema. He was transferred to a nursing home after 49 days and had permanent brain damage and reduced vision.

Conclusions.—Radiologists need to be aware of the radiologic findings associated with methanol poisoning. Abnormalities on DWI were correlated with cytotoxic edema in the early stages and may provide prognostic information.

▶ I have managed a few methanol cases that were only established on clinical grounds well after the methanol level had fallen to close to 0. Perhaps this technology would be helpful in those types of cases: it could add weight to the consideration of methanol poisoning when the level is not available or is no longer elevated. In addition, this imaging modality may shed insights in the rare patient with cranial nerve abnormalities because of ethylene glycol poisoning.

R. J. Hamilton, MD

Subject Index

Author Index

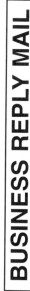

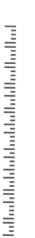

BUSINESS REPLY MAIL

FIRST-CLASS MAIL   PERMIT NO 7135   ORLANDO FL

POSTAGE WILL BE PAID BY ADDRESSEE

PERIODICALS ORDER FULFILLMENT DEPT
MOSBY
ELSEVIER
6277 SEA HARBOR DR
ORLANDO FL 32887-4800

VISIT OUR HOME PAGE!
www.us.elsevierhealth.com/periodicals

ELSEVIER
MOSBY